PHYSICAL REHABILITATION

OF THE

INJURED ATHLETE

PHYSICAL REHABILITATION
—— OF THE ——
INJURED ATHLETE

James R. Andrews, M.D.

Clinical Professor of Orthopaedics and Sports Medicine, University of Virginia
Medical School, Richmond, Virginia; Orthopaedic Surgeon,
Alabama Sports Medicine and Orthopaedic Center, Birmingham, Alabama

Gary L. Harrelson, M.S., A.T.,C.

Institute for Wellness and Sports Medicine, School of Human Performance
and Recreation, College of Health and Human Sciences,
University of Southern Mississippi, Hattiesburg, Mississippi

W.B. SAUNDERS COMPANY
Harcourt Brace Jovanovich, Inc.
Philadelphia London Toronto Montreal Sydney Tokyo

W.B. SAUNDERS COMPANY

Harcourt Brace Jovanovich, Inc.

The Curtis Center
Independence Square West
Philadelphia, Pennsylvania 19106

Library of Congress Cataloging-in-Publication Data

Physical rehabilitation of the injured athlete / [edited by] James R.
  Andrews, Gary L. Harrelson.
      p. cm.
    ISBN 0-7216-2689-0
      1. Sports—Accidents and injuries—Treatment.   2. Physical
  therapy.   3. Athletes—Rehabilitation.   I. Andrews, James R.
  II. Harrelson, Gary L.
      [DNLM: 1. Athletic Injuries—rehabilitation.   2. Physical Therapy.
  QT 260 P5786]
    RD97.P49   1991
    617.1'027—dc20
  DNLM/DLC   90-9231

Editor: W.B. Saunders Staff
Developmental Editor: Kathleen McCullough
Designer: Bill Donnelly
Production Manager: Bill Preston
Manuscript Editors: Tina K. Rebane and Louise Robinson
Illustrators: Glenn Edelmayer and Joseph Kulka
Illustration Coordinator: Brett MacNaughton
Page Layout Artist: Bill Donnelly
Indexer: Roger Wall

Physical Rehabilitation of the Injured Athlete   ISBN 0-7216-2689-0

Printed in Mexico

Last digit is the print number: 9   8   7   6   5   4   3   2   1

To my wife

Lisa

for her love and

understanding during the

drafting of this manuscript

and to

my parents,

who have always encouraged

me to make my

dreams and goals

a reality.

G.L.H.

CONTRIBUTORS

◆

Maggie Cooper, M.S., P.T.

Instructor, School of Physical Therapy, Medical College of Georgia, Augusta, Georgia

Use of Modalities in Rehabilitation

Ron Courson, P.T., A.T.,C.

DCH Regional Medical Center, University of Alabama, Tuscaloosa, Alabama

Role of Evaluation in the Rehabilitation Program

James B. Gallaspy, M.Ed., A.T.,C.

Associate Professor, School of Human Performance and Recreation, College of Health and Human Sciences, University of Southern Mississippi, Hattiesburg, Mississippi

Hamstring, Quadriceps, and Groin Rehabilitation

Gary L. Harrelson, M.S., A.T.,C.

Institute for Wellness and Sports Medicine, School of Human Performance and Recreation, College of Health and Human Sciences, University of Southern Mississippi, Hattiesburg, Mississippi

Physiologic Factors of Rehabilitation; Introduction to Rehabilitation; Knee Rehabilitation; Shoulder Rehabilitation; Elbow Rehabilitation

Glenn McWaters, B.S.

Formerly Director, The Sports Medicine and Fitness Institute, Birmingham; President, Bioenergetics, Inc., Pelham, Alabama

Aquatic Rehabilitation

Karen Middleton, P.T., A.T.,C.

Stanford University Sports Medicine Staff, Stanford, California

Goniometry; Range of Motion and Flexibility

Ed Mulligan, P.T., A.T.,C., S.C.S.

Clinical Coordinator, HealthSouth Sports Medicine and Rehabilitation Center, Fort Worth, Texas

Lower Leg, Ankle, and Foot Rehabilitation

Dale G. Pease, Ph.D.

Associate Professor and Chairman, Department of Health and Human Performance, University of Houston; Adjunct Associate Professor, Baylor College of Medicine, Houston, Texas

Psychologic Factors of Rehabilitation

PREFACE

◆

Therapeutic rehabilitation has long been a product of philosophies based on tradition handed down through the years from clinician to clinician. These concepts have usually been based on the premise, "Well, it has always worked for me," with the subsequent blending of these philosophies and/or exercises into therapeutic rehabilitation programs without an underlying scientific rationale for their implementation. Many early rehabilitation concepts and exercises were extrapolated from scientific models using biomechanical principles without empirical research data to support the theories. Over the past decade, rehabilitation research, specifically orthopedic sports medicine, has begun to "catch up" to the ever-expanding profession of orthopedic surgery. And we are forever indebted to the researchers who have contributed to the scientific base for rehabilitation.

The material within this book is based on a thorough review of the scientific literature. A scientific premise for rehabilitation and the vital importance of early motion are addressed. Emphasis is placed on closed-chain rehabilitation, proprioception restoration, specificity of rehabilitation movements, functional progression, and movement at functional speeds. Stress is placed on the need to treat the entire kinematic chain rather than independently to treat one joint within the chain. Protocols are used throughout the book as guidelines for rehabilitation and are by no means "the only way to do it." Rather, advancement through a rehabilitation program should be based on known healing restraint time of injured structures, the patient's pain tolerance level, joint effusion, and achievement of specific criteria before the rehabilitation program is advanced. Surgeons vary their surgical techniques for specific lesions, and this must be considered when developing a rehabilitation regimen. Rehabilitation can by no means be "cookbooked," with a program developed for every injury for every athlete, since individuals heal at varying rates and tolerate pain differently. Each patient brings a unique set of personal qualities that must be addressed by the clinician to facilitate the patient's rehabilitation. More than anything else, this book attempts to bring together an abundance of rehabilitation research upon which to base the advancement of an injured athlete through a rehabilitation protocol and implementation of specific exercises.

Physical Rehabilitation of the Injured Athlete is not intended to be all-inclusive, but rather addresses common problems specific to the athlete. Areas of vital importance in implementing a rehabilitation regimen are examined, including the psychological aspect of the injured athlete, goniometry, joint mobilization, evaluation of the injured athlete and how it relates to program implementation, types of exercise, crutch fitting and ambulation, the kinematic chain, components of rehabilitation, and aquatic therapy. Exercises are presented that the clinician can use in the implementation of a rehabilitation program, with contraindications for exercises for specific problems. The rehabilitation protocols outlined in this book are based on scientific rationales and have proved effective in clinical trials. Rehabilitation of such areas as the low back, neck, and wrist and hand are outside the scope of this book, and are adequately addressed in other texts.

It is our hope that *Physical Rehabilitation of the Injured Athlete* will serve as a reference for clinicians as well as a text for students interested in the area of athletic rehabilitation. We further hope that this book will serve as a clinician's reference source to enhance patient care and will provide students with the basic knowledge for the development and implementation of rehabilitation programs for the injured athlete.

JAMES R. ANDREWS, M.D.

GARY L. HARRELSON, M.S., A.T.,C.

CONTENTS

◆

CHAPTER 1

Psychologic Factors of Rehabilitation

Dale G. Pease, Ph.D.

Although coaches, athletes, and spectators involved in sport have recognized that physical injury is an inherent risk factor of participation, the psychologic aspects of participation and injury have often been overlooked. Until recently, many individuals in sport treated the body and mind as a dichotomous unit, resulting in the development of training programs that focused on the body and, in some cases, that treated the mind with scorn. Following the lead taken by those in other fields of medicine, practitioners of sports medicine are now moving toward a more holistic approach. It has been recognized that the psychologic state of the athlete is as important, and sometimes more important, than the athlete's physical state (Fig. 1–1).

With the growth and recognized importance of the field of sport psychology, there has been increasing interest in the relationship between psychologic factors and the occurrence and treatment of sports injuries. This chapter intends to help the clinician understand this relationship, especially in regard to the following: (1) potential risk factors; (2) responses to injury; (3) influence on the recovery period; and (4) "slumps" resulting from injury.

PSYCHOLOGIC RISK FACTORS

Are there psychologic factors that could help identify athletes who are more injury-prone than others? Early attempts to investigate this question used the "trait" approach, in which specific and enduring personality dispositions were identified in athletes with a history of injury. The personality studies included such traits as introversion–extroversion,* locus of control,† self-concept, anxiety, aggressiveness, and domi-

---

* Introverts tend to withdraw into themselves (introversion), whereas extroverts extend or seek out external stimulation (extroversion).

† Locus of control is the responsibility people feel for their behavior by referring to internal causes (e.g., attributed to their own actions) or to external causes, in which they have little control over the events in their lives.

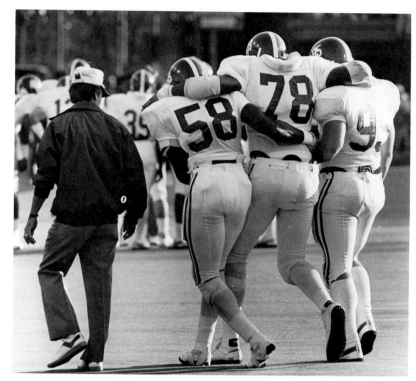

FIGURE 1—1   Risk factors have been recognized as inherent with sport participation. Until recently, the athlete's body and mind were treated as a single unit, with the latter receiving little or no attention. (From Philpot, D. (1986): Evaluation of the injured ankle. Sports Med. Update, 1(4):5.)

nance, which could be identified by using written tests. For example, it was believed that an athlete high in trait anxiety would have greater body tension and be less able to focus effectively on critical information involving performance, thus becoming more susceptible to injury.

A second example involves athletes with an external locus of control, who would perceive themselves as having less control over the events around them and thus have a greater potential for injury. By identifying certain psychologic traits as factors contributing to potential injury, an athlete with such traits might be advised to select sports with a low-injury risk factor or to take special precautions if participating in a sport with a high-injury risk factor.

Results of research using the trait approach have shown limited significant findings involving the relationship of psychologic traits and the occurrence of athletic injuries. It was found that football players who were more "tender-minded" and reserved were more susceptible to injury.[7, 8] Female basketball players with a higher incidence of injury scored more positively on self-concept and identity and on physical and personal self-factors than noninjured female players.[16] It was believed that these injured basketball players were more likely to take risks because of greater self-confidence and consequently increased their potential for injury. Although some studies have given limited support to the notion that there is a direct relationship between personality traits and the occurrence of injury, most researchers believe that other factors need to be investigated.

As a result of findings from these trait studies, research focus has shifted to exploring the relationship of stress to injury. The concept that stressful life events may be related to the occurrence of athletic injuries was initially based on reports in the general medical literature. Studies have shown a positive relationship between stressful life events, especially those with high negative stress, and the occurrence of injury and disease. Using these reports, Anderson and Williams[1] developed a theoretic model showing factors that could contribute to the stress-injury relationship in the sports setting (Fig. 1–2). Although this model includes the personality traits previously discussed, it uses these traits as contributors to an individual's history of stress events or as factors that have a direct impact on the stress response. Their model also includes the coping resources and interventions that can serve as modifiers of a potential stress response. The model should be reviewed to understand the contributing factors to the stress response and the proposed relationship among the factors. It is also referred to later in this chapter.

Several studies have investigated the life stress relationship to sports injuries. Bramwell and associates[3] studied the life changes of 79 varsity college football players for 1- and 2-year periods prior to their playing season, and found that a greater percentage of injuries occur in those in the high life change group. In their study of two college football teams, Passer and Seese[13] found a significant relationship between negative life stress and injury on one team but not on the other. Studies of elite female gymnasts revealed that stressful life events are related significantly to both the number and severity of injuries.[9] In this study,

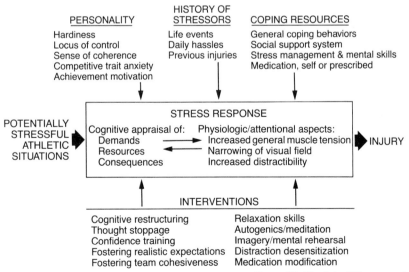

FIGURE 1–2   A model of stress and athletic injury. (From "A Model of Stress and Athletic Injury: Prediction and Prevention" by M. B. Andersen and J. M. Williams, 1988, *Journal of Sport and Exercise Psychology, 10,* p. 297. Copyright 1988 by Human Kinetics Publishers, Inc. Reprinted by permission.)

factors such as anxiety, locus of control, and self-concept were not significant predictors of injury. Although several studies have noted a relationship between high life stress (especially negative stress) and injuries, a study involving male and female intercollegiate volleyball players showed no relationship between life stress and injury.[15] The type of sport and the predominate types of injuries found in a sport may be important variables in the stress-injury relationship, but at present no published reports have addressed this hypothesis.

To explore the stress-injury relationship further, the physiologic and psychologic changes in response to stress must be understood, as shown in a model by Nideffer[12] (Fig. 1–3). In regard to physiologic changes, there is increasing concern about the muscle tension produced as a result of the stress response. Increased tension in the antagonistic and agonistic muscle groups results in a reduction of flexibility and loss of motor coordination. Another significant factor related to increased muscular tension is a slowed reaction time, which reduces the athlete's ability to respond to environmental events. Therefore, the maintenance of appropriate muscle tension to achieve a desired result appears to be essential in the prevention of injuries.

Studying the Nideffer model (see Fig. 1–3), it is seen that an important psychologic variable is the ability of the athlete to select and process information, because stress has been shown to narrow or switch the attentional focus. For example, a player under heavy stress in football might not process information in the peripheral areas of the visual field, resulting in a lack of response to oncoming physical contact

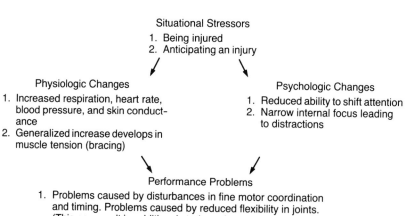

Situational Stressors
1. Being injured
2. Anticipating an injury

Physiologic Changes
1. Increased respiration, heart rate, blood pressure, and skin conductance
2. Generalized increase develops in muscle tension (bracing)

Psychologic Changes
1. Reduced ability to shift attention
2. Narrow internal focus leading to distractions

Performance Problems
1. Problems caused by disturbances in fine motor coordination and timing. Problems caused by reduced flexibility in joints. (This can result in additional strain and aggravation of existing injury.)
2. Decision problems and concentration disturbances. Feelings of being overloaded and confused. Inability to attend to stimuli relevant to the task because of physiologic distractions. Inability to shift attention from one focus to another.

FIGURE 1–3   Physical and psychologic changes accompany increases in pressure as a result of injury or the fear of injury. Problems in performance resulting from stress and reduced physiologic and psychologic flexibility can become chronic. Disturbances in physical flexibility affect concentration and, as the athlete becomes upset at his or her own failure (frustration or anxiety increases), the attentional and physiologic disturbances become stronger and more intractable. (Modified from Nideffer, R.M. (1983): The injured athlete: Psychological factors in treatment. Orthop. Clin. North Am., 14:373–385.)

(e.g., greater potential for a blind side hit). Another important aspect of attentional focus involves what the athlete was thinking at the time of injury. Using the Nideffer model, it is proposed that an athlete under stress, especially negative stress, might be thinking about the events causing the stress and not thinking about what is currently happening in the environment. Therefore, the athlete does not process relevant information that could result in a protective response. For example, a linebacker in football who has just learned of the divorce plans of his parents might be thinking of what his future holds (internal focus) and not attending well to information involving what is happening on the field (external focus). Hence, there would be a greater potential for injury for this athlete.

The importance of attentional focus in athletic injuries must include interest in recent studies involving the psychologic phenomenon of mood congruence. It has been shown that we attend, encode, and retrieve information that is congruent with our mood state.[2] For example, if the mood state of the athlete described above is depression, resulting from knowledge of the parents' divorce, the information he attends to probably contains affect-congruent information. In this case, it is negative information from the environment (external focus) and negative thoughts (internal focus) that are affecting his thought process.

If the mood state is anger as a result of the divorce plans, high levels of activation would be expected, which also disrupt the attentional ability and the processing of relevant information. With the occurrence of either emotion, depression or anger, the ability to control attention and process correct information is inhibited, thus increasing the potential for injury. The ability to control attention and block out irrelevant information depends greatly on the individual, with wide variation among athletes.

For the athlete returning to competition following recovery from injury, the role of attentional focus and muscular tension can be a major problem. Fear and/or worry about a second injury can place an athlete's thought processing in an internal mode, causing increased muscular tension. There has been interest in the role of psychologic hardiness as it relates to return from injury. Hardiness can be defined as a combination of commitment, control, and challenge on the part of an individual, and seems to be a moderating factor in the stress-illness relationship.[10] It is believed that athletes who exhibit greater qualities of this trait are better able to control the attentional processing of information and in turn reduce the potential for occurrence of a second injury. At present, however, not enough studies have been done on hardiness and its relationship to injury to be able to reach definite conclusions.

Fatigue, the final factor to be discussed here, has been recognized as a contributor to injury from the physical aspect. Usually, however, fatigue has been regarded as only a physical factor, and mental fatigue may be more important. The ability to maintain a high level of concentration (attention) requires a large amount of energy and, combined with a demanding training program, attention is reduced as both physical and mental fatigue sets in. Reduced attention results in slowed response times, and, combined with the loss of neuromuscular coordination, the potential for injury is increased.

Thus, although few studies have been done involving psychologic risk factors and injury, current evidence supports the importance of the stress response (as presented in the Anderson and Williams model, Fig. 1−2).

OCCURRENCE OF INJURY

When an athlete is injured, the primary focus of trainers, coaches, teammates, doctors, parents, and even the spectator is generally on tangible evidence of the injury. "How severe is the injury?" "Will surgery be required?" These questions are followed by others. "How long will the athlete be out of competition?" "Who will replace this athlete in the lineup?" And, if the athlete is in a critical position (e.g., quarterback, pitcher), many of the significant people working with this athlete might think of the season "going down the drain."

Immediate treatments, such as cryotherapy and immobilization, are usually provided quickly, followed by a rehabilitation program that includes a regimen for regaining strength and flexibility. Although the physical needs of an injured athlete are taken care of, other major needs that may create more pain than the physical aspect of the injury are often overlooked. If an athlete is injured, the thoughts and feelings of the athlete are often disregarded or given a low priority. These thoughts and feelings, reflecting on past experiences involving injury to self or others and how this injury may change the future, can produce psychologic pain that is greater and lasts longer than the physical pain. Well-intended comments to an injured athlete (e.g., "you will be okay" or "just hang in there") are often heard, but these do not really address the psychologic problems the athlete is experiencing.

As the initial physical pain of the injury subsides, the athlete encounters an array of psychologic reactions. Emotional responses, such as "why me?," "why now?," and "this can't be happening," take over the thoughts of the athlete. Other emotions, such as anger, depression, anxiety, and panic, are common responses.

Sometimes these emotions cannot be expressed overtly by the athlete, because this type of behavior is unacceptable in the "macho" world of athletics. When an athletic career is interrupted or perhaps terminated as a result of an injury, the years of expectations and hard work seem wasted and a strong emotional response, overt or hidden, must be expected.

Although an injury can be psychologically devastating to many athletes, some athletes view the injury with relief. For some athletes, the injury provides them with attention and support from others that they may not have been receiving prior to the injury. For others, the injury relieves the pressure to perform, and the respite from training and competition may be welcomed. This gives the athlete a chance to enjoy other aspects of life and provides time for re-evaluating the commitment to the sport. The idea that an athlete may obtain satisfaction from an injury, however, is often difficult for a trainer, especially a coach, to understand. With the emphasis on sports in today's society, resulting in enormous pressure on the athlete to perform and be successful, there is increasing evidence that more athletes are using this method of coping with some of these pressures.

As stated previously, various psychologic responses can be observed immediately following injury and can continue long after recovery. The nature and intensity of these responses depend on several factors, such as the type of injury, its importance to performing the skills essential to the sport, the time of injury in regard to the season and major competitive events, and the importance of participation to the athlete. The major variable related to these factors seems to be the athlete's perception of the injury and its effect on the future. Although the injury might seem minor to the trainer or physician, the athlete might believe that it is more severe and therefore could exhibit emotional responses that seem unwarranted to others. Of significance here is acceptance by the athlete of the trainer's or physician's appraisal of the injury. If the athlete lacks confidence in the ability of medical personnel to appraise and treat the injury properly, the athlete can reject and ignore the medical advice, resulting in a stronger negative emotional response.

Lynch[11] has reported that severely injured athletes go through stages of denial, anger, bargaining, depression, and acceptance. Athletes alternate among these stages and reflect feelings of fear, panic, and even learned helplessness.

These psychologic responses, coupled with the physical pain resulting from the injury, result in a threat to self-esteem and feelings of incompetence, and may have a major influence on the recovery period. This seems to be especially true if the athlete has no strong social support system available. During recovery the stress resulting from the injury can be a major problem—it is the perceived stress experienced by the athlete that is important. For example, the coach may plan for the injured athlete to return to his or her starting position following recovery and may discuss these plans with the athlete. If the athlete perceives the starting role to be in jeopardy, however, there can be additional stress on the athlete that others may not observe or understand. This stress, from whatever source, causes increased muscle tension and can reduce the circulatory system's ability to supply blood to the injured area. This stress can also reduce the ability of the athlete to perform the simple physical movement patterns necessary for rehabilitation.

Of prime importance in providing medical services to an athlete during recovery is the availability of a strong social support system. Extensive medical research has shown the value of support systems as buffers or moderators of the negative stress resulting from disease or injury. Results of studies involving sports settings have also suggested a positive relationship between desired athlete behaviors during the recovery period and the support provided by significant others.[5, 6] Weiss and Troxell[14] have presented a strong case for the role of the athletic trainer in the support system. The presence and positive support of others who understand the needs of the athlete and why certain behaviors are occurring are valuable in helping the athlete cope with various problems during the recovery period. This understanding is especially necessary because the injured athlete might be depressed and, as a result, could reject the efforts of people close to him or her. Within a short period, however, this same athlete may be seeking assurance and reinforcement from these same individuals.

Those in the support system, which must include the athletic trainer, physical therapist, and physician, therefore play an extremely important role in understanding and guiding the athlete through these emotional times during recovery.

ADHERENCE AND RECOVERY PROBLEMS

During the recovery period a disturbing behavior on the part of the athlete sometimes emerges. The athlete misses assigned therapy sessions or, when attending the session, does not put forth the necessary effort for effective rehabilitation. This becomes extremely disturbing to coaches, trainers, teammates, and others who are influenced by this lack of adherence and commitment on the part of this athlete. Some athletes may regard the occurrence of an injury as a positive event, in that it may relieve them of the pressures of competition, gain them attention, or allow them time to re-evaluate the importance of sports participation. Why don't athletes adhere to rehabilitation programs?

Research by Duda and colleagues[5] represents one of the few studies investigating why athletes do not adhere to rehabilitation programs. Their study involves 40 intercollegiate athletes who had sustained a sports injury of at least second-degree severity that resulted in scheduled rehabilitation sessions for 3 weeks or more. They measured the attendance, completion of exercise protocol, and observed exercise intensity of the injured athletes. The study showed that perceived value of the treatment, social support, degree of self-motivation, and task involvement in sports are significant predictors of adherence behaviors.

How do these factors relate to the participation of a sports medicine team in treatment of an injury? Educating the athlete about the nature and value of the treatment is a responsibility of the trainer and physician, with the aid of the coach and parents. Often, treatments and drug therapy are prescribed without providing the person receiving the treatment with information about how it influences the rehabilitation process.

This problem arises because it is often assumed that the athlete already knows why a treatment is prescribed or because, when large numbers of players are involved, such as a football team, there is not enough time to provide individual attention. The educational process is part of the responsibility of those who provide social support in the recovery period. Two factors—self-motivation and task involvement— are sometimes the most misunderstood variables when working with athletes, because most people assume that highly successful athletes have high levels of self-motivation and a high degree of involvement and commitment to their sport. This assumption is not true, however— for example, some athletes with great natural abilities have low-need achievement levels and a limited commitment to the sport for which they are recognized. Such athletes usually lack self-directed goals that can help provide the intrinsic drive necessary to gain maximum value from their natural abilities. Therefore, when this type of athlete is injured, the lack of internal drive and goals results in problems in regard to adherence to a prescribed rehabilitation program, which takes time and effort to complete. Also, the lack of adherence could be the result of the athlete's not viewing the reward system (extrinsic motivation) as providing the necessary returns for overcoming that lack of internal motivation to complete the rehabilitation program successfully.

These adherence variables are consistent with those found in the medical literature.[4] Sports adherence studies are limited, and many questions need to be answered to understand this problem better. These include type of sport, gender of athlete, time during the season when the injury occurs, and perceived cause of the injury. Injury is an inherent variable in sports participation, so factors that influence the adherence to rehabilitation programs are important for the effective functioning of a sports medicine team.

A behavioral observation reported by coaches and trainers following an injury and on returning to competition is that the athlete does not have the same intensity and dedication to the sport as observed before the injury. This loss of focus and intensity can contribute to adherence problems but becomes more serious on return to practice and competition.

It is generally believed that the athlete has a fear of being reinjured, and to some extent this is true. It may also be the case, however, that the athlete has had time to reflect on the role of sports in his or her life,

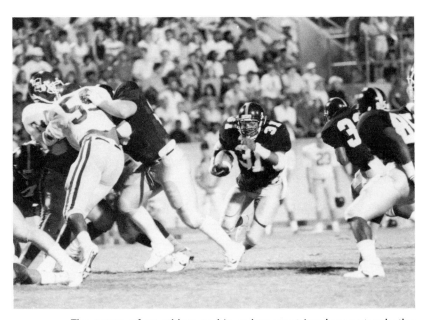

FIGURE 1–4 The return of an athlete to his or her sport involves not only the physical rehabilitation program, but also the athlete's mental health. Of the support personnel available, the athletic trainer can be the best qualified to address these concerns. (Photo by John Rawlston, News-Free Press.)

has questioned its importance and rewards, and, as a result, has established new priorities. One athlete, currently in her middle teens, after having to take time off from swimming because of a car accident injury, reported that "I never thought there were so many other fun things to do." This swimmer had been attending twice-a-day workouts for the past 10 years of her life, and everything she did was related to swimming. The "time out" gave her a chance to participate in other activities and changed her thinking about the importance of sports in her life.

Trainers, coaches, and significant others play important roles in the recovery period. It is their understanding of the problems that an athlete can encounter during this period that is critical to satisfactory recovery. They can provide the motivation to help the athlete adhere to rehabilitation programs and to return to practice and competition with a positive mental attitude (Fig. 1–4).

SLUMPS AND INJURIES

Most athletes at some time experience declines in performance, commonly referred to as "slumps." These can result from physical, technical, or psychologic problems or from some combination of these. The prescription for a slump can range from "work harder and work your way through it" to a "time out," during which the athlete has a period of total rest from the sport. How do athletic injuries and psychologic variables further relate to slumps?

Probably the most frequent cause of a slump is the physical component. Fatigue caused by overtraining and injury, especially nagging minor injuries that receive little attention, creates problems in the execution of the skill and results in a lower performance level. As the athlete senses the declining physical performance, psychologic factors resulting in anxiety, loss of concentration, and confidence become a major source of future problems.

The increased anxiety results in greater muscle tension, which interferes with coordination in the muscular system and results in a lower performance level and in increased risk of further injury. Because a slump can be extremely draining it can further add to the general fatigue factor, and the athlete's ability to concentrate on important information can be hindered still more.

Sometimes slumps are the result of problems that are not directly related to sport participation. Marital or financial problems or family illness could be the cause of a slump. Again, the problem of lack or loss of concentration increases the potential for injury to occur. In some cases the athlete may use the injury as a means of explaining the slump and to escape the pressure of performance and the need to explain the real problem to others.

It is therefore important that the members of the sports medicine team do not write off a slump as only a psychologic problem related to athletic performance. Often the antecedents to the observed psychologic responses, such as injury, fatigue, or outside influences, are the true source of the slump.

COPING STRATEGIES

The Anderson and Williams model (see Fig. 1—2) has two parts that show the importance of coping strategies. The first is listed under coping resources, where the importance of social support systems, stress management and mental skills, and general coping behaviors is shown to mediate the life stress factors and to interact directly with the stress response. The second aspect of the model deals with the interventions that can be used in response to stress. Although this model was designed to explain the psychologic phenomena involved as antecedents of an injury, the model can also be useful for understanding the psychologic components of postinjury responses. Therefore, it is important for the athlete to have coping strategies available both before and after injury.

Space limitations here prevent a detailed discussion of the many coping resources and interventions available, but one example is provided. Because many athletes and coaches are concerned about stress management, it can be important for an athlete to know some basic relaxation techniques. Athletes who know such skills as breathing techniques, ways of detecting and reducing muscular tension, and use of imagery can help prevent or reduce the severity of injury. If injury does occur, their knowledge of relaxation techniques can be useful during the recovery period.

Only recently have coaches shown an interest in having their athletes taught such psychologic skills as relaxation and imagery. Sometimes the coach has had the proper training for teaching such skills, but often the acquisition of these techniques is left to the athlete or some other interested person. Many teams do not have access to a sports psychologist or cannot afford to have one on staff. In such cases it is believed that the athletic trainer, who has the best general relationship with the athletes, can implement and carry out psychologic development programs most effectively.

SUGGESTIONS

Some suggestions for members of a sports medicine team to handle some of the problems discussed in this chapter include the following:

1. We must educate the athlete about the importance of the mind-body connection as part of the daily training program. This is based on the assumption that athletes who have developed cognitive strategies (e.g., relaxation, imagery, concentration) along with their physical skills have a better chance of preventing injury and are better equipped to cope with an injury if it does occur.
2. We must establish communication and support structures. In many sports communication between the coach and athlete is limited and, at best, superficial. Some athletes do not feel confident in regard to talking with the coach about their thoughts and feelings. It is in this regard that the trainer and other mem-

bers of the sports medicine team can be extremely important in providing a means for athletes to express their thoughts and feelings.

3. The athletic trainer already has major responsibilities for the prevention and care of the physical aspect of injuries and thus may be the best person to be involved in a psychologic training program if other resources are not available. The relationship of the athletic trainer to the athlete may be more flexible, open, and less threatening, and the athlete may feel more comfortable in discussing his or her mental needs with the trainer. Therefore, the athletic trainer should have knowledge and training about the psychologic aspects involved in sports participation.

References

1. Anderson, M.B., and Williams, J.M. (1988): A model of stress and athletic injury: Prediction and prevention. J. Sport Exerc. Psychol., 10:294–306.
2. Blaney, P.H. (1986): Affect and memory: A review. Psychol. Bull., 99:229–246.
3. Bramwell, S.T., Masuda, M., Wagner, N.N., and Holmes, T.H. (1975): Psychosocial factors in athletic injuries: Development and application of the social and athletic readjustment rating scale. J. Human Stress, 1:6–20.
4. Dishman, R.K. (1986): Exercise compliance. A new view for public health. Physician Sportsmed., 14:127–145.
5. Duda, J.L., Smart, A.E., and Tappe, M.K. (1989): Predictors of adherence in the rehabilitation of athletic injuries: An application of personal investment theory. J. Sport Exerc. Psychol., 11:367–381.
6. Fisher, A.C., Domm, M.A., and Wuest, D.A. (1988): Adherence to sports-injury rehabilitation programs. Physician Sportsmed., 16:47–52.
7. Irwin, R.F. (1975): Relationship between personality and the incidence of injuries to high school football participants. Dissertation Abstr. Int., 36:4328A.
8. Jackson, D.W., Jarrett, H., Bailey, D., et al. (1978): Injury prediction in the young athlete: A preliminary report. Am. J. Sports Med., 6:6–14.
9. Kerr, G., and Minden, H. (1988): Psychological factors related to the occurrence of athletic injuries. J. Sport Exercise Psychol., 109:167–173.
10. Kobasa, S.C., Maddi, S.R., and Puccetti, M.C. (1982): Personality and exercise as buffers in the stress–illness relationship. J. Behav. Med., 5:391–404.
11. Lynch, C.P. (1988): Athletic injuries and the practicing sport psychologists: Practical guidelines for assisting athletes. Sport Psychologist, 2:161–167.
12. Nideffer, R.M. (1983): The injured athlete: Psychological factors in treatment. Orthop. Clin. North Am., 14:373–385.
13. Passer, M.W., and Seese, M.D. (1983): Life stress and athletic injury: Examination of positive versus negative events and three moderator variables. J. Human Stress, 9:11–16.
14. Weiss, M.R., and Troxell, R.K. (1986): Psychology of the injured athlete. Athletic Training, 21:104–110.
15. Williams, J.M., Tonymon, P., and Wadsworth, W.A. (1986): Relationship of stress to injury in intercollegiate volleyball. J. Human Stress, 12:38–43.
16. Young, M.L., and Cohen, D.A. (1981): Self-concept and injuries among high school basketball players. J. Sports Med., 21:55–61.

CHAPTER 2

♦

Physiologic Factors of Rehabilitation

Gary L. Harrelson, M.S., A.T.,C.

The effects of immobilization on bone and connective tissue have been widely reported in the literature. The use of early range-of-motion exercises to prevent the deleterious effects of immobilization has become accepted practice in the orthopedic community. The proper use of exercise can speed up the healing process, whereas the lack of exercise during the early stages of rehabilitation can result in permanent disability. Caution must be observed, however, because exercise that is too vigorous can also result in permanent damage. Immobilization initially results in loss of tissue substrate, with a subsequent loss of basic tissue components. The reversibility of these changes appears to be dependent on the length of immobilization.

To understand the body's response to immobilization and remobilization, its normal reaction to injury must be addressed. The enzymes released when trauma occurs to a joint can cause cartilage degradation, chronic joint synovitis, and stretching of the joint capsule as a result of increased effusion.

REACTION TO INJURY

Inflammation is the body's response to injury and optimally results in injury healing and replacement of damaged and destroyed tissue, with an associated restoration of function.[36] Continued injury or microtrauma to an area, however, can cause a chronic inflammatory response that results in adverse effects to the joint and its surrounding structures. Regardless of the location and nature of the injurious agent, the inflammatory response is the same, consisting of chemical, metabolic, permeability, and vascular changes, followed by some form of repair.[52]

Figure 2–1 illustrates the primary and secondary injuries affiliated with trauma and the associated inflammation and repair processes. Primary injury occurs from the trauma that directly injures the cells themselves. Secondary injury (sometimes referred to as secondary

13

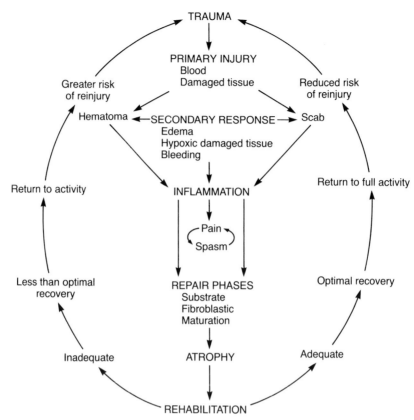

FIGURE 2–1 Cycle of athletic injury. (Reproduced by permission from Booher, James M., and Thibodeau, Gary A.: Athletic Injury Assessment. St. Louis, 1989, Times Mirror/Mosby College Publishing.)

hypoxia) is precipitated by the body's response to trauma. This response includes decreased blood flow to the traumatized region as a result of vasoconstriction, which decreases the amount of oxygen to the injured area. Thus, additional cells die because of secondary hypoxia; these dead cells organize and ultimately form a hematoma.

Cell degeneration or cell death perpetuates the release of potent substances that can induce vascular changes. The most common of these substances is histamine, which increases capillary permeability and allows the escape of fluid and blood cells into the interstitial spaces. In the non-injured state, plasma and blood proteins escape from capillaries by osmosis and diffusion into the interstitial spaces, but are reabsorbed. This homeostasis is maintained by colloids found within the blood system. Trauma results in increased capillary permeability as a result of the release of cell enzymes, however, allowing blood plasma and proteins to escape into surrounding tissues. Concurrently, the amount of colloids greatly increases in the surrounding tissues, thus reversing their effect. Rather than the colloids pulling fluid back into the capillaries, their presence outside the vessels causes additional fluid to be pulled into the interstitial tissues, resulting in swelling and edema.

The body's reaction postinjury is mobilization and transport of the defense components of the blood to the injured area. Initially, blood flow is reduced, allowing white blood cells to migrate to the margin of the vessel. These cells adhere to the vessel wall and eventually travel into the interstitial tissues. Once in the surrounding tissues, the white cells remove irritating material by the process of phagocytosis. Neutrophils are the first white blood cells to arrive, and they normally destroy bacteria. Because the presence of bacteria is not usually associated with athletic injuries, however, these neutrophils die.[52] Secondly, macrophages appear and phagocytize the neutrophil carcasses, cellular debris, fibrin, red cells, and other debris that may impede the repair process.[52] Unfortunately, the destruction of the neutrophils results in the release of active proteolytic enzymes (i.e., enzymes that hasten the hydrolysis of proteins into simpler substances) into the surrounding inflammatory fluid,[43] which can attack joint tissues. Although this is the natural response of ridding the body of toxic or foreign materials, prolonged continuation of this response can damage surrounding joint structures.

Once the inflammatory debris has been removed, repair can begin. Cleanup by the macrophages and repair often occur simultaneously. For repair to occur, however, enough of the hematoma must be removed to permit ingrowth of new tissue. Thus, the hematoma size or amount of exudate is directly related to total healing time. If hematoma size is minimized, healing can begin earlier and total healing time is reduced.[52]

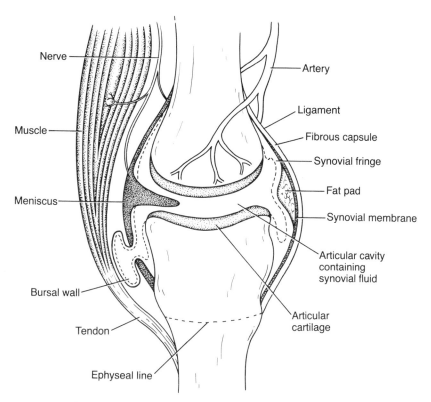

FIGURE 2–2   Synovial joint structures. (From Wright, V., Dowson, D., and Kerr, J. (1973): The structure of joints. Int. Rev. Connect. Tissue Res., 6:105–125.)

Response of Joint Structures to Injury

As a result of the inflammatory process, each joint component responds differently to injury (Fig. 2–2). The reaction of the synovial membrane to injury causes the proliferation of surface cells and an increase in vascularity and gradual fibrosis of the subsynovial tissue. Posttraumatic synovitis is not an uncommon entity with most injuries, if they occur only once. Continued mechanical irritation can produce chronic synovitis, resulting in the reversal of normal synovial cell ratios.[43, 83] Changes in synovial fluid occur as a result of synovial membrane alterations. As a consequence of the synovitis, cells are destroyed; the white blood cells ingest lysosomes and proteolytic enzymes. This ingestion and the subsequent death of white blood cells in the transudate result in the release of proteolytic enzymes. The overall consequence is the spawning of a vicious inflammatory cycle, which can keep reactive synovitis alive for some time, even without further trauma (Fig. 2–3).[9] As chronic posttraumatic effusions occur, the synovial membrane can continue with a sequel of progressing sclerotic alterations.[95] If conservative treatment consisting of anti-inflammatory medications, rest, aspiration, and cold applications does not relieve the symptoms, a synovectomy may be necessary.

Meniscus lesions within the knee invariably are accompanied by increased synovial effusion. Once corrected, the synovial irritation usually subsides. If left uncorrected, however, tissues not injured by the original trauma can be damaged from the prolonged inflammation, resulting in progressive degradation of the synovial membrane.

Fortunately, once the inflammation begins to abate, synovial tissue has a remarkable ability to regenerate, possibly stemming from its

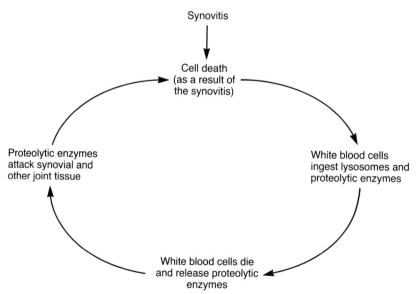

FIGURE 2–3   Continued mechanical irritation of a joint can result in chronic synovitis that is perpetuated by a vicious inflammatory cycle. This keeps the reactive synovitis alive for awhile, even without further trauma.

excellent blood supply and origin. Synovium regenerates completely within several months into tissue that is indistinguishable from the normal.[43]

Acute and chronic synovitis directly affects the amount and content of synovial fluid produced. Synovitis can result in an increased protein count within the synovial fluid. In addition, chronic synovitis can cause a decrease in synovial fluid viscosity and a decrease in the concentration of hyaluronic acid.[15] The concentration of hyaluronic acid has a direct relationship to the synovial fluid viscosity. Minor joint trauma results in no change in concentration or molecular weight of the hyaluronic acid.[15] As trauma severity increases, however, the hyaluronic acid concentration decreases below normal, and when the inflammatory process becomes sufficiently disruptive, joint lining cells not only fail to maintain hyaluronic acid concentration but also fail to maintain normal polymer weight.[15]

A hemarthrosis can result in the synovial fluid having a lower sugar concentration; blood clots can be detected in the synovial fluid; and fibrogen, which normally is not found in synovial fluid, can be detected as a result of bleeding into the joint. Because blood is quickly absorbed by phagocytic cells in the synovial membrane, it may not be evident in the synovial fluid until several days posthemarthrosis.[43]

The effect of a hemarthrosis on the synovial lining results in synovium proliferation and an increased rate of blood absorption with each repeated hemarthrosis. The stimulus for the production of this proliferative synovitis appears to be the iron released from the red blood cells.[43]

The absorption rate of solutions from the joint space is inversely proportional to the size of the particles; the larger the molecules, the slower the clearance. Clinically, absorption from a joint is increased by active or passive range of motion, massage, intra-articular hydrocortisone, or acute inflammation, whereas the effect of external compression is variable.[101]

The joint capsule reacts to injury in a manner similar to that of the synovial membrane. If the inflammatory process continues, the joint capsule eventually becomes a more fibrous tissue, and effusion into the joint cavity can lead to stretching of the capsule and associated ligaments. The higher the hydrostatic pressure and volume of effusion, the faster the fluid reaccumulates after aspiration.[43, 44] Conversely, a significant rise in intra-articular hydrostatic pressure contributes to joint damage by stretching the capsule and associated ligaments.

The load-carrying surfaces of the synovial joint are covered with a thin layer of specialized connective tissue, referred to as articular cartilage. The articular cartilage response to trauma is not unlike that of its counterparts within the joint. The mechanical properties of articular cartilage are readily susceptible to enzymatic degradation. This can occur after acute inflammation, synovectomy, immobilization, or other seemingly minor insults.[94] When articular cartilage loses its content of proteoglycan (protein aggregate that helps establish the resiliency and resistance to deformation of articular cartilage), the physical properties of the cartilage are changed; this renders the collagen fibers susceptible to mechanical damage.[94] As a result of this enzymatic degradation,

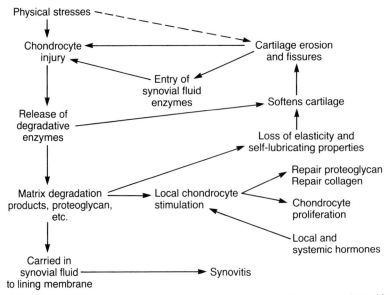

FIGURE 2–4   Postulated final pathway of cartilage degeneration. (Reproduced by permission from Howell, David S.: Osteoarthritis—etiology and pathogenesis. In American Academy of Orthopaedic Surgeons: Symposium on osteoarthritis, St. Louis, 1976, The C. V. Mosby Co.)

articular cartilage can erode and leave denuded bone, resulting in early, irreversible osteoarthritis or degenerative joint disease (Fig. 2–4).

The decrease of posttraumatic joint effusion is paramount in the early rehabilitation process and is important in the restoration of joint kinematics. Prolonged effusion, if left unchecked, can result in a reactive synovitis, joint capsule damage, and degradation of articular cartilage. The early use of mobilization techniques, such as continuous passive motion, and of modalities consisting of cryotherapy and vasopneumatic compression can aid in reducing joint effusion.

EFFECTS OF IMMOBILIZATION

Muscle

One of the first and most obvious changes that occurs as a result of immobilization is loss of muscular strength. This correlates with a reduction in muscle size and a decrease in tension per unit of muscle cross-sectional area.[6, 66, 67] MacDougall and colleagues[67] have reported that 6 weeks of elbow cast immobilization results in a more than 40% decrease in muscular strength. In addition, this strength deficit is correlated with a loss of fiber cross-sectional area and therefore with a decrease in muscle mass. Animal studies have confirmed a general correlation among muscle strength loss and volume and maintenance of specific strength; this can be measured as functional muscle strength for cross-sectional area in a muscle.[6] The rate of loss appears to be most rapid in the initial days of immobilization. Lindboe and Platou[62] have reported that muscle fiber size is reduced by 14 to 17% after 72 hours of immobilization in humans. After 5 to 7 days of immobilization, the absolute loss in muscle mass appears to slow considerably.[6]

It appears that there is a greater degeneration of slow-twitch (type I) versus fast-twitch (type II) fibers with immobilization.[8, 39, 40, 68, 99] Other researchers,[67] however, have shown there to be no selective loss of muscle mass in slow- versus fast-twitch fibers. It appears that both fast- and slow-twitch fibers atrophy. Whether atrophy is differential between fast- and slow-twitch muscle fibers or whether one fiber type is involved more than the other is still unclear.[18, 34]

In addition to the muscle size and volume changes that occur, immobilization also results in histochemical changes. These include a reduction in the levels of adenosine triphosphate (ATP), adenosine diphosphate (ADP), creatine, creatine phosphate (CP), and glycogen, and a greater increase in lactate concentration with work. Furthermore, the rate of protein synthesis decreases within 6 hours of immobilization.[6, 8, 67, 68, 106]

Immobilization also causes an increase in muscle fatigability as a result of decreased oxidative capacity. Reductions occur in maximum oxygen consumption, glycogen levels, and high-energy phosphate levels.[6, 7, 16, 67, 71] Rifenberick and Max[82] have reported fewer mitochondria in atrophic muscle and a significant decrease in mitochondrial activity by day 7 postimmobilization, causing a reduction in cell respiration and contributing to decreased muscle endurance. The following is a summary of the effects of immobilization on muscle:

1. Decrease in muscle fiber size
2. Decrease in mitochondria size and number
3. Decrease in total muscle weight
4. Increase in muscle contraction time
5. Decrease in muscle tension produced
6. Decrease in resting levels of glycogen and ATP
7. More rapid decrease in the ATP level with exercise
8. Increase in lactate concentration with exercise
9. Decrease in protein synthesis

It appears that there is selective muscle atrophy with immobilization. For example, immobilization of the thigh is often associated with selective atrophy of the quadriceps femoris muscle.[47] It was traditionally believed that the vastus medialis atrophies more than the other three heads of the quadriceps. Of the studies available, however, none supports this theory, and their results are more suggestive of a uniform atrophy.[61, 124] Clinically, it is observable that quadriceps atrophy is greater than that of the hamstrings. This observation is supported by muscle biopsy, which shows that the loss in muscular bulk is virtually confined to the quadriceps muscle. This has been further supported by computed tomography (CT) studies.[47, 64, 89]

Also, investigators using CT and ultrasound to measure quadriceps atrophy have reported that thigh circumference measurements, even if supplemented by caliper measurements of subcutaneous fat, underestimate the amount of quadriceps atrophy.[99, 125] Although the knee is

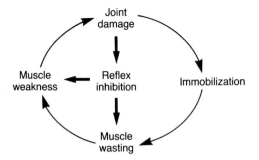

FIGURE 2–5 "Vicious cycles" of arthrogenous muscle weakness. (From Stoke, M., and Young A. (1984): The contribution of reflex inhibition to arthrogenous muscle weakness. Clin. Sci., 67:7.)

the most traditional area noted for selective atrophy, this phenomenon can also be noted in the triceps brachii of an immobilized elbow.[66]

Reflex inhibition can also lead to selective atrophy, particularly in the quadriceps. This type of muscle atrophy is referred to as "arthrogenous muscle wasting," which refers to muscular weakness resulting from injury or an inflamed joint (Fig. 2–5). This is commonly observed in the quadriceps muscle, and athletes describe it as their inability to contract their quadriceps muscle or as lack of control over that muscle ("quad shutdown"). This condition was originally ascribed to pain[25] but can have various underlying causes, the least common of which is pain. Most researchers have postulated that this is a reflex phenomenon having several causes, with no one entity being responsible.

The level of quadriceps activation can be determined through electromyography (EMG). The degree of unilateral quadriceps inhibition can be judged by the difference in maximum voluntary activation (MVA) between the two limbs. Research has shown[99] that quadriceps recruitment (quadriceps setting) is severely inhibited after an arthrotomy (with or without a meniscectomy). Maximum voluntary contraction is reduced by 70 to 90% for 3 to 4 days and is usually still about 40% below its preoperative level 2 weeks after surgery. Quadriceps inhibition 24 hours after arthroscopy (with or without a meniscectomy), however, is only about half that seen following an arthrotomy (with or without a meniscectomy).[92, 99]

It has been postulated that the greater magnitude of quad shutdown following an arthrotomy is a result of the small amount of capsular damage from an arthroscopy versus the "taking down" of the capsule, as in an arthrotomy.[99] The tension in the arthrotomy suture line can evoke afferent impulses from the same receptors activated by an increase in intra-articular pressure that results from an effusion.[125]

Pain has traditionally been regarded as the general cause of reflex inhibition. The perception of fear of pain can greatly affect muscular strength. Athletes who fear that muscle contraction will result in pain may be very apprehensive about contracting those particular muscles, but severe inhibition of muscle strength is seen even after pain subsides.[90] Stokes and Young[99] have noted that, during the first 24 hours postmeniscectomy, pain during contraction can be severe but, unlike that of inhibition, it is usually only mild for 3 to 4 days.[91] Ten to 15 days postoperatively pain is mild or absent, but the athlete still may have quad shutdown. In addition, injection of the meniscal bed and surrounding tissues with an anesthetic temporarily blocks most of the pain, but no change can be detected in quadriceps inhibition.[126]

Tourniquet ischemia has also been thought to contribute to quad shutdown. A study involving tourniquet application on normal subjects,[98] however, revealed that quadriceps MVA is unaltered after voluntary ischemia.

Research has shown that a knee distended with plasma also results in quad shutdown and subsequent quadriceps weakening in normal individuals, even in the absence of pain.[17, 48, 51] Stimuli from a distended knee joint might reflexively inhibit muscle strength development by a central nervous system pathway.[17] Aspiration of the effusion may decrease the severity of inhibition but rarely abolishes it.[99] Young and associates[125] and others[51] have reported that injection of small volumes of fluid (20 to 30 ml) into normal knees results in a 60% quadriceps inhibition, with the quadriceps inhibition increasing as infusion increases.

Joint angle has also been shown not only to have an effect on quadriceps inhibition but also on selective atrophy of muscles in regard to the angle of immobilization. Stratford[100] has reported that effusion inhibits quadriceps contraction less when the knee is in 30° of flexion rather than being fully extended. Similar results are even found following arthrotomy with meniscectomy, in that isometric quadriceps contraction is inhibited less in flexion than in extension.[53, 90, 99] It has been postulated that this is because intra-articular pressure is less when the knee is in 30° of flexion versus full extension.[28, 48, 59, 60, 90]

The length at which the muscle is immobilized also affects selective atrophy. Tardieu and colleagues[103] have suggested that muscle fibers under stretch lengthen by adding sarcomeres in series, whereas those immobilized in a shortened position lose sarcomeres. Thus, when a muscle is immobilized in a lengthened position, the length of the muscle fibers increases to accommodate the muscle's new length, along with other connective tissue changes. A similar adjustment occurs with muscle immobilized in a shortened position. In this case fiber lengths decrease and sarcomeres are subtracted to achieve the physiologic change.[116] Immobilization of a muscle in a shortened position leads to increased connective tissue and reduced muscle extensibility.[103] Garrett[34] has pointed out that muscle immobilization in a lengthened position maintains muscle weight and fiber cross-sectional area better than a shortened muscle, which may explain quadriceps selective atrophy. Because the knee is usually immobilized in an extended or slightly flexed position, the hamstrings are placed in a lengthened position and the quadriceps are in a shortened position.

Although effusion and periarticular damage are plausible reasons for quadriceps inhibition, it appears that it also may be a multifocal phenomenon, with an additional neurophysiologic basis involving the H reflex. The H reflex is a monosynaptic reflex that produces a small muscle contraction in response to low-intensity stimulation of mixed nerves. Infusion of sterile saline solution into the normal knee inhibits the quadriceps H reflex at rest[46, 96] and more severely during submaximal voluntary contraction.[46]

The measured muscular strength output during a large portion of the rehabilitation period following injury is less a function of innate muscle strength than of the amount of voluntary effort. Various factors appear to affect muscle inhibition in producing a maximal voluntary effort.[34]

Periarticular Connective Tissue

Periarticular connective tissue consists of ligaments, tendons, synovial membrane, fascia, and joint capsule. As a result of immobilization, biochemical and histologic changes occur in periarticular tissue around synovial joints, resulting in arthrofibrosis. Fibrous connective tissue is composed of two main components, cells and an extracellular matrix. The matrix primarily consists of collagen and elastin fibers and a nonfibrous ground substance. Fibrocytes, located between the collagen fibers in fibrous connective tissue, are the main collagen-producing cells. As collagen fibers mature, intra- and intermolecular bonds or cross links are formed and increase in number, thereby providing tensile strength to the fibers.[31, 32, 79] Based on the arrangement of its collagen fibers, connective tissue is commonly classified into two types, irregular and regular.[41] The irregular type of collagen is characterized by fibers running in different directions in the same plane.[20] This is functional for capsules, aponeuroses, and sheaths, which are physiologically stressed in many directions.[20, 41] Conversely, in the regularly arranged tissues, collagen fibers run more or less in the same plane and same linear direction.[20] This arrangement affords great tensile strength to ligaments and tendons, which physiologically receive primarily unidirectional stress.[20]

The extracellular matrix is often referred to as ground substance and is composed of glycoaminoglycans (GAGs) and water. To understand the changes that occur with immobilization it is important to be familiar with GAGs and their effect on connective tissue extensibility.[20] Four major GAGs are found in connective tissue: hyaluronic acid, chondroitin-4-sulfate, chondroitin-6-sulfate, and dermatan sulfate. Generally, GAGs are bound to a protein and are collectively referred to as proteoglycans. In connective tissue, proteoglycans combine with water to form a proteoglycan aggregate.

Water constitutes 60 to 70% of the total connective tissue content. GAGs have an enormous water-binding capacity and are responsible for this large water content. Together, GAGs and water form a semifluid viscous gel in which collagen and fibrocytes are embedded. Hyaluronic acid with water is thought to serve as a lubricant between the collagen fibers.[4, 41, 102] This lubricant maintains a distance between the fibers, thereby permitting free gliding of the fibers past each other and perhaps preventing excessive cross linking. Such free gliding is essential for normal connective tissue mobility.[4]

Arthrofibrosis is primarily induced by immobilization, which results in a significant reduction in GAG content with subsequent water loss, contributing to abnormal cross link formation and joint restriction. In addition, within the joint space and recesses, there is excessive connective tissue deposition in the form of fatty fibers, which later mature to form scar tissue that adheres to intra-articular surfaces and further restricts motion.[20]

The most significant change in GAG content reduction occurs within the matrix. Akeson and associates[1-4] have reported a 40% decrease in hyaluronic acid and a 30% decrease in chondroitin-4-sulfate and chondroitin-6-sulfate; collagen mass decreases by about 10%, and collagen turnover increases, with accelerated degradation and synthesis.[2]

The effects of immobilization on connective tissue can be summarized as follows:

1. Reduction in water and GAG content, decreasing the extracellular matrix
2. Reduction in extracellular matrix associated with decrease in lubrication between fiber cross links
3. Reduction in collagen mass
4. Increase in collagen turnover, degradation, and synthesis rate
5. Increase in abnormal collagen fiber cross links

The pathophysiology of arthrofibrosis appears to be the reduction in the semifluid gel as a result of loss of GAG and water, causing a decrease in the critical fiber distance between collagen fibers.[20] Friction is created between fibers, thus reducing collagen extensibility. Furthermore, with joint immobilization, the lack of movement perpetuates a random orientation of newly synthesized collagen fibrils, facilitating the development of irregular cross links in strategic regions of the collagen weave pattern (Fig. 2–6).

Early recognition of arthrofibrosis is paramount and its prevention is the most important consideration. Arthrofibrosis can be divided into three phases (see Table 2–1). Decreasing joint effusion, early muscle turn-on, and pain modulation are key components affecting the arthrofibrotic loop (Fig. 2–7). Arthrofibrotic lesions can usually be prevented by the following:[69] (1) early muscle turn-on; (2) control of the hemarthrosis; (3) control of pain; (4) control of postsurgical scarring; and (5) preoperative patient education to increase rehabilitation compliance.

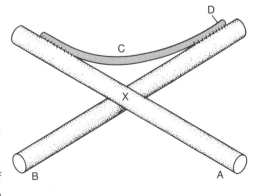

FIGURE 2–6 Idealized model of the interaction of collagen cross links at the molecular level. *A, B*, Pre-existing fibers. *C*, Newly synthesized fibril. *D*, Cross links created as the fibril becomes incorporated into the fiber. *X* represents the nodal point at which adjacent fibers are normally freely movable past each other. (Reprinted with permission of Pergamon Press from Akeson, W.H., Amiel, D., and Woo, S. (1980): Immobility effects of synovial joints: The pathomechanics of joint contracture. Biorheology, 17:95.)

TABLE 2–1   **STAGES OF ARTHROFIBROSIS**

Stage	Phase	Comments
I	Acute (first 3 weeks)	*Goal:* Prevention of complications 1. Early identification of a problem that could lead to complications 2. Early muscle turn on to avoid "shutdown" 3. Reduction of hemarthrosis
II	Subacute (weeks 3 to 8)	1. Constant evaluation is necessary because 10% of patients may enter the fibrosis stage as early as 10 days postoperatively 2. Rehabilitation is geared toward controlling stress on contracted tissues; includes joint mobilization techniques, low-force overpressure, isometrics in the shortened position, and a home program for motion restoration 6–8 times daily 3. Neurophysiologic response of the muscle is increased through electrical muscle stimulation and proprioception techniques
III	Chronic (week 10 plus)	The patient, through a conservative program or lack of compliance, enters a dangerous period, during which reversibility in 10% of patients may not occur *Goal:* Reversing loss of motion and scar tissue build-up 1. Characterized by ingrowth of tissue into the joint and tightness of periarticular structures 2. Treatment consists of careful manipulation or surgical lysis, followed by NSAIDs and careful implementation of a rehabilitation program

Data from: Mangine, R. (1990): The complicated knee: A loss of motion. *In:* 1990 Advances on the Knee and Shoulder. Cincinnati, Cincinnati Sports Medicine and Deaconess Hospital, Symposium held April 2–4, 1990.

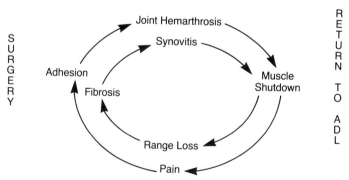

FIGURE 2–7   Arthrofibrotic loop. *Outer loop,* Acute phase. *Inner loop,* Subacute phase. (From Mangine, R. (1990): The complicated knee: A loss of motion. *In:* 1990 Advances on the Knee and Shoulder. Cincinnati, Cincinnati Sports Medicine and Deaconess Hospital, Symposium held April 2–4, 1990.)

Movement is essential in the prevention of contractures and adhesion formation within joints. Physical forces and motion modulate the synthesis of proteoglycans and collagen in normal joints. Stress and motion also influence the deposition of newly synthesized collagen fibers, allowing for proper collagen orientation to resist tensile stress. Motion appears to inhibit periarticular tissue contractures by the following mechanisms:[121]

1. Stimulation of proteoglycan synthesis, thereby lubricating and maintaining a critical distance between existing fibers
2. Ordering the disposition of new collagen fibers (rather than randomization) to resist tensile stress
3. Prevention of anomalous cross links in the matrix by preventing a stationary fiber-fiber attitude at intercept points

The matrix changes associated with immobilization (noted above) are relatively uniform in ligament, capsule, tendon, and fascia. These changes involve extracellular water loss and GAG depletion, along with collagen cross link changes.

Articular Cartilage

Articular cartilage is a thin covering on the ends of bones that creates the moving surfaces of synovial joints.[115] It varies from 1 to 7 mm in thickness, with the articular cartilage covering larger, weight-bearing joints (e.g., hip and knee) being thicker than that covering smaller, nonweight-bearing joints.[115, 122] Articular cartilage consists of fibers, ground substance, and cells. The fibers are composed of collagen and make up 57 to 75% of the cartilage's dry weight.[109] The ground substance is similar to that of periarticular tissue. It is composed of 70 to 80% water and 15 to 50% proteoglycans.[22, 109, 114] The amount of proteoglycans present depends on joint location. Weight-bearing joints have a higher proteoglycan content than nonweight-bearing joints.[108] Both collagen and proteoglycans are produced by chondrocytes.

Articular cartilage is avascular, and its nutritional requirements are met through diffusion and osmosis. The diffusion process occurs through a hydraulic pressure gradient. Low hydraulic pressure has no effect, whereas constant pressure interferes with nutrition.[115] High intermittent pressure loading does not contribute much to the diffusion rate.[70] Joint motion, however, increases the diffusion rate three to four times above static levels,[70] but joint motion in the absence of loading fails to maintain articular cartilage nutrition.[78]

The various effects of immobilization appear to depend on the length of immobilization, the position of immobilization, and joint loading. Cartilage degradation has been reported in rabbits as early as 1 week after immobilization,[14, 48] with a gradual progression of the degenerative process as immobilization continues.[106] Prolonged knee joint immobilization in forced full extension results in full-thickness loss of articular cartilage and infiltration of intra-articular adhesions.[86] Even periodic short-term immobilization results in cumulative, harmful joint effects.[111] Periodic immobilization longer than 30 days can lead to progressive osteoarthritis.[112]

The effects of immobilization on articular cartilage can be separated into contact and noncontact effects. In contact areas, the seriousness of the changes depends mainly on the degree of compression and, in non-contact areas, on the ingrowth of connective tissue on the articular surface.[50] Compression of articular cartilage decreases the synovial fluid diffusion rate and leads to pressure necrosis and chondrocyte death as a result of constant joint compression.[80, 110] Whether the lesions are reversible depends directly on the duration of continuous compression.[86] Also, loss of contact between opposed articular surfaces in weight-bearing and nonweight-bearing joints appears to lead to degenerative changes, suggesting a functional relationship between joint motion and normal articular cartilage surface contact.[40, 110]

The effects of immobilization on articular cartilage can be summarized as follows:

1. Decrease in proteoglycan synthesis
2. Softening of articular cartilage
3. Decrease in articular cartilage thickness
4. Adherence of fibrofatty connective tissue to cartilage surfaces
5. Pressure necrosis at points of cartilage–cartilage contact
6. Chondrocyte death

Intermittent joint loading appears to have a critical role in maintaining healthy articular cartilage. The formation and circulation of synovial and interstitial fluids are stimulated with intermittent joint loading and retarded in its absence. Because synovial fluid is important in cartilage nourishment and lubrication, intermittent pressure can facilitate chondrocyte nourishment and is important for cell function.[10, 21, 23] Conversely, joint immobilization in which the joint is constantly loaded or unloaded can compromise the metabolic exchange necessary for proper structure and function, eventually leading to cartilage degradation and eburnation.[26, 56, 86, 106] Knees immobilized in extension produce irreversible and progressive osteoarthritis. The compression between articular surfaces increases in the immobilized knee and reaches a level three times greater than the initial level after 4 weeks of immobilization.[111] Further evidence supporting the concept of intermittent joint compression is that joint motion without loading during the immobilization period does not prevent deterioration of the articular cartilage.[40]

Immobilized articular cartilage reveals structural, biochemical, and physiologic changes at the cellular and ultrastructural levels.[115] Consistently reported changes include the following: fibrillation, fraying, cyst formation, and loss of staining characteristics of the extracellular ground substance; varying degrees of chondrocyte degeneration, causing cell death and necrosis; cartilage proliferation at joint edges; atrophy in weight-bearing areas and regional bony eburnation; sclerosis; and cartilage resorption after 2 weeks of immobilization. These changes are generally irreversible, but the length of immobilization is important in determining whether the articular changes are irreversible.

Ligaments

Ligaments, like other connective tissue, undergo the same changes in structure as those in periarticular tissue. Because of their function and the bone—ligament interface, however, additional factors must be considered to understand ligaments' response to immobilization.

Like bone, a ligament appears to remodel in response to the mechanical demands placed on it. Stress results in a stiffer, stronger ligament, whereas inactivity yields a weaker, more compliant structure.[13] These changes in ligament properties appear to be caused more by an alteration in their mechanical properties and by subperiosteal resorption at the bone—ligament junction than by actual ligament atrophy.[58, 76] The alterations result in decreased tensile ligament strength, thus reducing the ligaments' ability to provide joint stability. Research has shown that ligaments respond to immobilization by various mechanisms:[2, 5, 33, 75, 119]

1. Significant decrease in linear stress, maximum stress, and stiffness
2. Decrease in ligament fibril cross-sectional area, resulting in a reduction in fibril size and density
3. Decrease in synthesis and degradation of collagen
4. Haphazard arrangement of new collagen fibers
5. Reduction in load and energy-absorbing capabilities of the bone—ligament complex
6. Decrease in the GAG level
7. Increase in osteoclastic activity at the bone—ligament junction, causing an increase in bone resorption in that area

Chemical changes in the medial collateral ligament (MCL) of the knee can be detected as early as 2 weeks following immobilization. By 9 weeks there is significant collagen degradation, with an additional decline in mechanical properties again at 12 weeks postimmobilization.[33, 119, 120] This results in a decrease of tensile properties, with an increased time to failure. Immobilization of primates' lower limbs showed a 40% decrease in maximum load to failure and a significant decrease in energy absorbed before failure in their anterior cruciate ligaments.[75] Most of these failures occurred at the bone—ligament junction.[75, 105] Furthermore, 5 months of postimmobilization reconditioning proved ineffective in restoring the ligament complex to its original state.[75, 76] At 12 months, however, strength and stiffness characteristics of the ligament were equal, but increased strength at the insertion site may be restored more slowly.[75, 76]

High-frequency, low-duration endurance exercises have been shown to have a positive influence on ligament mechanical properties.[13] These might even result in ligament hypertrophy as a result of increased collagen production and fiber bundle hypertrophy.[1] It appears, though, that an isometric exercise program during immobilization cannot stimulate or substitute for the normal physiologic loading of weight-bearing and therefore cannot prevent ligaments from decreasing in strength.[9]

Bone

The effects of immobilization on bone are similar to those on other connective tissues. Bone loss in response to diminished weight-bearing and muscle contraction is a consistent finding. Bone changes can be detected as early as 2 weeks following immobilization.[42, 73, 108] Although the pathogenesis of immobilization osteoporosis is unclear, animal studies have shown decreased bone formation and increased bone reabsorption.[12, 30, 35, 55] Similar findings were noted in patients on total bed rest.[19]

Bone hardness steadily decreases with the duration of immobilization. By 12 weeks it is 55 to 60% of normal.[97] There is also a decline in elastic resistance—the bone becomes more brittle and thus more susceptible to a fracture.

It appears that mechanical strain influences osteoblastic and osteoclastic activity on the bone surface.[24] Bone loss as a result of disuse atrophy occurs at a rate 5 to 20 times greater than that of metabolic disorders affecting bone.[72] The primary cause of this immobilization osteoporosis appears to be the mechanical unloading, which may be responsible for the inhibition of bone formation during immobilization.[123] Therefore, nonweight-bearing immobilization of an extremity should be limited to as short a period as possible.

CONTINUOUS PASSIVE MOTION

Salter,[85] in 1970, originated the biologic concept of continuous passive motion (CPM) of synovial joints to stimulate healing, regenerate articular tissue, and avoid the harmful affects of immobilization.[63] In 1978, Salter and Saringer (an engineer) collaborated to develop the first CPM device for humans (Fig. 2–8).[85] A continuous passive motion machine is an electrical, motor-driven device that helps support the injured limb. It is used to flex and extend a joint at variable rates through progres-

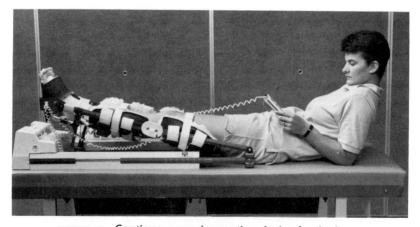

FIGURE 2–8   Continuous passive motion device for the knee.

sively increasing ranges of motion; no muscular exertion is required of the patient.

Salter and colleagues[75, 85, 86] have provided the first histologic evidence in support of CPM. They reported[85, 88] that CPM has a significant stimulus effect on healing articular tissue, including cartilage, tendons, and ligaments; it prevents adhesions and joint stiffness; it does not interfere with healing of incisions over the moving joint; and it can influence the regeneration of articular cartilage through neochondrogenesis.

When compared to immobilized tendons, CPM has proved effective in increasing linear and maximum stress, linear load, and ultimate strength for tendons.[63] Salter and Minster[87] have also reported preliminary results of semitendinous tenodesis for medial collateral ligament reconstructions in experimental animals, in which increased strength was reported after CPM. The application of early tensile forces appears to facilitate the proper alignment of collagen fibers during the initial healing process. Also, decreases in medication requests and decreases in wound edema and effusion in operative knees were reported in CPM patients.[76, 77] The greatest benefit of CPM appears to be the prevention of articular cartilage degradation. Salter[85] has reported that there appears to be more rapid and complete healing in cartilage defects in rabbits when CPM is used.

Continuous passive motion units are considered an acceptable practice following most orthopedic surgeries. Although initially designed for the lower extremity, CPM units are now available for the upper extremity as well. The advent of CPM has helped deter the deleterious effects of immobilization by allowing early motion, even in a protected range. Some indications for the use of CPM include ligament reconstructions or repairs, total joint replacement, release of joint contractures, tendon repairs, open reduction of fractures, and articular cartilage defects.

EFFECTS OF REMOBILIZATION

Physical forces provide important stimuli to tissue for the development and maintenance of homeostasis.[118] The lack of or denial of mobilization results in deleterious effects on bone, muscle, connective tissue, and articular cartilage. The advent of CPM in the late 1970s and early 1980s provided an impetus for initiating early motion to repaired tissues and for using early electrical muscle stimulation to aid in decreasing atrophy and promoting early muscle reeducation. In addition, the emergence of hinged braces, which allow for early protective motion, has helped foster early mobilization.

Early motion and the loading and unloading of joints through partial weight-bearing promote the diffusion of synovial fluid to nourish articular cartilage, meniscus, and ligaments. Moreover, research has shown that motion enhances this transsynovial nutrient flow.[60, 70, 81] Regardless of the cell-stimulating mechanism, it is clear that the fibroblasts and chondrocytes interpret physical forces so as to influence their rate of synthesis, and extracellular degradation of matrix components is similarly controlled.[2]

Immobilization through casting techniques is still used, however, in the treatment of many ligamentous reconstructions and fractures. It is not known whether the deleterious effects of prolonged immobilization can be reversed with remobilization techniques. These structural changes generally appear to depend on the duration and angle of immobilization and on the weight-bearing status.

Muscle

Muscle responds to remobilization more readily than other connective tissue structures. Muscle regeneration begins within 3 to 5 days after initiation of a reconditioning program.[16, 128] By 6 weeks postimmobilization it appears that both fast- and slow-twitch muscle fibers can recover completely.[117] Protein synthesis responds quickly to major changes in muscle contractile activity by a rapid increase in synthesis.[107] Booth and Seider[8] have reported that in rats ATP, glycogen, and protein concentrations following 90 days of immobilization return to control levels by recovery day 60. Soleus muscle wasting and protein content return to control levels by day 14. Maximum isometric tension does not return to normal, however, until day 120. Thus, the biochemical and physiologic changes that result in skeletal muscle immobilization do return to normal, but at differing times following termination of immobilization.

It has been theorized that electrical muscle stimulation (EMS) can provide enough muscle activity to deter atrophy and the deleterious muscle effects of immobilization. Most studies on the effects of EMS have been on normal muscle, and investigations concerning effects on diseased, traumatized, or immobilized muscle have not been as well reported. Initial investigations yielded promising results, but more recent studies have been less encouraging. Sisk and colleagues[93] have reported that EMS following anterior cruciate ligament reconstruction has no significant effect over 6 weeks of immobilization. Also, EMS to the quadriceps muscle appears not to be of significant magnitude to alter quadriceps atrophy,[37-39, 74] nor to affect the muscle enzyme changes that occur as a result of immobilization.[38, 39]

Although research has shown that EMS produces no significant changes in the muscle atrophy process, it has been postulated that use of this modality may be better than performing no exercise at all.[54, 74] EMS can be most helpful in regard to muscle reeducation, pain and spasm abatement, and decreasing effusion through the pumping action of the muscle as it contracts.

Unfortunately, it appears that neither EMS nor isometric exercise can help enough to prevent disuse atrophy.[37-39] Although the use of EMS and braces that allow for early limited range of motion can decrease atrophy somewhat, they do not adequately replace the amount and type of contractile activity.[6] It appears that the only way to prevent muscle atrophy in immobilized limbs is to replace the muscle usage removed by limb immobilization with an equivalent quantity and quality of muscle contraction.

Articular Cartilage

The effects of remobilization on articular cartilage seem to be time-dependent. Many studies have examined the effects of remobilization following immobilization on articular cartilage. Evans and co-workers[27] have reported cartilage alterations such as matrix fibrillation, cleft formation, and ulceration that are not reversible in rats with immobilization up to 90 days. They noted, however, that soft tissue changes are reversible if the period of immobilization does not exceed 30 days. Finsterbush and Friedman[29] also noted similar irreversible damage in remobilization experiments. Articular cartilage generally responds favorably to mechanical stimuli, with structural modifications noted after exercise.[45, 84] Furthermore, studies have shown that exercising on a treadmill from 1 to 6 hours daily did not contribute to an increased incidence of joint degeneration in mice.[57] This observation has been further supported by Jurvelin and colleagues,[49] whose animal studies revealed remarkable changes in articular cartilage within the first week of immobilization; running exercises up to 8 weeks, however, elicited only transitory to minor alterations in articular surface.

It has been speculated that the limitation of joint movement, whether there is contact or loss of contact between joint surfaces, produces changes by interfering with cartilage nutrition, which relies on loading and unloading of a joint for nourishment and diffusion. This is supported by research showing that articular cartilage changes still occur, even in joints that are mobilized, if weight-bearing is not allowed.[40]

Bone

Immobilization results in disuse osteoporosis, which may not be reversible on remobilization of the limb. The reversibility is related to the severity of changes and to the length of immobilization. Permanent osseous changes appear to occur with an immobilization period exceeding 12 weeks.[127] Even though bone loss in the first 12 weeks is regained, the period of recovery is at least as long and may be many times longer than the immobilization period.[11] The most effective method of modifying osteoporosis caused by reduced skeletal loads appears to be through exercise. Isotonic and isometric exercises have been shown to decrease bone loss in subjects who were exposed to prolonged periods of weightlessness and bed rest.[65, 113] Activity increases bone formation in these situations and can hasten recovery following the return to a normal loading environment. If an appropriate environment can be maintained during immobilization of a limb, the deleterious effects of disuse on bone can be partially prevented, and rehabilitation can be accelerated.[11]

Ligaments

Remobilization following immobilization of ligaments occurs in an asynchrous fashion. It appears that the bone—ligament junction recovers at a much slower rate than the mechanical or midsubstance properties of the ligament.[119, 120] Cabaud and colleagues[13] have reported that ligament strength and stiffness in rat anterior cruciate ligaments can increase with endurance-type exercises. Others have noted similar results.[49, 50] Moreover, not only does the injured ligament result in weaker mechanical properties at midsubstance and at the bone—ligament complex, but nontraumatized ligaments become weaker as a result of immobilization. These weakened mechanical ligament properties must be considered when planning a rehabilitation program.

Recovery from immobilization depends on the duration of immobilization. Woo and associates[119] have noted that 1 year of immobilization is required before the architectural components of the medial collateral ligament—tibia junction return to normal following 12 weeks of immobilization. Noyes[75] has reported that in primates after 5 months of remobilization, followed by total body immobilization, there is only partial recovery in ligament strength, although ligament stiffness and compliance parameters return to control values. It was reported that 12 months are required for complete recovery of ligament strength parameters.[75] Tipton and co-workers[104] have observed 50% of normal strength in a healing ligament by 6 months, 80% after 1 year, and 100% after 1 to 3 years, depending on the type of stresses placed on it and the prevention of repeated injury.

It appears that ligament properties return to normal with remobilization, but this depends on the duration of the immobilization, with the bone—ligament junction requiring longer to return to normal following immobilization.

Connective Tissue

Few studies have documented the effects of remobilization following immobilization on cross link formation.[20] Evidence has shown that movement maintains lubrication and critical fiber distance within the matrix and ensures an orderly deposition of collagen fibrils, thereby preventing abnormal cross link formation.[20] Often, for range of motion to be restored, forceful manipulation that breaks the intracapsular fibrofatty adhesions may have to be performed.[20] Although range of motion is restored, it has been speculated that there is peeling of the fibrofatty tissue from the bone ends, with these ragged edges of adhesions remaining in the joint.[23, 27] There is also increased joint inflammation from the manipulation, resulting in an increased potential for chronic synovitis.

Motion problems should be detected early, joint end-feel assessed by palpation, and the reason for the motion problem determined. If manipulation is the treatment of choice, it should be performed early in the recovery process to decrease the amount of joint damage resulting from a manipulation and to prevent the connective tissue changes from becoming morphologic changes.

The deleterious effects of immobilization on bone and connective tissue have been widely reported. The efficacy of early, controlled mobilization to allow orderly organization of collagen in lines of stress and to promote healthy joint arthrokinematics is supported by many studies. Acute injury that is not treated adequately with an early concentration on decreasing joint effusion and pain, with restoration of normal joint arthrokinematics, can result in a vicious inflammatory cycle, perpetuating the degradation of articular cartilage by the enzymes released with cell death. This articular cartilage damage is a secondary injury induced by inadequate attention to decreasing the severity of the early inflammatory process.

The harmful effects of immobilization on muscle are the most obvious changes. Muscle atrophy can be detected as early as 24 hours after immobilization. Muscle responds to immobilization by a decrease in muscle fiber size, total muscle weight, mitochondria size and number, the muscle tension produced, resting levels of glycogen and of ATP, and protein synthesis. With exercise there is an increase in muscle contraction time and the lactate level.

Muscle shutdown is also a phenomenon generally seen following immobilization, but it can readily be detected after most surgeries. It is observed in the quadriceps muscle following knee surgery. Although many reasons for muscle shutdown have been postulated, it appears to be affected by one or more of the following factors: joint effusion, angle of joint immobilization, periarticular tissue damage from surgery or trauma, and the H reflex.

Immobilization causes biochemical and histochemical changes in the periarticular tissue, ultimately contributing to arthrofibrosis. Immobilization-induced arthrofibrosis has been widely documented, although the exact mechanism is still speculative. Connective tissue usually responds to immobilization by a reduction in water and glycoaminoglycans; a decrease in the extracellular matrix, which leads to a reduction in the lubrication between fiber cross links; a decrease in collagen mass; and an increase in collagen turnover, degradation, and synthesis rate and in abnormal collagen fiber cross links.

Ligaments are affected by immobilization similarly. It appears that the bone–ligament interface undergoes an increase in osteoclastic activity, resulting in a weaker bone–ligament junction. There is also ligament atrophy, with a corresponding decrease in linear stress, maximum stress, and stiffness.

The greatest insult from immobilization appears to be on the articular cartilage. The intermittent loading and unloading of synovial joints promote the metabolic exchange necessary for the proper structure and function of articular cartilage. Joint immobilization, in which articular cartilage is in constant contact with opposing bone ends, can cause pressure necrosis. Conversely, noncontact between joint surfaces can promote ingrowth of connective tissue into the joint. Diminished weight-bearing and the loading and unloading of an extremity also cause an increase in bone resorption in that area.

Continuous passive motion (CPM) devices allow for early joint motion, with no detrimental side effects. Continuous passive motion provides a significant stimulus effect on healing articular tissue, including cartilage, tendon, and ligament, as well as preventing joint adhesions and stiffness. Patients using CPM devices have shown a decrease in joint hemarthrosis and pain medication requests.

Most tissue appears to recover at different rates with mobilization following immobilization, with muscle recovering the fastest. Although few studies on the effects of mobilization on immobilized connective tissue have been reported, it has been proved that early mobilization maintains lubrication and critical fiber distance among collagen fibrils in the matrix, thus preventing abnormal cross link formation. Articular cartilage and bone respond the least favorably to mobilization following immobilization. Articular cartilage changes depend on the length and angle of immobilization. Prolonged immobilization can result in irreversible articular cartilage changes.

To avoid the deleterious effects of immobilization, early protected motion and weight-bearing as healing restraints allow are advocated. These help deter the secondary problems perpetuated by immobilization.

References

1. Akeson, W.H., Woo, S.L.-Y., Amiel, D., et al. (1984): The chemical basis of tissue repair. *In:* Hunter, L.Y., and Funk, F.J. (eds.): Rehabilitation of the Injured Knee. St. Louis, C.V. Mosby, pp. 93–148.
2. Akeson, W.H., Amiel, D., Abel, M.F., et al. (1987): Effects of immobilization on joints. Clin. Orthop., 219:28–37.
3. Akeson, W.H., Amiel, D., and LaViolette, D. (1967): The connective tissue response to immobility: A study of the chondroitin-4- and 6-sulfate and dermatan sulfate changes in periarticular connective tissue of control and immobilized knee of dogs. Clin. Orthop., 51:183–197.
4. Akeson, W.H., Amiel, D., and Woo, S. (1980): Immobility effects of synovial joints: The pathomechanics of joint contracture. Biorheology, 17:95–110.
5. Binkley, J.M., and Peat, M. (1986): The effects of immobilization on the ultrastructure and mechanical properties of the medial collateral ligament of rats. Clin. Orthop. Rel. Res., 203:301–308.
6. Booth, F.W. (1987): Physiologic and biochemical effects of immobilization on muscle. Clin. Orthop. Rel. Res., 219:15–20.
7. Booth, F.W., and Kelso, J.R. (1973): Effect of hindlimb immobilization on contractile and histochemical properties of skeletal muscle. Pflugers Arch., 342:231–238.
8. Booth, F.W., and Seider, M.J. (1979): Recovery of skeletal muscle after 3 months of hindlimb immobilization in rats. J. Appl. Physiol., 47:435–439.
9. Bozdech, Z. (1976): Posttraumatic synovitis. Acta Chir. Orthop. Traumatol. Cech., 43:244–247.
10. Broom, N.D., and Myers, D.B. (1980): A study of the structural response of wet hyaline cartilage to various loading situations. Connect. Tissue Res., 7:227.
11. Burr, D.B., Frederickson, R.G., Pavlinch, C., et al. (1984): Intracast muscle stimulation prevents bone and cartilage deterioration in cast-immobilized rabbits. Clin. Orthop. Rel. Res., 189:264–278.
12. Burdeaux, B.D., and Hutchinson, W.J. (1953): Etiology of traumatic osteoporosis. J. Bone Joint Surg. [Am.], 35:479.
13. Cabaud, H.E., Chatty, A., and Gildengorin, V. (1980): Exercise effects on the strength of the rat anterior cruciate ligament. Am. J. Sports Med., 8:79.
14. Candolin, T., and Videman, T. (1980): Surface changes in the articular cartilage of

rabbit knee during immobilization. A scanning electron microscopic study of experimental osteoarthritis. Acta Pathol. Microbiol. Immunol. Scand., 88:291.

15. Castor, C.W., Prince, R.K., and Hazelton, M.J. (1966): Hyaluronic acid in human synovial effusions: A sensitive indicator of altered connective tissue cell function during inflammation. Arthritis Rheumatol., 9:783–794.

16. Cooper, R.R. (1972): Alternatives during immobilization and regeneration of skeletal muscle in cats. J. Bone Joint Surg. [Am.], 54:919.

17. DeAndrade, J.R., Grant, C., and Dixon, A. (1965): Joint distension and reflex inhibition in the knee. J. Bone Joint Surg. [Am.], 47:313–322.

18. Dickinson, A., and Bennett, K.M. (1985): Therapeutic exercise. Clin. Sports Med., 4:417–429.

19. Donaldson, C.L., Hulley, S.B., Vogel, J.M., et al. (1970): Effect of prolonged bed rest on bone mineral. Metabolism, 19:1071.

20. Donatelli, R., and Owens-Burkhart, A. (1981): Effects of immobilization on the extensibility of periarticular connective tissue. J. Orthop. Sports Phys. Ther., 3: 67–72.

21. Ekholm, R. (1955): Nutrition of articular cartilage: A radioautographic study. Acta Anat., 24:329.

22. Elliot R.J., and Gardner, D.L. (1979): Changes with age of the glycosaminoglycans of human cartilage. Ann. Rheum. Dis., 38:371–377.

23. Enneking, W.F., and Horowitz, M. (1972): The intra-articular effects of immobilization on the human knee. J. Bone Joint Surg. [Am.], 54:973.

24. Epker, B.N., and Frost, H.M. (1965): Correlation of bone resorption and formation behavior of loaded bone. J. Dent. Res., 44:33.

25. Eriksson, E. (1981): Rehabilitation of muscle function after sports injury—major problem in sports medicine. Int. J. Sports Med., 2:1–6.

26. Eronen. I., Videman, T., Friman, C., and Michelesson, J.E. (1978): Glycosaminoglycan metabolism in experimental osteoarthritis caused by immobilization. Acta Orthop. Scand., 49:329.

27. Evans, E.B., Egger, G.W.N., Butler, M., and Blumel, J. (1960): Experimental immobilization and remobilization of rat knee joints. J. Bone Joint Surg. [Am.], 42:737–758.

28. Eyring, E.J., and Murray, W.R. (1964): The effect of joint position on the pressure of intra-articular effusion. J. Bone Joint Surg. [Am.], 46:1235.

29. Finsterbush, A., and Friedman, B. (1975): Reversibility of joint changes produced by immobilization in rabbits. Clin. Orthop., 111:290–298.

30. Fleisch, H., Russell, R.G., Simpson, B., and Muhlbauer, R.C. (1969): Prevention by a diphosphonate of immobilization osteoporosis in rats. Nature, 223:221.

31. Freeman, M.A.R. (1979): Adult Articular Cartilage, 2nd ed. Tunbridge Wells, England, Pitman Medical, pp. 183–196.

32. Fujimoto, D., Moriquichi, T., Ishida, T., and Hayashi, H. (1978): The structure of pyridinoline, a collagen cross link. Biochem. Biophys. Res. Commun., 84:52–57.

33. Gamble, J.G., Edwards, C.C., and Max, S.R. (1984): Enzymatic adaptation in ligaments during immobilization. Am. J. Sports Med., 12:221–228.

34. Garrett, G.E. (1989): Effects of injury on muscle and the patellofemoral joint. In: 1989 Advances on the Knee and Shoulder. Cincinnati, Cincinnati Sports Medicine and Deaconess Hospital, Symposium held March 6–8, 1989.

35. Geiser, M., and Trueta, J. (1985): Muscle action, bone rarefaction, and bone formation. J. Bone Joint Surg. [Br.], 40:282.

36. Golden, A. (1980): Reaction to injury in the musculoskeletal system. In: Rosse, C., and Clawson, D.K. (eds.): The Musculoskeletal System in Health and Disease. New York, Harper & Row.

37. Halkjaer-Kristensen, J., and Ingemann-Hansen, T. (1985): Wasting of the human quadriceps muscle after knee ligament injuries. I. Anthropometrical consequences. Scand. J. Med. [Suppl.], 13:5–11.

38. Halkjaer-Kristensen, J., and Ingemann-Hansen, T. (1985): Wasting of the human quadriceps muscle after knee ligament injuries. II. Muscle fibre morphology. Scand. J. Med. [Suppl.], 13:12–20.

39. Halkjaer-Kristensen, J., and Ingemann-Hansen, T. (1985): Wasting of the human quadriceps muscle after knee ligament injuries. III. Oxidative and glycolytic enzyme activities. Scand. J. Med. [Suppl.], 13:21–28.

40. Hall, M.C. (1963): Cartilage changes after experimental relief of contact in the knee of the mature rat. J. Bone Joint Surg. [Am.], 95:36.

41. Ham, A.C., and Cormack, D. (eds.) (1979): Histology, 8th ed. Philadelphia, J.B. Lippincott.

42. Hardt, A.B. (1972): Early metabolic responses of bone to immobilization. J. Bone Joint Surg. [Am.], 54:119.

43. Hettinga, D.L. (1979): I. Normal joint structures and their reaction to injury. J. Orthop. Sports Phys. Ther., 1:16–22.

44. Hettinga, D.L. (1979): II. Normal joint structures and their reaction to injury. J. Orthop. Sports Phys. Ther., 1:83–88.

45. Holmdahl, D.E., and Ingelmark, B.E. (1948): Des Gelenkknorpels unter verschiedenen funktionellen Verhältnissen. Acta Anat. (Basel), 7:309–375.

46. Iles, J.F., Stokes, M., and Young, A. (1985): Reflex actions of knee joint receptors on quadriceps in man. J. Physiol., 360:481.

47. Ingemann-Hansen, T., and Halkjaer-Kristensen, J. (1980): Computerized tomographic determination of human thigh components. The effects of immobilization in plaster and subsequent physical training. Scand. J. Rehabil. Med., 12:27.

48. Jayson, M.I.V., and Dixon, A. (1970): Intra-articular pressure in rheumatoid arthritis of the knee. III. Pressure changes during joint use. Ann Rheum. Dis., 29:401–408.

49. Jurvelin, J., Helminen, H.J., Laurisalo, S., et al. (1985): Influences of joint immobilization and running exercise on articular cartilage surfaces of young rabbits. Acta Anat., 122:62–68.

50. Jurvelin, J., Kiviranta, I., Tammi, M., and Helminen, J.H. (1986): Softening of canine articular cartilage after immobilization of the knee joint. Clin. Orthop. Rel. Res., 207:246–252.

51. Kennedy, J.C., Alexander, I.J., and Hayes, K.C. (1982): Nerve supply of the human knee and its functional importance. Am. J. Sports Med., 10:329–335.

52. Knight, K. (1976): The effects of hypothermia on inflammation and swelling. Athletic Training, 11:7–10.

53. Krebs, D.E., Staples, W.H., Cuttita, D., and Zickel, R.E. (1983): Knee joint angle: Its relationship to quadriceps femoris activity in normal and post-arthrotomy limbs. Arch. Phys. Med. Rehabil., 64:441.

54. Kubiak, R.J., Whitman, K.M., and Johnston, R.M. (1987): Changes in quadriceps femoris muscle strength during isometric exercise versus electrical stimulation. J. Orthop. Sports Phys. Ther., 8:537–541.

55. Landry, M., and Fleisch, H. (1964): The influence of immobilization on bone formation as evaluated by osseous incorporation of tetracyclines. J. Bone Joint Surg. [Br.], 46:764.

56. Langenskiold, A., Michelsson, J.E., and Videman, T. (1979): Osteoarthritis of the knee in the rabbit produced by immobilization. Attempts to achieve a reproducible model for studies on pathogenesis and therapy. Acta Orthop. Scand., 50:1.

57. Lanier, R.R. (1946): The effects of exercise on the knee joints of inbred mice. Anat. Rec., 94:311–319.

58. Laros, G.S., Tipton, C.M., and Cooper, R.R. (1971): Influence of physical activity on ligament insertions in the knees of dogs. J. Bone Joint Surg. [Am.], 53:275.

59. Levick, R.J. (1983): Joint pressure-volume studies: Their importance, design and interpretation. J. Rheumatol., 10:353.

60. Levick, R.J. (1983): Synovial fluid dynamics: The regulation of volume and pressure. In: Holborrow, E.J., and Maroudas, A. (eds.): Studies in Joint Disease. London, Pitman Medical, pp. 153–240.

61. Lieb, F.J., and Perry, J. (1968): Quadriceps function. An anatomical and mechanical study using amputated limbs. J. Bone Joint Surg. [Am.], 50:1535–1548.

62. Lindboe, C.F., and Platou, C.S. (1984): Effects of immobilization of short duration on muscle fibre size. Clin. Physiol., 4:183.

63. Loitz, B.J., Zernicke, R.F., Vailas, A.C., et al. (1989): Effects of short-term immobilization versus continuous passive motion on the biomechanical and biochemical properties of the rabbit tendon. Clin. Orthop., 244:265–271.

64. LoPresti, C., Kirkendall, D., Street, G., et al. (1984): Degree of quadriceps atrophy on a 1-year postanterior cruciate repair. Med. Sci. Sports Exerc., 16:204.

65. Lynch, T.N., Jensen, R.L., Stevens, D.M., et al. (1967): Metabolic effects of prolonged bed rest: Their modification by simulated altitude. Aerospace Med., 38:10.

66. MacDougall, J.D., Elder, G.C.B., Sale, D.G., et al. (1980): Effects of strength training and immobilization on human muscle fibers. Eur. J. Appl. Physiol., 43:25.

67. MacDougall, J.D., Ward, G.R., Sale, D.G., and Sutton, J.R. (1977): Biochemical adaptation of human skeletal muscle to heavy resistance training and immobilization. J. Appl. Physiol., 43:700–703.

68. Maier, A., Crockett, J.L., Simpson, D.R., et al. (1976): Properties of immobilized guinea pig hindlimb muscles. Am. J. Physiol., 231:1520–1526.

69. Mangine, R.E. (1990): The complicated knee: A loss of motion. In: 1990 Advances on the Knee and Shoulder. Cincinnati, Cincinnati Sports Medicine and Deaconess Hospital. Symposium held April 2–4, 1990.

70. Maroudes, A., Bullough, P., Swanson, S., and Freeman, M. (1968): The permeability of articular cartilage. J. Bone Joint Surg. [Br.], 50:166–177.

71. Max, S.R. (1972): Disuse atrophy of skeletal muscle: Loss of functional activity of mitochondria. Biochem. Biophys. Res. Commun., 46:1394–1398.

72. Mazess, R.B., and Whedon, G.D. (1983): Immobilization and bone. Calcif. Tissue Int., 35:265.

73. Minaire, P., Meunier, P., Edouard, C., et al. (1974): Quantitative histological data on disuse osteoporosis. Calcif. Tissue Res., 17:57.

74. Morrissey, M.C., Brewster, C.E., Shields, C.L., and Brown, M. (1985): The effects of electrical stimulation on the quadriceps during postoperative knee immobilization. Am. J. Sports Med., 13:40–45.

75. Noyes, F.R. (1977): Functional properties of knee ligaments and alterations induced by immobilization. Clin. Orthop. Rel. Res., 123:210–242.

76. Noyes, F.R., Mangine, R.E., and Barber, S. (1974): Biomechanics of ligament failure. II. An analysis of immobilization, exercise, and reconditioning effects in primates. J. Bone Joint Surg. [Am.], 56:1406.

77. O'Driscoll, S.W., Kumar, A., and Salter, R.B. (1983): The effect of continuous passive motion on the clearance of a hemarthrosis from a synovial joint: An experimental investigation in the rabbit. Clin. Orthop., 176:305.

78. Palmoski, M.J., Colyer, R.A., and Brandt, K.D. (1980): Joint motion in the absence of normal loading does not maintain articular cartilage. Arthritis Rheum., 23:325–334.

79. Peacock, E.E., Jr. (1981): Wound Repair, 3rd ed. Philadelphia, W.B. Saunders.

80. Radin, E.L., Paul, I.L., and Pollock, D. (1970): Animal joint behavior under excessive loading. Nature, 266:554–555.

81. Renzoni, S.A., Amiel, D., Harwood, F.L., and Akeson, W.H. (1984): Synovial nutrition of knee ligaments. Trans. Orthop. Res. Soc., 9:277.

82. Rifenberick, D.H., and Max, S.R. (1974): Substrate utilization by disused rat skeletal muscles. Am. J. Physiol., 226:295–297.

83. Roy, S., Ghadially, F.N., and Crane, W.A.J. (1966): Synovial membrane and traumatic effusion: Ultrastructure and autoradiography with tritiated leucine. Ann. Rheumatol. Dis., 25:259–271.

84. Saaf, J. (1950): Effect of exercise on adult cartilage. Acta Orthop. Scand. [Suppl.], 7:1–83.

85. Salter, R.B. (1989): The biologic concept of continuous passive motion of synovial joints. Clin. Orthop., 242:12–25.

86. Salter, R.B., and Field, P. (1960): The effects of continuous compression on living articular cartilage. J. Bone Joint Surg. [Am.], 42:31–49.

87. Salter, R.B., and Minster, R.R. (1982): The effect of continuous passive motion on a semitendinous tenodesis in the rabbit knee (abstr.). Orthop. Trans., 6:292.

88. Salter, R.B., Simmonds, D.F., Malcolm, B.W., et al. (1975): The effect of continuous passive motion on the healing of articular cartilage defects: An experimental investigation in rabbits (abstr.). J. Bone Joint Surg. [Am.], 57:570.

89. Sargeant, A.J., Davies, C.T.M., Edwards, R.H.T., et al. (1976): Functional and structural changes after disuse of human muscle. Clin. Sci., 52:337.

90. Shakespeare, D.T., Stokes, M., Sherman, K.P., and Young, A. (1983): The effect of knee flexion on quadriceps inhibition after meniscectomy. Clin. Sci., 65:64.

91. Sherman, K.P., Shakespeare, D.T., Stokes, M., and Young, A. (1983): Inhibition of voluntary quadriceps activity after meniscectomy. Clin. Sci., 64:70.

92. Sherman, K.P., Young, A., Stokes, M., and Shakespeare, D.T. (1984): Joint injury and muscle weakness. Lancet, 2:646.

93. Sisk, D.T., Stralka, S.W., Deering, M.B., and Griffin, J.W. (1987): Effect of electrical stimulation on quadriceps strength after reconstructive surgery of the anterior cruciate ligament. Am. J. Sports Med., 15:215–220.

94. Sledge, C.B. (1975): Structure, development, and function of joints. Orthop. Clin. North Am., 6:619–628.

95. Soren, A., Rosenbauer, K.A., Klein, W., and Huth, F. (1973): Morphological examinations of so-called posttraumatic synovitis. Beitr. Pathol., 1950:11–30.

96. Spencer, J.D., Hayes, K.C., and Alexander, I.J. (1984): Knee joint effusion and quadriceps reflex inhibition in man. Arch. Phys. Med. Rehabil., 65:171.

97. Steinberg, F.U. (1980): The Immobilized Patient: Functional Pathology and Management. New York: Plenum Press.

98. Stokes, M., Mill, K., Shakespeare, D., et al. (1984): Post-operative inhibition: Voluntary ischemia does not alter quadriceps function in normal subjects. In: Wittle, M.W., and Harris, J.D. (eds.): Biomechanical Measurement in Orthopaedic Practice. New York, Oxford University Press.

99. Stokes, M., and Young, A. (1984): The contribution of reflex inhibition to arthrogenous muscle weakness. Clin. Sci., 67:7–14.

100. Stratford, P. (1981): Electromyography of the quadriceps femoris muscles in subjects with normal knees and acutely effused knees. Phys. Ther., 62:279.

101. Stravino, V.D. (1972): The synovial system. Am. J. Phys. Med., 51:312–320.

102. Swann, D., Radin, E., and Nazimiec, M. (1976): Role of hyaluronic acid on joint lubrication. Ann. Rheum. Dis., 33:318–326.

103. Tardieu, C., Tabary, J.C., Tabary, C., and Tardieu, G. (1982): Adaptation of connective tissue length to immobilization in the lengthened and shortened positions in cat soleus muscle. J. Physiol., 78:214.

104. Tipton, C.M., James, S.L., Mergner, W., et al. (1970): Influence of exercise on strength of medial collateral knee ligament of dogs. Am. J. Physiol., 218:894.

105. Tipton, C.M., Marrhes, R.D., Maynard, J.A., and Carey, R.A. (1975): The influence of physical activity on ligaments and tendons. Med. Sci. Sports, 7:165–175.

106. Trias, A. (1961): Effects of persistent pressure on articular cartilage. J. Bone Joint Surg. [Am.], 43:376–386.

107. Tucker, K.R., Sider, M.J., and Booth, F.W. (1981): Protein synthesis rates in atrophied gastrocnemius muscles after limb immobilization. J. Appl. Physiol., 51:73–77.

108. Uhthoff, H.K., and Jaworski, Z.F.G. (1978): Bone loss in response to long-term immobilization. J. Bone Joint Surg. [Br.], 60:420.

109. Venn, M.F. (1979): Chemical composition of human femoral head cartilage: Influence of topographical position and fibrillation. Ann. Rheum. Dis., 38:57–62.

110. Videman, T. (1981): Changes of compression and distances between tibial and femoral condyles during immobilization of rabbit knee. Arch. Orthop. Trauma Surg., 98:289.

111. Videman, T. (1982): Experimental osteoarthritis in the rabbit. Comparison of different periods of repeated immobilization. Acta Orthop. Scand., 53:339.

112. Videman, T. (1987): Connective tissue and immobilization. Clin. Orthop. Rel. Res., 221:26–32.

113. Vogt, F.B., Mack, P.B., Beasley, W.G., et al. (1965). The effect of bed rest on various parameters of physiological function. Part XII. The effect of bed rest on bone mass and calcium balance. Washington, DC, National Aeronautics and Space Administration, Publ. No. CR-182.

114. Weiss, C. (1979): Normal and osteoarthritic articular cartilage. Orthop. Clin. North Am., 10:175–189.

115. Westers, B.M. (1982): Review of the repair of defects in articular cartilage: Part I. J. Orthop. Sports Phys. Ther., 3:186–192.

116. Williams, P.E., and Goldspink, G. (1978): Changes in sarcomere length and physiological properties in immobilized muscle. J. Anat., 127:459.

117. Witzmann, F.A., Kim, D.H., and Fitts, R.H. (1982): Recovery time course in contractile function of fast and slow skeletal muscle after hindlimb immobilization. J. Appl. Physiol., 52:677–682.

118. Wolff, J. (1982): Das Gesetz der Transformation der Knochen. Berlin, A. Hirschwald.

119. Woo, S., Gomez, M.A., Sites, T.J., et al. (1987): The biomechanical and morphological changes in the medial collateral ligament of the rabbit after immobilization and remobilization. J. Bone Joint Surg. [Am.], 69:1200–1211.

120. Woo, S., Inoue, D.M., McGurk-Burleson, E., and Gomez, M.A. (1987): Treatment of the medial collateral ligament injury. II: Structure and function of canine knees in response to differing treatment regimes. Am. J. Sports Med., 15:22–29.
121. Woo, S., Matthew, J.V., Akeson, W.H., et al. (1975): Connective tissue response to immobility. Arthritis Rheum., 18:257–264.
122. Wright, V., Dowson, D., and Kerr, J. (1973): The structure of joints. Int. Rev. Connect. Tissue Res., 6:105–125.
123. Wronski, T.J., and Morey, E.R. (1982): Skeletal abnormalities in rats induced by simulated weightlessness. Metab. Bone Dis., 4:69.
124. Young, A., Hughes, I., Round, J.M., and Edwards, R.H.T. (1982): The effect of knee injury on the number of muscle fibers in the human quadriceps femoris. Clin. Sci., 62:227–234.
125. Young, A., Stokes, M., and Iles, J.F. (1987): Effects of joint pathology on muscle. Clin. Orthop., 219:21–27.
126. Young, A., Stokes, M., Shakespeare, D.T., and Sherman, K.P. (1983): The effect of intra-articular bupivacaine on quadriceps inhibition after meniscectomy. Med. Sci. Sports Exerc., 15:154.
127. Young, D.R., Niklowitz, W.J., and Steele, C.R. (1983): Tibial changes in experimental disuse osteoporosis in the monkey. Calcif. Tissue Int., 35:304.
128. Zarins, B. (1982): Soft tissue injury and repair: Biomechanical aspects. Int. J. Sports Med., 3:19.

CHAPTER 3

◆

Role of Evaluation in the Rehabilitation Program

Ron Courson, P.T., A.T.,C.

One of the most challenging areas in the field of sports medicine is rehabilitation following athletic injury. The goals of any rehabilitation program include returning the athlete to optimal preinjury status and developing a preventive maintenance program to minimize the possibility of injury recurrence. The clinician should strive to return athletes to their activity without restriction as soon as possible, but within safe guidelines. Rehabilitation is challenging in that all athletes are different, as is every athletic injury, and have unique characteristics. Therefore, each athlete responds to injury in a unique and different manner. Rehabilitation protocols are frequently used by sports medicine care providers for guidance in treating specific pathologies. Although these protocols help provide consistency and continuity throughout the rehabilitation process, it must be remembered that they are only guidelines. The optimal rehabilitation program should be individualized to the athlete, the specific pathology, and the resultant problems that the athlete is experiencing. The initial injury evaluation and subsequent re-evaluations are therefore critical. A thorough evaluation provides the information needed to structure a rehabilitation program tailored to address identified problems.

The problem-solving approach best addresses the challenge of athletic injury rehabilitation. The evaluation provides the foundation from which the problem-solving approach is constructed. A proper evaluation depends on a detailed and accurate athlete history; knowledge of anatomy, kinesiology, and applied biomechanics; diligent observation; and a thorough physical examination. The examiner should establish an orderly and sequential method for ensuring that nothing is overlooked. On completion of the evaluation, a list of specific problems should be identified. A plan of care should be developed to address each problem and, on implementation, regular re-evaluations should be performed to gauge progress and ascertain the effectiveness and efficiency of administered treatments. The problem-solving approach can be summarized as follows:

1. Evaluation: subjective history, objective findings
2. Identification of specific problems
3. Development of plan of care for addressing specific problems, short- and long-term goals, and criteria for return to functional activity
4. Initiation of plan of care
5. Periodic re-evaluation and adaptation of plan of care, as appropriate
6. Return to functional activity following successful completion of identified rehabilitation goals and discharge parameters

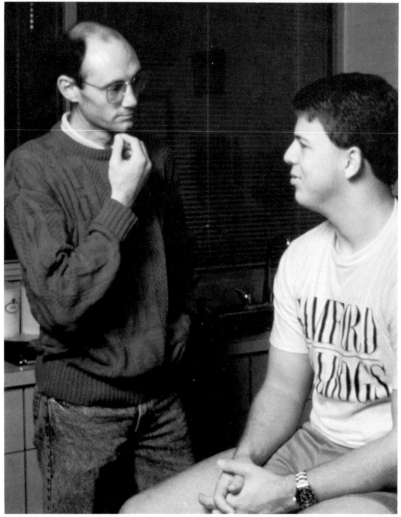

FIGURE 3–1   The examiner must obtain a detailed and complete history from the athlete. (From Doronzo, J.F., and Van Dilen, T. (1990): Mild head injuries in football players. Sports Med. Update, 5(1):12–14.)

7. Development of preventive maintenance rehabilitation program and use of prophylactic devices, as needed, to reduce the incidence of injury recurrence

EVALUATION FORMAT

Subjective History

It is important to obtain a detailed and complete history from the athlete during the evaluation (Fig. 3–1). The evaluator, similarly to an investigator, seeks the answers to a number of questions and should obtain the following information:

1. What is the age, sex, race, and general body type or build of the athlete? Research has shown that certain populations may be predisposed to specific pathologies or conditions. The evaluator should be cognizant of these and observe for positive findings in the evaluation that might have a correlation (e.g., increased incidence of epiphyseal fractures in young, skeletally immature athletes; increased incidence of patellar–femoral pathology in female athletes secondary to a larger Q angle).
2. What is the athlete's activity or sport? What position does the athlete play? This information assists the evaluator in determining the stresses placed on the athlete when participating, and in determining functional activity parameters for discharge and return to activity.
3. What is the athlete's chief complaint?
4. What was the mechanism of injury? Knowledge of the mechanism of injury provides information about what type of trauma was incurred and what anatomic structures may be involved. In addition to the athlete's description, information obtained from other witnesses, film, or videotape, if available, can help ascertain the exact injury mechanism.
5. Does the athlete have a history of related previous injury? Muscle atrophy, ligamentous laxity, crepitus, or other pathologic findings can be a result of previous injury.
6. Is the injury of an acute nature or of insidious onset?
7. Did the athlete hear or feel an abnormal sound or sensation as the injury occurred?
8. Is the athlete experiencing pain, swelling, crepitus, change in sensation, loss of strength, loss of range of motion, instability, or any other reportable abnormal findings?
9. Was the athlete able to continue the activity following injury?
10. Does activity or rest change the athlete's perception of the pain?
11. Are the symptoms improving, worsening, or remaining the same? It is important to know the time of onset, as well as the duration and intensity of the symptoms.

12. What are the sites and boundaries of pain or abnormal sensation? The evaluator may elect to have the athlete complete a subjective pain survey or pain scale rating test.
13. Has the athlete attempted to treat the injury (e.g., with rest, support, assistive ambulation devices, therapeutic heat or cold, exercise)? If so, what has been the outcome?
14. Does the athlete have a history of any unrelated previous or current injuries or illnesses?
15. Is the athlete currently taking any type of prescription or over-the-counter medication?
16. Are there any etiologic considerations or precipitating factors that might predispose the athlete to an injury or to the exacerbation of an injury?

Obtaining an accurate and detailed history is important in the evaluation process. With experience, the evaluator can often make a "preliminary" assessment of the injury from the history. The information obtained from the athlete's history provides guidance and direction to the evaluator in proceeding with the evaluation. The evaluator should be careful, however, not to jump to hasty conclusions. The adage, "You see what you look for, you recognize what you know," should remind the evaluator to always proceed with an open mind and to be aware of all possible scenarios.

Objective Evaluation

The objective evaluation consists of documentable physical findings that the evaluator discovers through observation, palpation, range-of-motion assessment, muscle performance, neurovascular status, special testing, and functional and sport-specific testing.

Observation

The observation process begins when the evaluator first encounters the athlete. In an acute on-the-field injury, this involves noting the mechanism of injury and observing the athlete following injury. In a nonacute injury setting, the observation process begins when the athlete presents for evaluation. The evaluator should observe the athlete's general appearance. How does the athlete stand or walk? Does the athlete use crutches, cane, or other assistive devices? Does the athlete use a support, such as a brace or sling? Does the athlete experience difficulty in removing clothing or taking a place on the evaluation table?

With a lower extremity injury, the examiner should remember to compare the weight-bearing and nonweight-bearing postures. The weight-bearing stance reveals how the body compensates for structural abnormalities. The nonweight-bearing posture illustrates functional and structural ability without compensation.

Inspection

Following observation of the athlete's general appearance the examiner should perform a closer inspection, noting the following (Fig. 3–2):

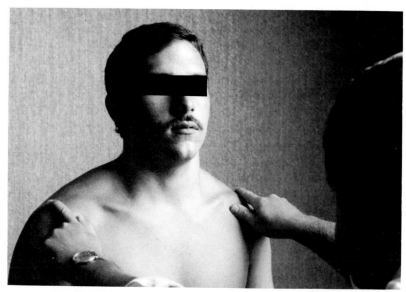

FIGURE 3–2   During the observation and inspection phase of the evaluation the examiner should make bilateral comparisons and note ecchymosis, symmetry, effusion, bleeding, and skin temperature. (From Gallaspy, J.B., and Poole, W.H. (1989): Evaluation of the acromioclavicular joint. Sports Med. Update, 4(3):28–30.)

(1) presence of discoloration or ecchymosis; (2) symmetry, using bilateral comparison where available; (3) skin appearance, noting color, texture, and temperature; (4) signs of trauma; (5) obvious deformity; (6) pain; (7) swelling; and (8) bleeding.

Palpation

Palpation is the process whereby the evaluator applies his or her hands to the athlete's body surface to detect evidence of injury or tenderness (Fig. 3–3). Palpation should be carried out systematically to ensure that all anatomic structures are examined. This procedure involves determining a starting point and working from that point to the surrounding tissues. The examiner should begin slowly and carefully, applying light pressure initially and gradually working into a deeper palpation pressure. Bilateral comparison should be used, if available. Palpable deformities, elicitation of pain or tenderness, crepitus, and any other differences or abnormalities should be noted.

Range-of-Motion Testing

As applicable to the injury situation the evaluator should measure range of motion, both passively and actively (Fig. 3–4). Passive range of motion is the amount of motion obtained by the evaluator without assistance from the athlete. Testing passive range of motion provides the evaluator with information regarding joint arthrokinematics, articular surface integrity, and extensibility of the joint capsule, associated ligaments, and muscles. Active range of motion is the amount of joint motion obtained by the athlete during performance of unassisted, vol-

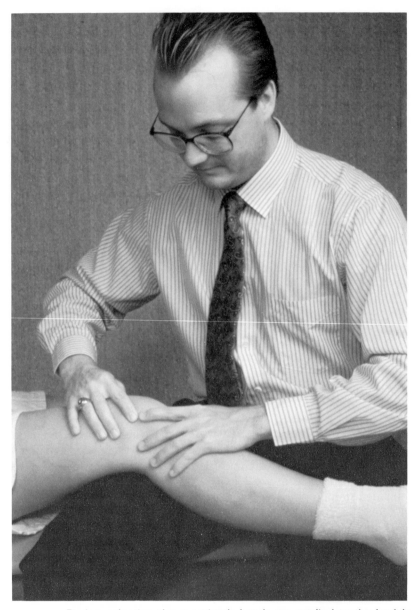

FIGURE 3–3   During palpation the examiner's hands are applied to the body's external surface to detect evidence of injury or tenderness. (From Mulligan E.P. (1989): Etiological considerations in the evaluation of patellofemoral dysfunction. Sports Med. Update, 4(3):3–6.)

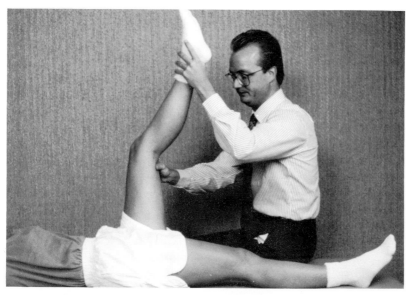

FIGURE 3–4 Range of motion should be assessed passively and actively to determine the reason(s) for its loss. (From Mulligan, E.P. (1989): Etiological considerations in the evaluation of patellofemoral dysfunction. Sports Med. Update, 4(3):3–6.)

untary joint motion. Testing active range of motion provides the examiner with additional information regarding a joint, including muscle strength and movement coordination. Assessment of active range of motion is important for providing information regarding the athlete's functional ability.

Range-of-motion deficits can have a number of causes, including the following: (1) a mechanical block within the joint caused by a loose body or osteophyte formation; (2) muscular tightness; (3) adaptive shortening of the capsular and/or ligamentous structures; (4) swelling; (5) pain inhibition; or (6) a combination of two or more of these factors. It is important to determine the reason for the range-of-motion deficiency to plan the appropriate course of treatment in the rehabilitation program.

A goniometer should be used to obtain objective range-of-motion measurements (see Chap. 4). Goniometric measurements of active and passive ranges of motion obtained on a regular basis provide objective data regarding the effectiveness of rehabilitation treatment and the athlete's progress.

Muscle Performance Assessment

The evaluator should also assess muscle performance as applicable to the injury situation. This can include assessment of the quality, recruitment, and isolation of an isometric muscle contraction with an acute musculoskeletal injury, a postsurgical evaluation, and performance of specific manual muscle testing techniques or isokinetic testing. Muscle performance testing provides the evaluator with information regarding the integrity of the contractile tissues, neuromuscular status, and movement coordination.

Resistive isometric tests can be performed to assess the status of musculoskeletal tissues (Fig. 3–5). Isometric contractions are performed to stress muscle and tendon without stressing accessory tissues. Careful observation, palpation, and correct positioning are essential for testing validity. A knowledge of functional anatomy and kinesiology is paramount. When performing resistive tests, the evaluator should note the strength of the muscle contraction, symmetry to the contralateral side, and whether the contraction elicits pain, and should observe for crepitus, muscle deformation, and any other abnormal findings.

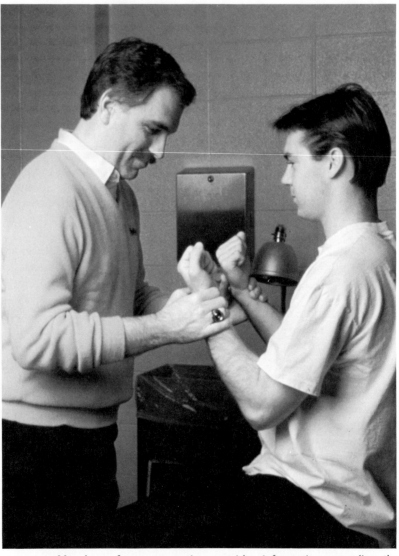

FIGURE 3–5 Muscle performance testing provides information regarding the integrity of the contractile tissues, neuromuscular status, and movement coordination. (Photo courtesy of Sports Medicine Update, Birmingham, AL. HealthSouth Rehabilitation.)

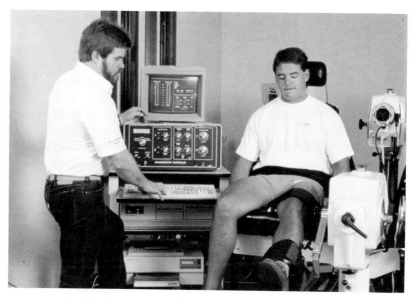

FIGURE 3–6 Isokinetic testing allows the examiner to load the muscle throughout the entire range of motion at speeds that are more comparable to those of athletic activities than isotonic contractions. (Photo courtesy of Sports Medicine Update, Birmingham, AL. HealthSouth Rehabilitation.)

With nonacute athletic injuries, isokinetic testing, if applicable, may provide a more objective analysis of muscle performance (Fig. 3–6). Isokinetic muscle performance testing can provide data regarding peak torque, angle of peak torque, agonist : antagonist muscle ratio, rate of tension development, reciprocal innervation time, and a power, work, and torque curve analysis. Isokinetic testing allows the examiner to load the muscle throughout the entire range of motion at speeds that are more functional to athletic activities than isometric or isotonic contractions.

Strength testing performed regularly, whether manual muscle or isokinetic testing, provides objective data regarding the effectiveness of the rehabilitation program and the athlete's progress.

Neurovascular Assessment

A neurovascular screening should be performed by the evaluator using tests that the evaluator believes are relevant to the suspected pathology. These may include balance assessment; motor function, deep tendon reflex, and dermatome sensation tests; pulse and blood pressure monitoring; and capillary refilling determination.

Special Testing

Once the evaluator has completed the subjective history and preliminary objective evaluation, special testing pertinent to the suspected pathology may be undertaken. This may include joint stability testing, circumferential measurements, and specific pathology tests.

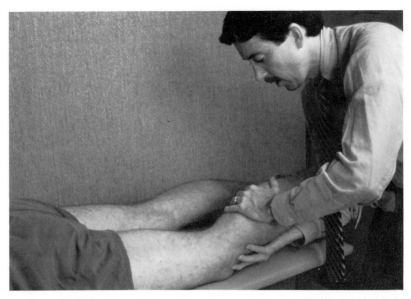

FIGURE 3–7   Stability testing helps determine the integrity of ligamentous struc-tures by placing a mechanical stress on the structure. (From Moran, D.J., and Floyd, R.T. (1990): The Lachman test: Alternative techniques and applications for anterior cruciate ligament evaluation. Sports Med. Update, 5(1):3–5.)

Stability testing is performed to determine the integrity of ligamen-tous structures by placing a mechanical stress on the structure. The examiner should possess a thorough knowledge of anatomy to be able to visualize each structure tested (Fig. 3–7). The evaluator should first

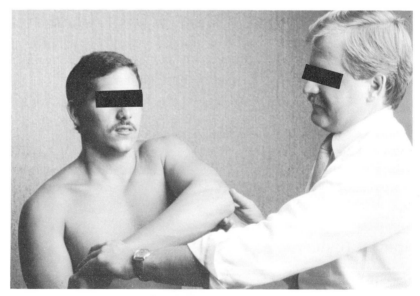

FIGURE 3–8   Special tests can help determine the presence or absence of sus-pected pathology. (From Gallaspy, J.B., and Poole, W.H. (1989): Evaluation of the acromioclavicular joint. Sports Med. Update, 4(3):28–30.)

perform stability testing of the uninvolved joint to obtain baseline data for comparison with the involved joint. In addition, allowing the athlete to experience the testing on the uninvolved joint first helps develop confidence and trust in the examiner and decrease apprehension. Correct positioning is essential for obtaining validity with stability testing. The athlete should be encouraged to relax, because muscle spasm could negate the validity of the test results. The evaluator should note any degree of instability, elicitation of pain or tenderness, crepitus, or evidence of other abnormalities during the stability testing.

Circumferential measurements can be taken to provide objective documentation of such problems as muscle atrophy or effusion. The evaluator should use anatomic landmarks and standard measurements to establish continuity and consistency.

Special tests can be performed, as indicated, to confirm or rule out suspected pathology (Fig. 3–8). Examples include testing for the rotator cuff impingement sign, the "labral clunk test" for a glenoid labrum tear, the Thompson test for a ruptured Achilles tendon, and the Finklestein test for DeQuervain's syndrome.

Functional Testing and Sport-Specific Testing

The evaluator may elect to perform a functional testing program, as applicable, to determine whether these sequential activities produce pain or other symptoms. For example, a functional testing program for an injured ankle may include the following: (1) squatting (both ankles should dorsiflex symmetrically); (2) standing on toes (both ankles should plantar flex symmetrically); (3) standing on one foot; (4) standing on the toes of one foot; (5) walking on the toes; (6) running straight ahead; (7) running with cutting movements; and (8) jumping.

If the athlete can perform functional tests without difficulty, the evaluator may elect to proceed with more advanced sports testing specific to the athlete's sport. For instance, the evaluator may ask a quarterback to simulate taking a snap and dropping back to pass; or may ask a baseball pitcher returning from a rotator cuff injury to pitch a simulated game.

Additional Considerations

The thorough evaluator must not only consider the pathology, but must go beyond it to uncover the possible cause. The evaluator must not examine only the specific site of pathology, but should visualize the entire kinetic chain and examine adjacent joints and other related structures. Biomechanics and kinesiology of the sport-specific skills that the athlete performs should be taken into consideration. On completion of the evaluation, the clinician should develop a plan of care that encompasses rehabilitation of the primary pathology and correction of any underlying problems that may have predisposed the athlete to the pathology.

IDENTIFICATION OF SPECIFIC PROBLEMS

Following completion of the evaluation process, the evaluator should compile a list of specific problems related to the athletic injury. For example, evaluation of a college football running back following an acute inversion ankle sprain might reveal the following problems:

1. Physiologic healing constraints with grade I injury to the anterior talofibular and calcaneofibular ligaments (recognizing a 3- to 5-week normal healing time frame for ligamentous injury)
2. Negative lateral ankle instability, but increased pain with mechanical stress placed on ligaments with stress testing
3. Point tenderness over lateral aspect of ankle, specifically centered over involved ligamentous structures
4. Inability to bear weight fully
5. Moderate effusion and ecchymosis of ankle and forefoot
6. Decreased range of motion in plantar flexion, dorsiflexion, inversion, and eversion
7. Decreased muscular strength in plantar flexion, dorsiflexion, inversion, and eversion
8. Decreased proprioception and kinesthetic awareness
9. Loss of function; decrease in athletic activities and activities of daily living (ADLs) secondary to pathology
10. Need for cardiovascular and well-limb maintenance program during rehabilitation and recovery process

DEVELOPMENT OF A PLAN OF CARE

Following identification of specific problems, a plan of care should be developed to address each problem. For example, in developing a plan of care for the athlete with the injury described above, the clinician might use the following:

1. Partial weight-bearing on two crutches, with the ankle placed in a prophylactic brace or strapping to relieve the weight-bearing problem, protection of injured ligamentous structures during recovery phase, and minimization of pain and discomfort
2. Cryotherapy, compression (through elastic bandaging or compression sleeve), elevation, intermittent compression, electrical muscle stimulation set at muscle pump contraction parameters, centripetal massage, and active or active-assisted range of motion to relieve effusion and ecchymosis
3. Cryotherapy and electrical muscle stimulation set at pain modulation parameters to relieve pain
4. Active, active-assistive, and passive range-of-motion program to deal with range-of-motion deficits
5. Submaximal progression to maximal multiple angle isometrics, manual resistance, proprioceptive neuromuscular facilitation (PNF) diagonal patterns, and submaximal progression to maximal isotonic exercise implemented, as applicable, to treat strength deficits

6. Balance, proprioception, and kinesthetic awareness activities implemented, as appropriate, to manage deficits
7. Implementation of well-limb maintenance program
8. Implementation of upper body ergometer, stationary cycle, and aquatic rehabilitation exercises for cardiovascular maintenance

The components of the rehabilitation program should be directed toward achieving modulation of pain, normal range of motion and joint arthrokinematics, normal muscular flexibility and strength, and the balance, power, coordination, endurance, accuracy, and timing necessary to return to the preathletic activity level without restriction. Through the use of therapeutic exercise, therapeutic modalities, and patient education, a structured rehabilitation program can be designed and individualized to the athlete's specific pathology and problems identified. When establishing a plan of care, two questions should be asked:

1. What goals and types of treatment comprise a well-designed program? The clinician should have a scientific rationale underlying each treatment technique.
2. Do the proposed treatments safely and effectively accomplish the intended goals? Objective measurements recorded periodically can assist the clinician in monitoring the progress of the rehabilitation program.

GOAL SETTING AND ESTABLISHMENT OF DISCHARGE PARAMETERS

Along with the plan of care, specific rehabilitation goals should be developed. As with any project, goals help provide a sense of purpose and direction. Goals should be set up on both a short-term (7 to 10 days) and long-term basis. Discharge parameters and return to athletic activity criteria should also be established. Consideration must be given to the nature of the pathology, the athlete's sport and position, and the physical demands placed on the athlete.

The decision to release an athlete recovering from injury for a progressive return to athletic activity is the final stage of the rehabilitation and recovery process. The decision should be carefully considered by each member of the sports medicine team involved in the rehabilitation process. In considering return to activity, the following concerns should be addressed: recognition of physiologic healing constraints; pain status; presence of swelling; range-of-motion status; strength status; balance, timing, proprioception, and kinesthetic awareness; sport-specific demands; conditioning; prophylactic strapping, bracing, or padding; responsibility of the athlete; predisposition to injury; psychologic factors; gradual, progressive return to activity; athlete education and preventive maintenance program; and functional testing.

PERIODIC RE-EVALUATION

Periodic re-evaluations of the athlete should be performed to monitor the effectiveness of the rehabilitation program. Objective data recorded on a regular basis, such as range-of-motion measurements, manual muscle testing grades, and circumferential measurements, provide information regarding the effectiveness and efficiency of treatment. Following re-evaluation, the original goals of treatment should be re-examined and modified as needed, and the plan of care adapted accordingly.

The area of athletic rehabilitation is among the most challenging and exciting in the field of sports medicine. The clinician works with the other members of the sports medicine team to achieve a common goal: return of the injured athlete to the preinjury athletic activity level as soon as possible, within safe guidelines. The success of rehabilitation depends directly on the evaluation process. By performing a thorough evaluation, identifying specific problems, developing a plan of care, and performing subsequent re-evaluations to determine the efficiency and effectiveness of treatments, the clinician can help the injured athlete return to the playing arena.

The following forms represent the steps in a hypothetic evaluation and rehabilitation process for a right ankle sprain.

REHABILITATION: INITIAL EVALUATION

Name: Smith, John   Sport: Football   Date: 9/10/90

Identification # 41024   Age: 20 D.O.B. 7/14/70 Sex: M Physician: Jones

SUBJECTIVE

Present History/Chief Complaint/Mechanism of Injury Athlete presents c/o Rt. ankle pain, swelling, LOF, inability to bear weight. Athlete leapt to catch pass, landing on and forcibly inverting Rt. ankle. Evaluated on football practice field; assisted to T.R.

Past Medical History Athlete states Rt. ankle sprain approximately 2 yrs. ago. Neg. Fx. Returned to athletic activity without further problems until present. PMH otherwise unremarkable.

Medical Tests Rt. ankle x-rays by Dr. Jones at Medical Center, Neg.

Medications None

Treatment to Date I.C.E. NWB with 2 crutches.

OBJECTIVE

Presentation NWB with 2 crutches. Compress. wrap Rt. ankle

Observation Moderate effusion/ecchymosis Rt. ankle, localized over lateral ankle and forefoot.

Palpation Point tenderness elicited over ant. talofibular & calcaneofibular lig. Neg. palpable deformity or crepitus

Range of Motion PF 25°, DF -10°, Inv. 8°, Ever. 2° Toe ext./flex. WNL

Muscle Performance MMT deferred at present 2° to ↑pain with active movement, inability to perform normal active movement patterns.

Neurovascular Bilateral achilles DTR WNL. Intact sensation to light touch. Distal foot pulses WNL.

Special Testing Neg. ligamentous instability, however,↑ pain with inversion stress and anterior drawer tests.

Area of Injury

Circumferential Measurements

Left	Right	Reference Landmarks
26	29	Med. Mall (MM)
23	24.5	5cm prox. MM
25	27	5cm distal MM

Initial Rehabilitation Program:

1) I.C.E. 2)EMS, pain modulation parameters, 3)Intermittent compression @ 80mmHg 60 sec. on/15sec. off x 20 min 4)Application of felt over forefoot & felt horseshoe pad over lat. mall., lat. aspect of ankle with elastic wrap from base of toes to mid-calf. Fitted with crutches & review NWB gait on level surface & ↓↑stairs.

ASSESSMENT

Clinical Impression: Grade I inversion ankle sprain: ant. talofibular and calcaneofibular ligaments.
Tolerated initial Rx. well.

Rehabilitation Problems Identified: ☒ Physiological Healing Constraints ☒ Pain ☒ Swelling ☒↓ ROM ☒↓ Muscle Performance ☒↓ Balance/Proprioception ☒ Loss of Function ☒ Other Inability to FWB

Rehabilitation Potential Good

Rehabilitation Goals STG (7-10 days): 1)FWB without assistive device, 2)ROM WNL, 3)Minimal effusion, 4)No pain. LTG: Return to previous athletic activity level without restriction. ROM & strength WNL.

PLAN

Continue to monitor progress B.I.D. Advance weight bearing status as tolerable.

REHABILITATION PROGRAM

Name: Smith, John   Injury: Rt. Ankle Sprain   Sport: Football

Date of Rehabilitation Session	9/10	9/11	9/12	9/13	9/14	9/15	9/16	9/17	9/18	9/19	9/20	9/21	9/22
THERAPEUTIC EXERCISE													
Range of Motion A AA P	P/AA	P/AA	P/AA	AA/A	→								→
Flexibility	Passive DF with towel	→		Achilles Slant Board	Stretching		→						→
Towel Toe Curls			X	X	X	X							
Marble Pick-ups			X	X	X	X							
Isometric PF/DF			X	X	X	X							
Isom. Inv/Ever				X	X								
TheraBand PF		Blue 2x10	3x10	4x10	Black 3x10	→	5x10	Grey 3x10	→	5x10	→		→
TheraBand DF		Blue 2x10	3x10	4x10	Black 3x10	→	5x10	Grey 3x10	→	5x10	→		→
TheraBand Inv.				Blue 2x10	3x10	5x10	Black 3x10	5x10	Grey 3x10	5x10	→		→
TheraBand Ever.				Blue 2x10	3x10	5x10	Black 3x10	5x10	Grey 3x10	5x10	→		→
Pro-Fitter							X	X	X	X	X	X	X
One Foot Balance					X	X	X	X	X	X	X	X	X
Isokinetic PF/DF						VSRP X	X	X	X	X	X	X	X
Isokinetic Inv/Ever							VSRP X	X	X	X	X	X	X
Mini-Trampoline							X	X	X	X	X	X	X
PNF					X	X	X	X	X	X	X	X	X
Balance/Proprioception Activities			NWB BAPS	NWB BAPS	PWB BAPS	PWB BAPS	PWB BAPS	FWB BAPS	FWB BAPS	FWB BAPS	FWB BAPS	FWB BAPS	FWB BAPS
Cardiovascular Training		UBE	UBE	Fitron	→								→
Well Limb Maintenance	Continue well-leg, U.E. strength training under strength coach supervision												→
Aquatic Exercise			Wet-Vest	Wet-Vest	Wet-Vest	Wet-Vest	Pool Run	Pool Run	Pool Run	Pool Run	Spt. Skill	Spt. Skill	Spt. Skill
THERAPEUTIC MODALITIES													
Cryotherapy	with elev.	with elev.	with elev.	with elev.	with elev.	with elev.	X	X	X	X	X	X	X
Diathermy													
Elec. Stim. Current *	6	6	2	2	2	2							
Iontophoresis c̄___													
Intermittent Compression	c elev X	X	X	X	X								
Massage (centripetal)	X	X	X	X	X								
Mobilization													
Phonophoresis c̄___													
Thermotherapy													
Traction													
Ultrasound					Pulse 25%	Pulse 50%	Pulse 75%	Cont. 1.0w	Cont. 1.0w	Cont. 1.25w	Cont. 1.25w	Cont. 1.5w	Cont. 1.5w
Whirlpool (Contrast)				X	X	X							
Warm WP @ 100°F							X	X	X	X	X	X	X

* Electrical Stimulating Current Parameters:
1. Mm. re-ed.
2. Mm. pump contractions
3. Retard. of atrophy
4. Mm. Strengthening
5. Increase ROM
6. Pain Modulation

REHABILITATION: RE-EVALUATION

Name: Smith, John   Sport: Football   Date: 9/16/90

Identification # 41024   Age: 20   D.O.B. 7/14/70 Sex: M   Physician: Jones

SUBJECTIVE

Present Injury History S/P 1 wk. Rt. Grade I inversion ankle sprain. Athlete presents without c/o. States "Fell I'm progressing well with rehab... when do you think I'll be ready to go back to football practice.

OBJECTIVE

Presentation FWB with Air-Cast Ankle Brace, Rt.

Observation Minimal effusion Rt. ankle. Neg. effusion in foot. Pocket of swelling localized over anterior lateral aspect of ankle. Ecchymosis breaking up.

Palpation Minimal point tenderness elicited over anterior talofibular & calcaneofibular lig. Neg. deformity, crepitus

Range of Motion PF, Inv., Ever. = WNL
              DF = 5°

Muscle Performance MMT Grades:
              PF = 4+/5   DF = 4+/5
              Inv. = 4/5   Ever. = 4/5

Neurovascular NVI

Special Testing Neg. instability. Neg. pain with ligamentous stress testing

Area of Injury

Circumferential Measurements		
Left	Right	Reference Landmarks
26	27	Med. Mall. (MM)
23	23.5	5cm prox. MM
25	26	5cm distal MM

Overview: Rehabilitation Program To Date:

Progressed from NWB --- TDWB --- PWB --- FWB over past week. Initial rehab. concentrated on pain modulation, effusion, and strength & ROM. Working with strength & conditioning coach with wll-limb maintenance program & cont'd cardio-vascular maintenance program with UBE, Fitron, & aquatic rehab. Pt. has progressed well with initiation of proprioception & balance activities.

ASSESSMENT

Clinical Impression/Rehabilitation Progress: Progressing well at this time-frame with injury.

Rehabilitation Problems Identified: ☒ Physiological Healing Constraints ☒ Pain ☒ Swelling ☒↓ ROM
☒↓ Muscle Performance ☒↓ Balance/Proprioception ☒ Loss of Function
☐ Other

Rehabilitation Goals STG: 1) DF ROM WNL, 2)Neg. effusion, 3) Neg. pain, 4)MMT ankle strength levels WNL   LTG: Return to athletic activity level without restrictions. ROM/strength WNL. Prevenative maintenance program.

PLAN

Continue to monitor progress B.I.D. Advance strength, balance, proprioception activities as appropriate. Begin preparation for gradual return to functional activity.

REHABILITATION: DISCHARGE SUMMARY

Name: Smith, John   Sport: Football   Date: 9/22/90

Identification #: 41024   Age: 20 D.O.B. 7/14/70 Sex: M Physician: Jones

SUBJECTIVE	Present Injury History S/P 2 wks. Rt. Grade I inversion ankle sprain. Athlete presents without c/o. "I'm ready to go full-speed now".

OBJECTIVE

Presentation FWB

Observation Neg. effusion Rt. ankle/foot
    Neg. ecchymosis.

Palpation Neg. point tenderness.
    Neg. deformity, crepitus.

Range of Motion PF, Inv., Ever. = WNL
    DF = 10°

Muscle Performance MMT reveals 5/5 PF/DF/Inv/Ever.
Isokinetic testing reveals peak torque & total work WNL in PF/DF & Inv/Ever (enclosed in chart)

Neurovascular NVI

Special Testing Neg. ligamentous instability. Neg. pain with ligamentous stress testing.

Area of Injury

Circumferential Measurements

Left	Right	Reference Landmarks	
26	26	Med Mall	(MM)
23	23	5cm prox MM	
25	25	5cm distal MM	

Functional Testing/ Sports Specific Skills Perfromed following under supervision without pain, instability, or other symptoms, full squat, standing on toes, one foot balance, one foot hopping, forward/reverse running, cutting, figure 8 run, carioca, 5-10-5 lateral mobility run, sport simulated movemtnets (cuts, pass paterns).

ASSESSMENT

Clinical Impression: Progressing well at this time-frame since injury. Participating in 1/2 and 3/4 speed drills and non-contact activities over past 3 days without difficulty.

PLAN

☐ Return to athletic activity without restrictions

☒ Return to athletic activity with the following restrictions: Continue maintenance rehab. program & use of protective bracing.

☒ Performance of preventative maintenance program as follows: Achilles flexibility pre/post athletic activity Ankle PF/DF/Inv/Ever resistive ex. with Thera-Band 3x10 ea QD; proprioceptive/ balance activities with BAPS, Pro-Fitter, one foot balance QD; cryotherapy after athletic activity.

☒ Prophylactic strapping/bracing as follows: Taping, Air-Cast stirrup ankle brace for athletic activities.

☒ Other: Fitted with high top athletic shoes by equipment manager.

Bibliography

Arnheim, D. (1985): Modern Principles of Athletic Training. St. Louis, Times Mirror/Mosby.

Gould, J., and Davies, G. (1985): Orthopaedic and Sports Physical Therapy. St. Louis, C.V. Mosby.

Kessler, R.M., and Hertling, D. (1985): Management of Common Musculoskeletal Disorders. Philadelphia, Harper & Row.

Kisner, C., and Colby, L.A. (1985): Therapeutic Exercises: Foundations and Techniques. Philadelphia, F.A. Davis.

Magee, D.J. (1987): Orthopedic Physical Assessment. Philadelphia, W.B. Saunders.

Prentice, W.E. (1990): Rehabilitation Techniques in Sports Medicine. St. Louis, Times Mirror/Mosby.

Roy, S., and Irvin, R. (1983): Prevention, Evaluation, Management, and Rehabilitation. Englewood Cliffs, NJ, Prentice-Hall.

Torg, J.S., Vesgo, J.J., and Torg, E. (1987): Rehabilitation of Athletic Injuries. Chicago, Year Book Medical Publishers.

CHAPTER 4

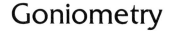

Goniometry

Karen Middleton, P.T., A.T.,C.

Goniometry is the use of instruments for measuring the range of motion in bodily joints. All clinicians should be competent in performing and interpreting objective measurements of joint motion. Initial range-of-motion measurements provide a basis for developing a treatment plan, and repeated measurements throughout the course of rehabilitation help determine whether improvement has been made and goals achieved. This chapter discusses the goniometric techniques for measuring basic joint motions of the upper and lower extremities.

HISTORICAL CONSIDERATIONS

The literature is extensive and describes many aspects of goniometric measuring. Gifford,[6] in 1914, was probably the first to have reported on goniometric devices in the United States. Historically, many articles have described and recommended various instruments and methods of measurement.[3,9,11,12,14-17] These instruments are generally of two types: (1) devices of universal application (i.e., full-circle manual universal goniometer), which remain the most versatile and popular (Fig. 4–1); and (2) goniometers designed to measure a single range of motion for a specific joint (Fig. 4–2).

As goniometry evolved, efforts were directed toward standardizing methods of measurement, including the need for common nomenclature and definition of terms; for a clear definition of movements to be measured; and for establishment of normal ranges of motion. In 1965 the American Academy of Orthopaedic Surgeons published a manual of standardized methods of measuring and recording joint motion; since then there have been numerous reprints.[1] Norkin and White[13] have provided a thorough description of goniometry.

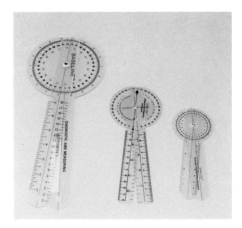

FIGURE 4–1 Full-circle manual universal goniometer.

GONIOMETRIC ASSESSMENT

Anatomic Zero Position

The anatomic zero position is the starting 0° orientation for most measurements.[11] The exceptions are shoulder rotation, hip rotation, and forearm pronation–supination, with the starting position between the two extremes of motion. If the individual to be measured cannot assume the starting position, the position of improvisation should be noted when recording joint motion. The degrees of joint motion are added in the direction of joint movement. Average ranges of motion for the upper and lower extremities are outlined in Table 4–1.[1]

Reliability of Measurement and Technical Considerations

The reliability of goniometric joint motion measurements has been studied. Several reports noted that joint range of motion can be mea-

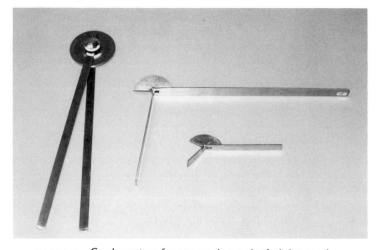

FIGURE 4–2   Goniometers for measuring a single joint motion.

TABLE 4–1   **AVERAGE RANGES OF MOTION FOR THE UPPER AND LOWER EXTREMITIES (IN DEGREES)**

Joint	Motion	Source of Data	
		AMERICAN ACADEMY OF ORTHOPAEDIC SURGEONS[1]	KENDALL AND McCREARY[8]
Shoulder	Flexion	0–180	0–180
	Extension	0–60	0–45
	Abduction	0–180	0–180
	Internal rotation	0–70	0–70
	External rotation	0–90	0–90
Elbow	Flexion	0–150	0–145
Forearm	Pronation	0–80	0–90
	Supination	0–80	0–90
Wrist	Extension	0–70	0–70
	Flexion	0–80	0–80
	Radial deviation	0–20	0–20
	Ulnar deviation	0–30	0–35
Thumb			
CMC*	Abduction	0–70	0–80
	Flexion	0–15	0–45
	Extension	0–20	0
MCP*	Flexion	0–50	0–60
IP*	Flexion	0–80	0–80
Digits 2 to 5			
MCP	Flexion	0–90	0–90
	Extension	0–45	
PIP*			
DIP*	Flexion		
	Extension		
Hip	Flexion	0–120	0–125
	Extension	0–30	0–10
	Abduction	0–45	0–45
	Adduction	0–30	0–10
	External rotation	0–45	0–45
	Internal rotation	0–45	0–45
Knee	Flexion	0–135	0–140
Ankle	Dorsiflexion	0–20	0–20
	Plantar flexion	0–50	0–45
	Inversion	0–35	0–35
	Eversion	0–15	0–20
Subtalar	Inversion	0–5	
	Eversion	0–5	

Adapted from Norkin, C.C., and White, D.J. (1985): Measurement of Joint Motion: A Guide to Goniometry. Philadelphia, F.A. Davis.
* CMC, carpometacarpal; MCP, metacarpophalangeal; IP, interphalangeal; PIP, proximal interphalangeal; DIP, distal interphalangeal.

sured with a high degree of reliability.[4,5,7,10] Boone and colleagues[2] have indicated that the same individual should perform goniometric measurements when the effects of treatment are evaluated. When the same tester measures the same movement, increases in joint motion of at least 3° to 4° determine improvement. When more than one tester measures the same movement, improvement is determined with more than a 5° measurement increase. Accurate reproducibility depends on careful measurement technique. Appropriate steps in measuring include the following: (1) positioning and stabilization of the joint; (2)

identification of anatomic landmarks; and (3) proper alignment and reading of the goniometer.

Positioning of the athlete should be consistent. The prone or supine position provides greater stabilization through the athlete's body weight. Measurements are acquired as passive range of motion when possible and the body part uncovered for better accuracy. The goniometer is placed next to or on top of the joint, whenever possible, and the goniometer arms are placed along the longitudinal axis of the bones of the joint after the motion has occurred. In evaluation of the joint and assessment of range of motion, the clinician should view the affected joint from above and below to determine if any additional limitations are present in the involved extremity. The opposite extremity must also be assessed to determine normal motion for that athlete.

APPLICATIONS

Upper Extremities

Shoulder

Flexion

SUGGESTED TESTING POSITION   The athlete is in the anatomic supine position (Fig. 4–3), with the forearm in midposition between supination and pronation.

GONIOMETER ALIGNMENT   The goniometer is aligned along (1) the head of the lateral humeral condyle and (2) the midaxillary line of trunk (Fig.4-4).

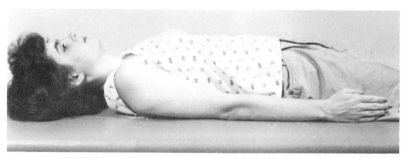

FIGURE 4–3

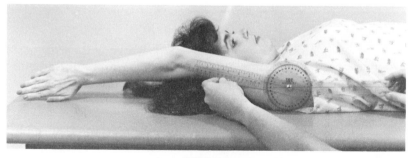

FIGURE 4–4

Extension

SUGGESTED TESTING POSITION   The athlete is in the anatomic prone position (Fig. 4–5), with the forearm in midposition between supination and pronation.

      GONIOMETER ALIGNMENT   The goniometer is aligned along (1) the head of the lateral humeral condyle and (2) the midaxillary line of trunk (Fig. 4–6).

Abduction

SUGGESTED TESTING POSITION   The athlete is in the anatomic supine position (Fig. 4–7), with the forearm in midposition between supination and pronation.

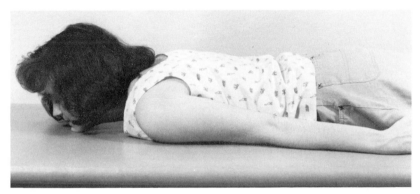

FIGURE 4–5

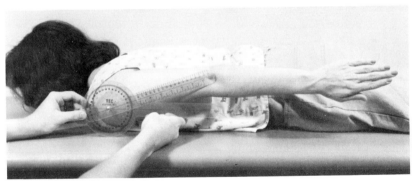

FIGURE 4–6

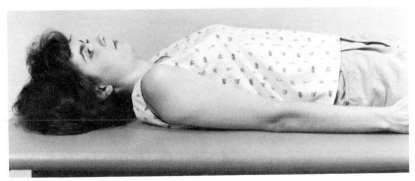

FIGURE 4–7

GONIOMETER ALIGNMENT   The goniometer is aligned (1) along the anterior longitudinal axis of the humerus and (2) parallel to the midline of the body (Fig. 4–8).

Adduction

SUGGESTED TESTING POSITION   The athlete is in the anatomic supine position, with the forearm in midposition between supination and pronation (see Fig. 4–7).

GONIOMETER ALIGNMENT   The goniometer is aligned (1) along the anterior longitudinal axis of the humerus and (2) parallel to the midline of the body (Fig. 4–9).

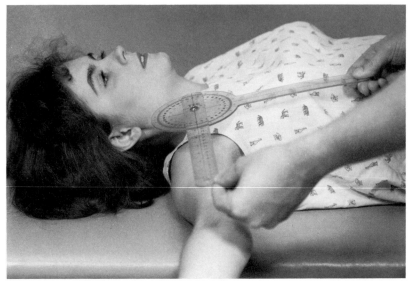

FIGURE 4–8

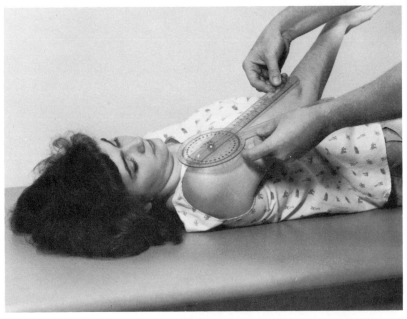

FIGURE 4–9

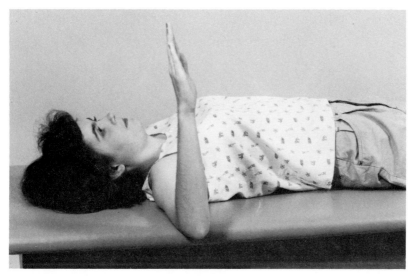

FIGURE 4–10

External Rotation

SUGGESTED TESTING POSITION   The athlete is supine, with the arm abducted to 90°, the elbow flexed to 90°, and the forearm pronated perpendicular to the table (Fig. 4–10).

GONIOMETER ALIGNMENT   The goniometer is aligned (1) along the ulna to the ulnar styloid process and (2) parallel to the table (Fig. 4–11).

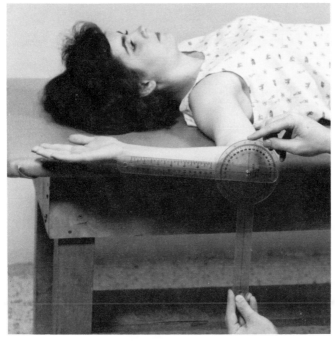

FIGURE 4–11

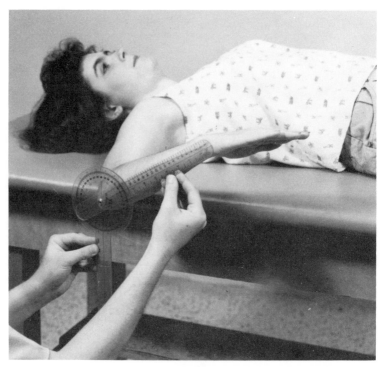

FIGURE 4–12

Internal Rotation

SUGGESTED TESTING POSITION   The athlete is supine, with the arm abducted to 90°, the elbow flexed to 90°, and the forearm pronated perpendicular to the table (see Fig. 4–10).

    GONIOMETER ALIGNMENT   The goniometer is aligned (1) along the ulnar styloid process and (2) parallel to the table (Fig. 4–12).

Elbow

Flexion

SUGGESTED TESTING POSITION   The athlete is in the anatomic supine position (see Fig. 4–7).

    GONIOMETER ALIGNMENT   The goniometer is aligned along (1) the lateral midline of the humerus, humeral head to lateral condyle, and (2) the lateral midline of the radius to the radial styloid process (Fig. 4–13).

Extension

SUGGESTED TESTING POSITION   The athlete is in the anatomic supine position (see Fig. 4–7).

    GONIOMETER ALIGNMENT   The goniometer is aligned along (1) the lateral midline of the humerus, humeral head to lateral condyle, and (2) the lateral midline of the radius to the radial styloid process (Fig. 4–14).

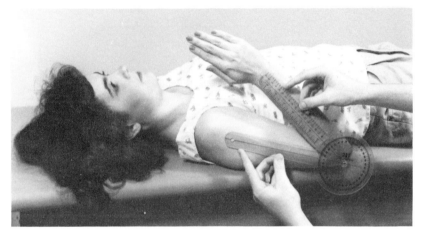

FIGURE 4–13

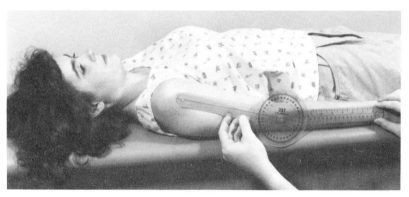

FIGURE 4–14

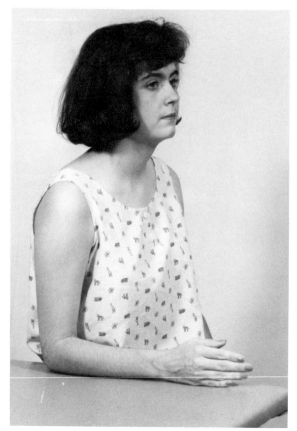

FIGURE 4—15

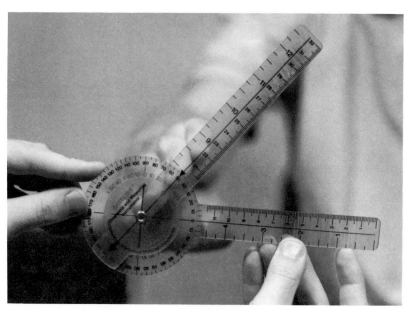

FIGURE 4—16

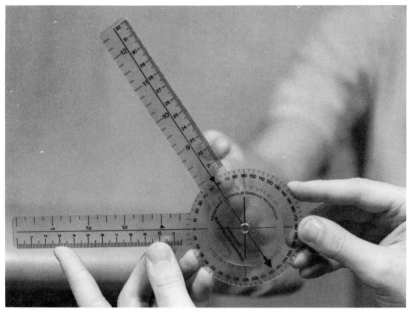

FIGURE 4—17

Forearm

Pronation

SUGGESTED TESTING POSITION   The athlete is seated, with the elbow flexed to 90° and the forearm midway between supination and pronation (Fig. 4—15).

GONIOMETER ALIGNMENT   (1) With the fingers straight, the goniometer is lined up with the line formed by the fingertips or, with the fingers flexed, lined up with the line formed by the proximal interphalangeal joints, and (2) parallel to the table (Fig. 4—16).

Supination

SUGGESTED TESTING POSITION   The athlete is seated, with the elbow flexed to 90° and the forearm midway between supination and pronation (see Fig. 4—15).

GONIOMETER ALIGNMENT   (1) With the fingers straight, the goniometer is lined up with the line formed by the fingertips or, with the fingers flexed, lined up with the line formed by the proximal interphalangeal joints, and (2) parallel to the table (Fig. 4—17).

Wrist

Flexion

SUGGESTED TESTING POSITION   The athlete is supine, with the arm abducted to 90°, the elbow flexed to 90°, and the forearm pronated (Fig. 4—18).

GONIOMETER ALIGNMENT   The goniometer is aligned with (1) the lateral midline of ulna and (2) the fifth metacarpal (Fig. 4—19).

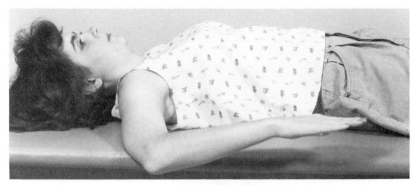

FIGURE 4—18

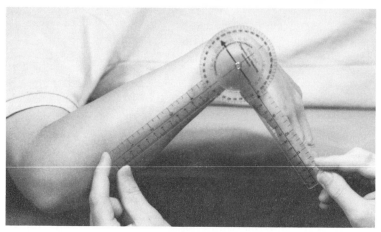

FIGURE 4—19

Extension

SUGGESTED TESTING POSITION   The athlete is supine, with the arm abducted to 90°, the elbow flexed to 90°, and the forearm pronated (see Fig. 4—18).

GONIOMETER ALIGNMENT   The goniometer is aligned with (1) the lateral midline of the ulna and (2) the fifth metacarpal (Fig. 4—20).

Radius and Ulna

Radial Deviation

SUGGESTED TESTING POSITION   The athlete is in the supine position, with the arm abducted to 90°, the elbow flexed to 90°, and the forearm pronated (see Fig. 4—18).

GONIOMETER ALIGNMENT   The goniometer is aligned (1) across the radial styloid process and (2) the third metacarpal (Fig. 4—21).

Ulnar Deviation

SUGGESTED TESTING POSITION   The athlete is supine, with the arm abducted to 90°, the elbow flexed to 90°, and the forearm pronated (see Fig. 4—18).

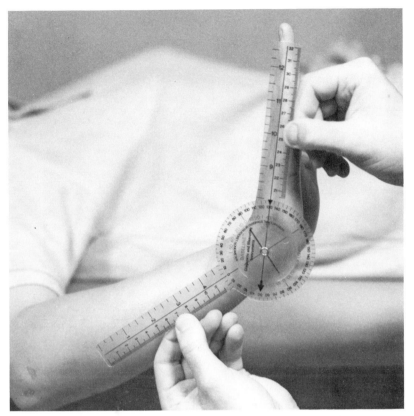

FIGURE 4–20

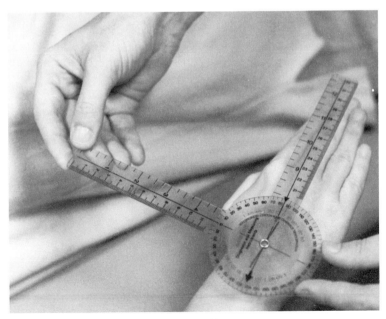

FIGURE 4–21

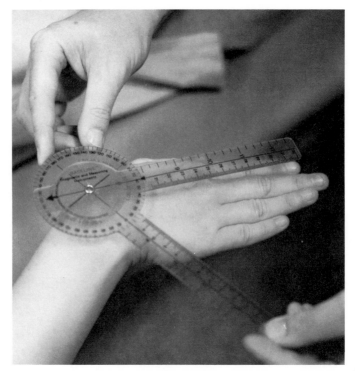

FIGURE 4—22

GONIOMETER ALIGNMENT   The goniometer is aligned (1) across the ulnar styloid process and (2) the third metacarpal (Fig. 4—22).

Fingers

Flexion

GONIOMETER ALIGNMENT   The goniometer is aligned along the (1) lateral side of the proximal phalanx and (2) the lateral side of the distal phalanx (Fig. 4—23).

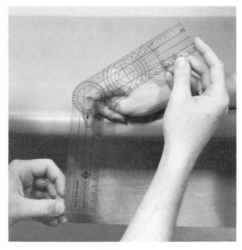

FIGURE 4—23

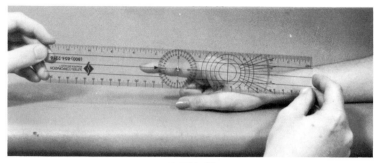

FIGURE 4–24

Extension

GONIOMETER ALIGNMENT   The goniometer is aligned along the (1) lateral side of the proximal phalanx and (2) the lateral side of the distal phalanx (Fig. 4–24).

Lower Extremities

Hip

Flexion

SUGGESTED TESTING POSITION   The athlete is in the anatomic supine position, with the knee bent to 90° when going through the motion (Fig. 4–25).

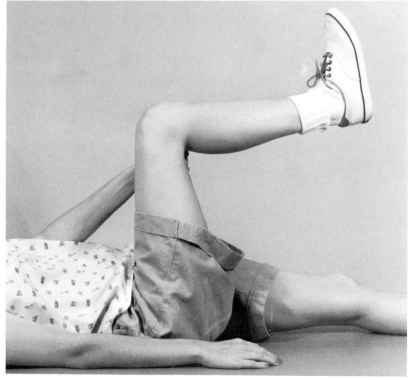

FIGURE 4–25

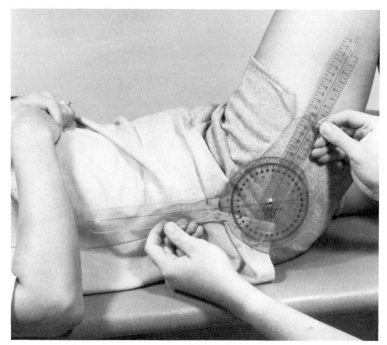

FIGURE 4—26

GONIOMETER ALIGNMENT   The goniometer is aligned (1) laterally along the long axis of the trunk, and (2) on the lateral side, along the longitudinal axis of the femur, greater trochanter to lateral femoral condyle (Fig. 4–26).

Extension

SUGGESTED TESTING POSITION   The athlete is in the anatomic prone position (Fig. 4–27).

GONIOMETER ALIGNMENT   The goniometer is aligned (1) laterally along the long axis of the trunk, and (2) on the lateral side, along the longitudinal axis of the femur, greater trochanter to lateral femoral condyle (Fig. 4–28).

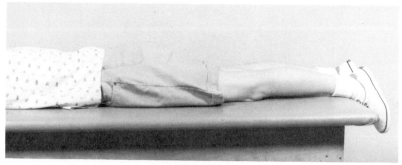

FIGURE 4—27

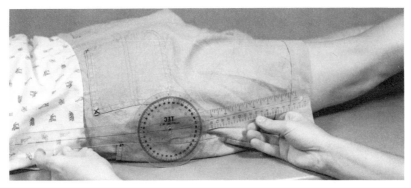

FIGURE 4-28

Straight Leg Raising

SUGGESTED TESTING POSITION   The athlete is in the anatomic supine position, with the knee straight through the motion and the ankle dorsiflexed.

GONIOMETER ALIGNMENT   The goniometer is aligned (1) laterally along the axis of the trunk, and (2) laterally along the longitudinal axis of the femur, greater trochanter to lateral femoral condyle (Fig. 4–29).

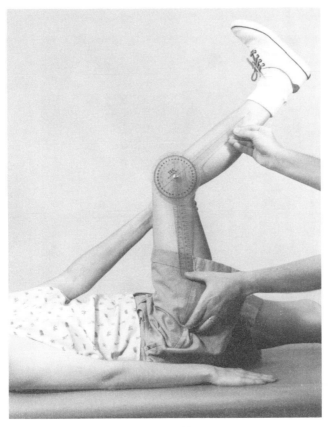

FIGURE 4-29

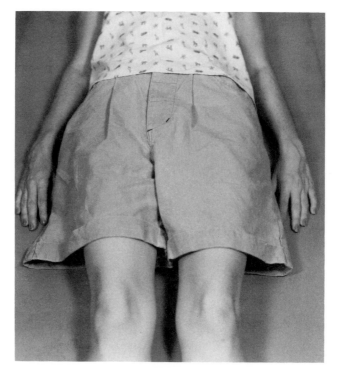

FIGURE 4–30

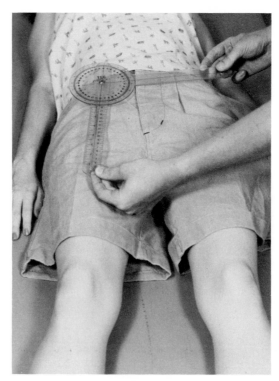

FIGURE 4–31

Abduction

SUGGESTED TESTING POSITION   The athlete is in the anatomic supine position (Fig. 4–30).

GONIOMETER ALIGNMENT   The goniometer is aligned (1) between the two anterior superior iliac spines, and (2) along the anterior thigh, with the midline of the thigh to the midline of the patella (Fig. 4–31).

Adduction

SUGGESTED TESTING POSITION   The athlete flexes the hip and knee in a supported position, with the lower extremity brought under the supported extremity.

GONIOMETER ALIGNMENT   The goniometer is aligned (1) between the two anterior superior iliac spines, and (2) along the anterior thigh, with the midline of the thigh to the midline of the patella (Fig. 4–32).

Internal Rotation

SUGGESTED TESTING POSITION   The athlete is seated, with the hip flexed to 90° and the knee flexed to 90° over the edge of the table (Fig. 4–33).

GONIOMETER ALIGNMENT   The goniometer is aligned (1) parallel to the table and (2) along the midline of the anterior tibia, with the patella to midposition between the malleoli (Fig. 4–34).

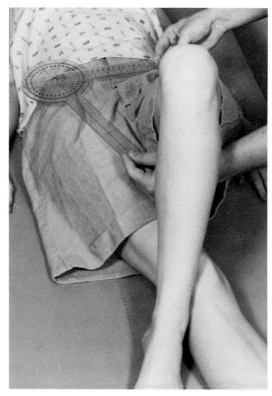

FIGURE 4–32

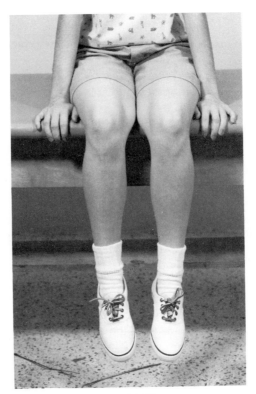

FIGURE 4–33

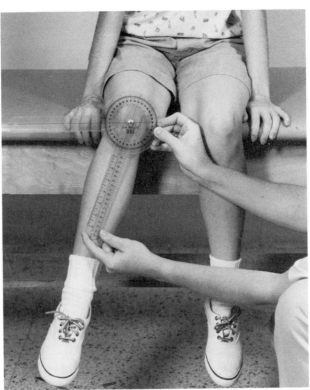

FIGURE 4–34

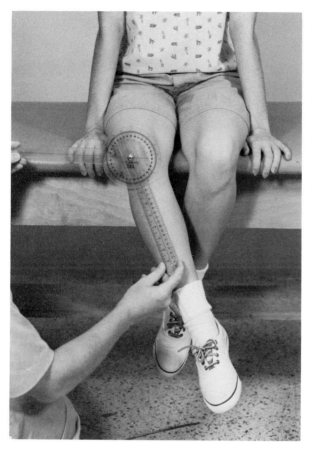

FIGURE 4—35

External Rotation

SUGGESTED TESTING POSITION   The athlete is seated, with the hip flexed to 90° and the knee flexed to 90° over the edge of the table (see Fig. 4—33).

GONIOMETER ALIGNMENT   The goniometer is aligned (1) parallel to the table and (2) along the midline of the anterior tibia, with the patella to midposition between the malleoli (Fig. 4—35).

Knee

Flexion

SUGGESTED TESTING POSITION   The athlete is in the supine position, with the hip flexed.

GONIOMETER ALIGNMENT   The goniometer is aligned along (1) the lateral femur, with the greater trochanter to lateral femoral condyle, and (2) the fibular head to lateral malleolus (Fig. 4—36).

Extension

SUGGESTED TESTING POSITION   The athlete is in the anatomic supine position.

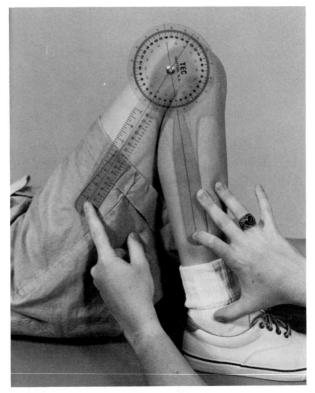

FIGURE 4—36

GONIOMETER ALIGNMENT   The goniometer is aligned along (1) the lateral femur, greater trochanter to lateral femoral condyle, and (2) the fibular head to lateral malleolus (Fig. 4—37).

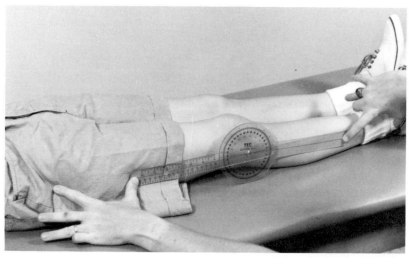

FIGURE 4—37

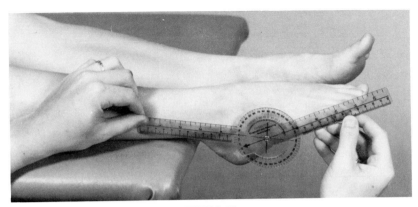

FIGURE 4–38

Ankle

Plantar Flexion

SUGGESTED TESTING POSITION   The athlete is in the anatomic supine position, with the knee flexed or straight.

    GONIOMETER ALIGNMENT   The goniometer is aligned (1) along the midline of the fibula, fibula head to lateral malleolus and along the midline of the fifth metatarsal; *or* (2) along the lateral malleolus to the bottom of the heel and parallel with the bottom of the heel (Fig. 4–38).

Dorsiflexion

SUGGESTED TESTING POSITION   The athlete is in the anatomic supine position, with the knee flexed or straight.

    GONIOMETER ALIGNMENT   The goniometer is aligned (1) along the midline of the fibula, fibula head to lateral malleolus and along the midline of the fifth metatarsal; *or* (2) along the lateral malleolus to the bottom of the heel and parallel with the bottom of the heel (Fig. 4–39).

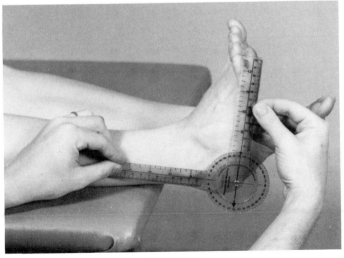

FIGURE 4–39

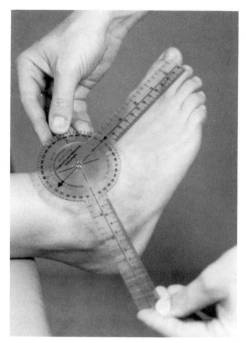

FIGURE 4—40

Inversion

SUGGESTED TESTING POSITION   The athlete is in the anatomic supine position.

GONIOMETER ALIGNMENT   The goniometer is aligned (1) across the two malleoli and (2) with the second metatarsal (Fig. 4—40).

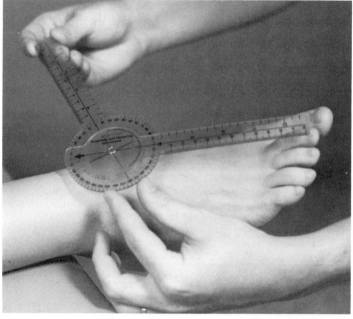

FIGURE 4—41

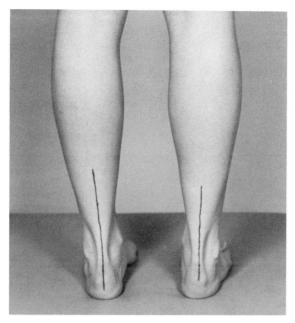

FIGURE 4—42

Eversion

SUGGESTED TESTING POSITION   The athlete is in the anatomic supine position.

GONIOMETER ALIGNMENT   The goniometer is aligned (1) across the two malleoli and (2) with the second metatarsal (Fig. 4—41).

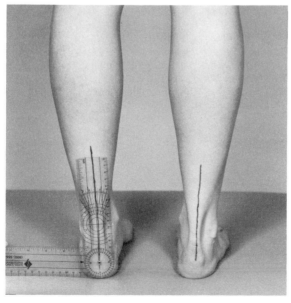

FIGURE 4—43

Subtalar Joint

Inversion/Eversion

SUGGESTED TESTING POSITION   The athlete is in the standing position (Fig. 4–42).

GONIOMETER ALIGNMENT   The goniometer is aligned (1) parallel to the floor and (2) bisecting the tendocalcaneus (Fig. 4–43).

References

1. American Academy of Orthopaedic Surgeons (1965): Joint Motion: Method of Measuring and Recording. New York, Churchill-Livingston.
2. Boone, D.C., Azen, S.P., Linn, C.N., et al. (1978): Reliability of goniometric measurements. Phys. Ther., 58:1355–1360.
3. Clark, W.A. (1921): A protractor for measuring rotation of joint. J. Orthop. Surg., 3:154–155.
4. Ekstuand, J., Wiktorsson, M., and Oberg, B. (1982): Lower extremity goniometric measurements: A study to determine their reliability. Arch. Phys. Med., 63:171–175.
5. Gajdosik, R.L., and Bohannon, R.W. (1987): Clinical measurement of range of motion —review of goniometry emphasizing reliability and validity. Phys. Ther., 67:1867–1872.
6. Gifford, H.D. (1914): Instruments for measuring joint movements and deformities in fracture treatment. Am. J. Surg., 28:237–238.
7. Gogia, P.P., Braatz, J.H., Rose, S.J., and Norton, B. (1987): Reliability and validity of goniometric measurements of the knee. Phys. Ther., 67:192–195.
8. Kendall, H.O., and McCreary, E.K. (1983): Muscles: Testing and Function, 3rd ed. Baltimore, Williams & Wilkins.
9. Leighton, J.R. (1955): An instrument and technic for the measurement of range of joint motion. Arch. Phys. Med., 36:571–577.
10. Low, J.L. (1976): The reliability of joint measurement. Physiotherapy, 62:7.
11. Moore, M.L. (1949): The measurement of joint motion. Part I: Introductory review of the literature. Phys. Ther. Rev., 29:195–205.
12. Moore, M.L. (1949): The measurement of joint motion. Part II: The technic of goniometry. Phys. Ther. Rev., 29:256–264.
13. Norkin, C.C., and White, D.J. (1985): Measurement of Joint Motion: Guide to Goniometry. Philadelphia, F.A. Davis.
14. Parker, J.S. (1929): Recording arthroflexometer. J. Bone Joint Surg., 11:126–127.
15. West, C.C. (1945): Measurement of joint motion. Arch. Phys. Med., 26:414–425.
16. Wiechec, F.J., and Krusen, F.H. (1939): A new method of joint measurement and a review of the literature. Am. J. Surg., 43:659–668.
17. Wilson, J.D., and Stasch, W.H. (1945): Photographic record of joint motion. Arch. Phys. Med., 27:361–362.

CHAPTER 5

◆

Use of Modalities in Rehabilitation

Maggie Cooper, M.S., P.T.

Because athletic trainers and physical therapists are frequently the first of the health care team to see the injured athlete, they can be extremely effective or damaging in the treatment of that athlete. A thorough evaluation, with proper consideration given to important clinical signs and symptoms, can enable the clinician to detect serious injuries in their early stages before the full extent of damage is evident, more minor problems that have the potential of developing into a more serious injury if not adequately prevented, and more chronic conditions that have not yet progressed to the point of interfering with performance and causing debilitation. Athletic trainers and physical therapists can be extremely effective in helping to modify the course of an athlete's injury. The judicious and timely use of therapeutic techniques, tailored specifically to the individual athlete's condition, can radically alter the events that follow. For example, trainers and therapists are in an excellent position to prevent the development of chronic edema, which can markedly interfere with later attempts at treatment, and to help prevent occurrence of an additional injury in the athlete who has attempted too much activity following prolonged immobilization.

Some of the most powerful therapeutic tools available to clinicians include cold, heat, electricity, compression, and massage, commonly known as modalities. Application of the appropriate modality at a particular stage of the healing process can act to prevent undue complications, and can help save much time, time that might otherwise be spent unnecessarily in a prolonged period of convalescence. This chapter describes these therapeutic modalities: how they act on the human body, their methods of application, and considerations for clinical use.

THERAPEUTIC COLD

Physiologic Effects

Therapeutic cold, or cryotherapy, when applied to the human body, elicits a number of physiologic responses including vasoconstriction, a decrease in the rate of chemical reactions involved in cellular metabolism, reduction in the conduction velocity of impulses in peripheral nerves, reactive hyperemia, and an increase in muscular strength. Following the application of a therapeutic cold modality to the body, the immediate physiologic response is vasoconstriction of the arterioles and venules, which significantly reduces blood flow to the area. It is thought that this action occurs by two indirect mechanisms—a cold stimulus acting through the sympathetic nervous system to increase the smooth muscle tone of the arteriole and venule walls, thus diminishing their circumference, and an increase of the viscosity of blood itself, so that it moves more sluggishly through the blood vessels.[39] Cold is thought to have a direct effect on the vessels themselves, but this action is seen only if the influence of the nervous system has been eliminated, and then only at low temperatures.

Cold also acts to slow the rate of the chemical reactions that occur as a part of tissue metabolism. In addition to slowing the formation of normal metabolic by-products, which would usually stimulate vasodilation, cold also acts to inhibit the release of histamine.[22] It is well known that, following an injury, damaged cells stimulate the release of histamine, a potent vasodilator that dramatically increases blood flow to an area. The histamine response is then maintained by mast cells.[16] The net effect of this process is the development and maintenance of large amounts of edematous fluid secondary to the increased blood flow. Although edema itself is not harmful to the body, some of its side effects are. If the amount of edema present in an area of tissue is sufficiently large, the exchange of nutrients and metabolites can be slowed to such a degree that an environment toxic to cells develops, or intracellular pressure can exceed the capillary hydrostatic pressure so that the blood supply is seriously diminished, resulting in cellular anoxia. Both processes act to stimulate the release of additional histamine, thus perpetuating the cycle.

Primarily because of its role in vasoconstriction and inhibition of histamine release, cold is the therapeutic agent of choice in the initial treatment of an acute, traumatic injury. As a therapeutic modality, however, cold has an additional property that is of clinical importance in the treatment of an acute athletic injury—it is an effective pain reliever. The precise mechanism by which the application of cold acts to reduce pain is not known, but it is speculated to arise from one of two sources, or possibly a combination of these sources. A number of authors have documented the slowing of nerve conduction velocity following the application of cold modalities.[15, 56] Transmission can be slowed by as much as 29.4% following a 20-minute cold application, with conduction continuing to be impaired to some degree for up to 30 minutes after the cold modality is removed.[39] According to the gate theory of pain control, it has also been speculated that cold acts to relieve pain by interfering with the transmission of pain impulses at the second-order neurons, located in the dorsal root ganglion of the spinal cord.[26] Thus, cold modalities are believed to relieve pain by slowing and reducing the number of pain impulses sent by the peripheral nerves, and by interfering with the transmission of those impulses into the brain as they synapse onto the second-order neurons in the spinal cord.

Following the removal of a cold modality, the body responds by flooding the area with blood and bringing the tissue temperature back to a more normal level.[43] This pouring of blood into the area brings with it greater than usual levels of oxygen and nutrients, a factor that is extremely important in the treatment of overuse injuries, in which the levels of tissue breakdown exceed those of tissue repair.[26] For those athletes whose high level of activity produces a chronic inflammatory condition, in which the body is continually failing in its attempts to heal itself, (e.g., tennis elbow or shin splints), regular cold applications can

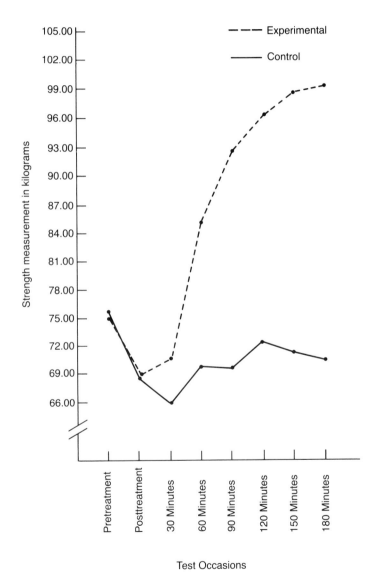

Test Occasions

FIGURE 5–1   Mean plantar flexion strength measurements during and after cold immersion. (From Oliver, R.A., Johnson, D.J., Wheelhouse, W.W., and Griffin, P.P. (1979): Isometric muscle contraction response during recovery from reduced intramuscular temperature. Arch. Phys. Med. Rehabil., 60:128.)

boost the healing process sufficiently to allow athletes to continue their high level of activity.

Finally, cold has the unusual property of actually increasing muscular strength.[24, 43] Measures of strength taken immediately after a 30-minute submersion of a leg into a cold bath of 10 to 20° C (50 to 68° F) have revealed strength to be significantly diminished (Figs. 5–1 and 5–2). Measures taken after this period, however, showed that muscle strength increased and eventually exceeded pretreatment levels.[43] In both studies, strength of the cooled muscle tissue began to exceed precooled or normal levels at 60 to 80 minutes following removal from

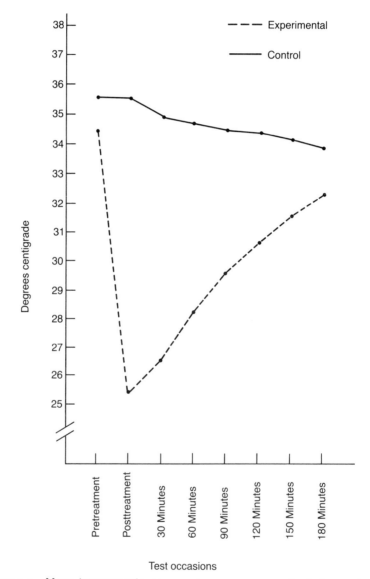

FIGURE 5–2   Mean intramuscular temperature measurements during and after cold immersion. (From Oliver, R.A., Johnson, D.J., Wheelhouse, W.W., and Griffin, P.P. (1979): Isometric muscle contraction response during recovery from reduced intramuscular temperature. Arch. Phys. Med. Rehabil., 60:128.)

the cold modality, and maintained remarkably high levels for up to 180 minutes.[24, 43] Both studies also noted the accompanying elevation of blood flow to the cooled muscle, with a consequent rise in tissue temperature. Johnson and Leider[24] have speculated that the mechanism by which muscle strength increases is a result of the elevated tissue temperature. Thus, less strength would be spent in overcoming the innate stiffness of the muscles and tendons that act to produce the movement. Oliver and colleagues[43] have suggested that the expanded blood flow to the area "disportionately" increases the excitability of muscle membranes, so that in response to a given neuronal stimulus more fibers are recruited.[43]

Indications and Contraindications

Knowledge of the physiologic effects of cold modalities automatically leads us to the types of conditions for which cryotherapy is indicated. Therapeutic cold is clearly an excellent choice in treating the early stages of acute trauma. It not only controls the formation of edema, but is also an outstanding pain reliever, especially that caused by muscle spasm or splinting and guarding. The vasodilatory properties of cold make it effective in helping to heal chronic overuse syndromes, such as rotator cuff, elbow extensor, or ankle dorsiflexor tendinitis. It can dramatically increase muscle strength, thus allowing for greater and earlier participation in excercise programs following a period of prolonged immobilization that has resulted in muscular atrophy.

Cryotherapy is contraindicated for Raynaud's disease, in which the application of cold causes the arteries of fingers and toes to narrow, with resultant tissue ischemia. It is also contraindicated for athletes with cold allergies, in whom cold modalities produce skin redness, wheal formation, flushing of the face, fainting, a decrease in blood pressure, and increased heart rate.[39] Other contraindications include individuals with multiple myeloma, leukemia, and systemic lupus erythematosus, who should be checked for cryoglobinemia. The presence of this protein causes blood to gel or a precipitate to form when cold is applied. The precipitate then shuts off the blood supply to tissues. Finally, athletes who have cold hemoglobinuria should not use cold modalities.[39] In these athletes, cold causes a breakdown of red blood cells, showing up as blood in the urine. Cryotherapy should be carefully considered and vital signs closely monitored in the athlete known to have pre-existing high blood pressure because of the vasopressor response most individuals experience to cold, in which blood pressure suddenly increases. These conditions are rare, however, and the athlete with Raynaud's phenomenon is most likely aware of the problems posed by the application of cold. Because of the severity of reaction in individuals who may not be aware that they have a cold allergy, cryoglobinemia, or cold hemoglobinuria, it is strongly recommended that athletes be monitored closely for abnormal reactions during their initial treatment sessions.

Cold should never be applied over areas of tissue that have a compromised circulatory supply or anesthetic skin. In both cases the tissue cannot protect itself from the potential damage of frostbite.

Specific Modalities and Their Application

Cold Packs

Cold packs used in clinics and training rooms are typically found in one of two forms—conventional packs made by the clinician or those commercially prepared and kept cold in a freezer.

Conventional Cold Packs   Conventional cold packs consist of chipped ice placed into a plastic bag, with the size determined by the area to be covered.

APPLICATION   A quantity of chipped ice is placed into a plastic bag, which is knotted to keep the ice in the bag. For hygienic and comfort reasons, a towel, washcloth, or paper towel should be placed between the pack and the skin. Because air is an effective insulator, the towel should be moistened prior to placement of the ice pack,[39] with the temperature of the towel being determined by the clinician's preference. A cold, wet towel speeds the removal of heat from the tissues, but a warm or room temperature towel is more comfortable for the athlete. The pack is placed over the towel and can be held in place by elastic straps, if necessary. A dry towel is placed over the ice pack to protect it from warming to room temperature (Fig. 5–3). The usual length of application is 20 to 30 minutes, with the skin being checked periodically for wheal or blister formation, especially during the first few treatment sessions. When finished, the pack is thrown away.

ADVANTAGES AND DISADVANTAGES   Probably the greatest advantage of conventional ice packs is their ability to maintain a constant temperature (ice remaining at 0°C or 32° F), which makes them more effective for cooling tissues. McMaster and colleagues[38] have found that, compared to other forms of cold packs, ice consistently produces the greatest decrease in tissue temperature over a 60-minute period of cooling in animal subjects (Table 5–1, Fig. 5–4). Additionally, the ice pack can be molded to those body parts of difficult configuration, such as the shoulder, elbow, and ankle. Finally, once the initial expense of an on-site ice machine has been met, the individual ice packs are not expensive to make.

Commercial Cold Packs   Commercial cold packs are usually composed of a silicon gel enclosed in a strong vinyl case (Fig. 5–5). They must be kept frozen at temperatures of at least $-5°$ C ($-23°$ F) for a minimum of 2 hours prior to use.[39]

TABLE 5–1   **MEAN DECREASE IN TEMPERATURE (°C) WITH ICE PACK APPLICATION**

Coolant device	Length of Exposure (min)			
	15	30	45	60
Ice	3.4	6.9	9.2	11.3
Gel	1.8	4.4	6.5	8.4
Chemical	1.6	2.9	3.0	3.5
Freon	0.2	0.9	1.2	1.7

From McMaster, W.C., Liddle, S., and Waugh, T.R. (1978): Laboratory evaluation of various cold therapy modalities. Am. J. Sports Med., 6:291–294.

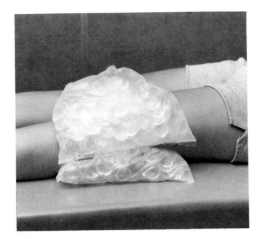

FIGURE 5–3 Conventional cryotherapy technique. Although not pictured, a moist towel can be used under the ice pack for comfort and a dry towel placed over the ice pack to protect it from warming to room temperature.

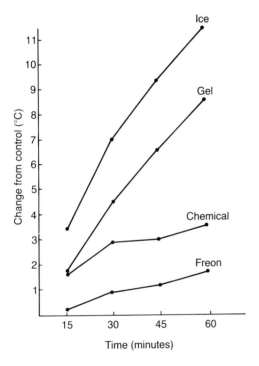

FIGURE 5–4 Average tissue temperature reduction achieved by the use of various modalities. (From McMaster, W.C., Liddle, S., and Waugh, T.R., (1978): Laboratory evaluation of various cold therapy modalities. Am. J. Sports Med., 6:291–294.)

FIGURE 5–5 Commercial cold pack. This is convenient but it does not cool as effectively as a conventional ice pack.

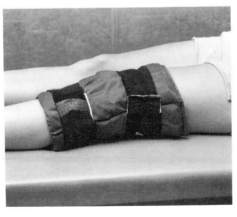

APPLICATION   Again, for reasons of hygiene and comfort, a towel can be placed between the athlete's skin and the cold pack, and, to ensure the transmission of energy between the body and the cold pack, the towel should be wet. The usual length of application is 15 to 20 minutes. With longer application, the pack becomes sufficiently warm to require replacement with a colder pack. The pack can be molded to the body and may need to be held in place with elastic straps or bandages. A dry towel is needed to protect the pack from warming to room temperature. When treatment is complete the pack is refrozen for subsequent use.

ADVANTAGES AND DISADVANTAGES   This is a convenient form of cold pack, and the initial cost is offset by the fact that the packs can be reused indefinitely. Also, the initial cost of these packs is not even close to that of a chipped ice machine. Although they do provide adequate cooling, however, they are not as effective as conventional cold packs (see Fig. 5–3) and must be frozen for a relatively long period (at least 2 hours) before they are cold enough to be used again. Finally, whereas the silicon gel can be reused indefinitely, if the vinyl covering is broken, it leaks gel and cannot be repaired.

Ice Bucket or Bath

When cooling of the entire surface of a distal extremity such as a hand, forearm, foot, or lower leg is desired, the use of an ice bucket or whirlpool filled with ice and water can be most effective (Fig. 5–6).

APPLICATION   The bucket or whirlpool is filled with a quantity of water, and ice is added until the temperature drops to the desired level. The temperature range is typically 13 to 18° C (55 to 64° F).[39] The limb is then placed in the bucket or bath, usually for 5 to 15 minutes.[44]

ADVANTAGES AND DISADVANTAGES   This particular method of cold application is ideal for treating the distal portions of the extremities—specifically the hands, feet, wrists, and ankle joints. If the goal is to reduce edema, however, placing the body part in a dependent position, in which gravity helps keep fluid in the limb, can diminish or even overcome the beneficial effects of the cold and thereby produce a limb that is more edematous following treatment than before. Prentice[44] has indicated that an excellent method for avoiding this outcome involves placing compression bandages on the body part prior to submersion.

Advocates of ice buckets and baths claim that this method has an enormous advantage over the application of other forms of cold because the athlete can actively move the body part while it is submerged; the combination of cold and movement is known as cryokinetics. For athletes who cannot harm themselves by excessive motion, such as an individual whose primary problem is restricted ankle motion following prolonged immobilization, exercising under the pain-relieving effects of cold is advantageous. For athletes who must use pain as their guideline to safe limits of movement, however, this method is obviously contraindicated. Cold interferes with the ability to perceive pain, thus placing them at risk for reinjury. For example, athletes with a second-degree lateral ankle ligament sprain would want to be able to judge accurately and acutely when they were inverting and plantar flexing

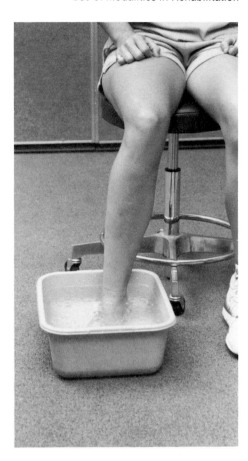

FIGURE 5–6 Ice bucket or bath. This is excellent for treating distal portions of extremities but is not indicated for those in whom edema reduction is warranted.

sufficiently to extend their injury. If their ability to perceive pain is dampened by the anesthetic effects of cold, they may unwittingly make their injury more severe or reinjure a partially healed ligament. Because of the effect of cold on peripheral nerves, it is advisable that, following an ice bath or bucket treatment, the athlete wait until sensation has completely returned before ambulating on a weight-bearing joint, such as the ankle.

Ice Massage

Ice is formed into the proper shape in a small paper or styrofoam cup.

APPLICATION When ready to use a section of the cup is peeled away, exposing the portion of ice to be rubbed against the athlete's skin. The clinician leaves a portion of the cup over the ice to protect his or her fingers or holds onto a tongue depressor placed into the cup before freezing to act as a handle. The ice is rubbed in a circular or lengthwise stroking fashion over a relatively small area, usually about a 4-inch square (Fig. 5–7). The athlete should experience several distinct sensations—intense cold, burning, aching and, finally, analgesia. When analgesia is reached, the massage is usually discontinued, although some clinicians recommend stopping at 5 to 7 minutes even if analgesia has not occurred. Continued icing after the skin is analgesic is not

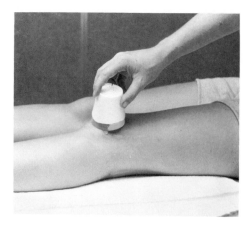

FIGURE 5–7 Ice massage. This effectively produces local cooling in discrete areas, making it an excellent treatment choice for overuse syndromes.

recommended because of the possibility of frostbite. For hygienic reasons the ice is thrown away and not reused after treatment.

ADVANTAGES AND DISADVANTAGES Although it remains controversial as to how much deep cooling this method of therapeutic cold produces, it clearly accomplishes dramatic cooling of the skin.[26] Thus, in conditions in which pain and muscle spasm are significant factors, use of this method can be extremely beneficial, resulting in pain relief and muscle relaxation. Additionally, it produces local cooling of discrete areas efficiently, with a large reactive hyperemia to the areas cooled once the treatment has ended. This makes it ideal for treating overuse syndromes, such as rotator cuff tendinitis, poorly perfused tissues (e.g., the ligaments of the ankle), and areas of local inflammation (e.g., as with bursitis). Finally, because skin temperature rarely drops below 15° C, or 59° F, in the course of administering this modality, it can be performed at home safely by the athlete.[39]

Its primary disadvantage is the discomfort the athlete experiences before analgesia is reached. It may be helpful to inform the athlete that, although initial treatment sessions of ice massage are uncomfortable, this perception lessens with continued use and habituation.[34]

Considerations for Use

In using the cold modalities, the athletic trainer or physical therapist must consider ways to avoid undercooling, which does not achieve the desired result, and overcooling, which risks tissue damage. Therapeutic cold modalities produce their effects by conducting higher-energy, warmer molecules out of the body tissues to the lower-energy, colder molecules of the modality, to which they transfer their energy. This removes heat energy from the body tissues, thus cooling them. To do this effectively, several factors must be taken into account; their interrelationship can be summarized by the following equation:

$$D = \frac{area \cdot k \cdot (T_1 - T_2)}{thickness\ of\ tissue}$$

where D is the rate of energy transfer, area equals the amount of surface area to which the cold modality is applied, k is the thermal conductivity of the tissue, (T_1-T_2) is the temperature difference between the skin and cold modality, and thickness of tissue is the depth of cooling to be achieved.[39] In other words, to cool a segment of tissue effectively, a modality must be applied that is cold enough, covers a sufficiently large area, and is located over tissue with a thermal conductivity that allows heat to be transferred to the surface. Therefore, chipped ice packs are strongly recommended, because they remain at 0°C (32° F) until all the ice has melted, a feature not found in commercial cold packs.[38]

Water, muscle, and bone all have thermal conductivities that allow cooling of tissues following topical cold application. Fat, however, is an excellent insulator, with a thermal conductivity less than half that of muscle or bone and almost one-third that of water.[39] Studies have shown that the thickness of the subcutaneous fat layer between the skin and muscle being cooled can have a dramatic effect on how cold the underlying muscle tissue becomes (Fig. 5–8).[35] Thus, for a patient with a substantial layer of subcutaneous fat, effective cooling can take a long time.[5] Some practitioners even recommend a full half-hour of cooling for the obese patient.

Assuming that the clinician has been able to cool the area effectively, we know that the athlete is experiencing at least some level of cold-induced analgesia. For this reason, and because the joints are now stiffer (which slows the ability of muscles to react to excessive and potentially damaging motions), it is strongly recommended that the athlete not exercise or play until 1 or 2 hours have passed since cooling.[39] Furthermore, the athlete should be cautioned to avoid situations of potential reinjury, such as walking or running on an uneven surface.

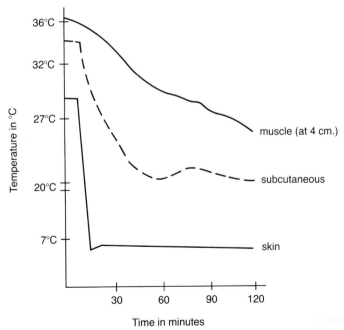

FIGURE 5–8 Tissue temperature changes during ice pack application to the calf. (From Michlovitz, S. (1986): Thermal Agents in Rehabilitation. Philadelphia, F.A. Davis, p. 75.)

Overcooling is accompanied by two primary hazards. When skin temperature drops below 15°C (59° F) the body ceases vasoconstriction to the area and initiates the "hunting reaction," in which the vascular system fluctuates between vasoconstriction to avoid loss of body core heat and vasodilation to avoid local tissue necrosis.[26] Extreme or excessive cooling stimulates this protective vasodilation, which has the effect of increasing edema in the limb.[37] Thus, whereas adequate cooling is needed to bring about the vasoconstriction required to control edema, excessive or prolonged cooling has the opposite effect. In fact, too much cooling can produce even more edema than if cold is not applied at all.[37] Generally, cold should be applied for 5 to 30 minutes, with shorter times being used when more moderate ranges of temperature are desired or for the athlete with only a thin layer of subcutaneous fat.

Even with periodic vasodilation and warming of tissues as a result of the hunting phenomenon, which floods the area with warm blood, the body might not be able to protect local tissues from frostbite and necrosis. Nerve tissue appears to be especially vulnerable to the effects of local cooling. Drez and associates[14] have reported five patients with nerve palsy secondary to cryotherapy, one of whom had not spontaneously recovered by 9 months following injury. They recommended that ice not be applied for more than 20 minutes, with 30 minutes being the absolute maximum length of treatment, and that areas of tissue where superficial nerves are located be avoided altogether.[14]

Finally, the clinician should exercise caution in applying vigorous cold over open wounds during the first 2 to 3 weeks of healing, because studies have reported that this practice significantly reduces the tensile strength of the wound.[39] Cold diminishes the rate of metabolic processes, thus slowing the rate of scar formation and healing.

THERAPEUTIC HEAT

Before discussing specific modalities of therapeutic heat and their actions, it is appropriate to divide them into two classes of heating agents, superficial and deep. Because the two groups share many common features, it could be argued that they merely occupy different positions on the same spectrum. This is certainly true in regard to the degree of vasodilation elicited by superficial and deep heating agents. The deep heating agents, however, have some unique differences, both in the effects they produce and the energy sources they use, so they actually represent a separate class. For our purposes therapeutic heating agents are presented as two distinct groups.

Superficial Heating Modalities

Physiologic Effects

Most superficial heating agents transfer their energy to the body in the same way as therapeutic cold modalities—by conduction. Energy in the form of heat is externally applied to the body. The energy is transferred from the object of highest energy (in this case, the modality) to the object of lowest energy (in this case, the body), which has the net effect of warming the tissues. Superficial heating agents are similar in certain ways to therapeutic cold modalities. Because they are both applied externally they have similar physiologic effects, although, because the heating agents are warmer than the body, the direction of heat transfer is reversed. Superficial heating modalities elicit vasodilation, relieve pain, diminish muscle tone and spasticity, increase the metabolic rate of cells, and diminish joint stiffness.

Superficial heating agents, when applied to the body, produce only mild increases in tissue temperatures. Generally, when a superficial heating agent is applied to the body, internal temperatures rise gradually, do not exceed 40°C (104° F), and the duration of temperature elevation at its peak level is relatively short.[29] As expected, an elevation in tissue temperature elicits an increase in local blood flow. This occurs primarily in the vessels of the skin and subcutaneous tissues.[39] Increases in blood flow to deeper tissues such as skeletal muscle usually appear to be produced by the metabolic demands of exercising muscle, and thus change little with the application of a superficial heating agent.[39] The vigor of this response is determined by the combined actions of reflexes to local axons and spinal cord, as well as by the prostaglandins and histamine released by the local tissues whose temperature is elevated.[39] In addition, secretion of perspiration releases kallikrein (a potent vasodilator) from sweat glands, which in turn acts on an intermediary globulin, stimulating bradykinin release. Bradykinin further vasodilates the blood vessels. The net effect is a mild inflammatory response, increases in intravascular pressure and permeability of vessel walls resulting in outward fluid filtration, and consequent edema formation.[39] For this reason, heating agents are usually contraindicated in the presence of an active inflammatory process or significant amounts of edema.

This increase in blood flow not only cools the tissues by drawing heat away to other areas of the body, where it can be dispersed, but also brings greater than normal amounts of oxygen and nutrients into the area. The rates of chemical reactions, especially those of cell metabolism, are dramatically increased by the rise in temperature.[39, 53] Thus, a sudden and large demand for both oxygen and nutrients is made by the cells. If this demand is not satisfied adequately, the cells die. Heating modalities are therefore always contraindicated for tissues with a restricted blood supply. Damaged tissues in the process of healing also increase the rate of their cellular processes, hopefully speeding their rate of repair.

Vasodilation occurs not only in the area being heated, but also in tissues distant to the heating agent through consensual or indirect vasodilation.[1] Thus, an area of the body opposite to that being directly heated shows evidence of vasodilation and increased blood flow, even though neither the temperature of the tissue nor its metabolic demands have changed from the resting state. Because increased blood flow occurs reflexively instead of being demanded by an increase in temperature or metabolism, no damage occurs in tissues with compromised circulation. In fact, for the geriatric athlete or younger individual recovering from trauma involving the circulatory system, consensual vasodilation is an excellent method for encouraging the development of collateral circulation.

It is thought that superficial heating agents act to relieve pain and diminish muscle spasm in the same ways as the cold modalities. Both Michlovitz[39] and Licht[34] have cited numerous studies indicating that muscle tone decreases by the topical application of heat. Although the precise neurologic mechanism by which this occurs remains controversial, it is widely accepted that the reaction does occur. The fact that muscle tone is reduced is well known by anyone who has ever felt their muscles relax under the effects of a hot shower, heating pad, or Jacuzzi. Also, topically applied heating agents are known to stimulate increased activity of skin thermoreceptors. According to the gate theory of sensory afferent modulation, the increased input from these receptors is believed to compete with pain impulses for transmission into the central nervous system, with fewer pain impulses making their way to the brain.[26]

Finally, the topical application of heating agents decreases joint stiffness.[55] In combination with the mild pain-relieving and vasodilatory properties of superficial heat, this makes it an ideal modality to use prior to exercise.

As might be concluded from this discussion, the use of superficial heating agents is indicated whenever a mild increase in blood flow, increased speed of healing, partial relief of pain, relaxation of muscles, or decreased joint stiffness is desired. In conditions such as relief of painful muscle spasms, nonacute muscle contusions, and tight joint capsules, superficial heating modalities can be useful components of the treatment regimen. The clinical use of hot packs, whirlpools, paraffin baths, contrast baths, and fluidotherapy is usually related to their pain-relieving and joint pliability properties. Alterations in blood flow brought about by superficial agents are restricted to the skin and subcutaneous tissues.

Superficial heating agents, as is true of all topically applied modalities, are contraindicated for use on anesthetic skin. Because of their vasodilatory and growth-promoting properties, they are contraindicated for use on areas of tissue not adequately supplied with blood and in the presence of internal infections, thrombophlebitis, cancers, rheumatoid arthritis during the active phase, and an ongoing inflammatory process or significant edema. Individuals with bleeding disorders should also avoid the use of heating agents.

Specific Modalities and Their Application

Hot Packs

Hydrocollator packs are composed of a silicate gel in a canvas cover. The packs are stored in a water bath maintained at a temperature of 71 to 79.4°C (160 to 175° F).[29] When in use the packs are wrapped in dry toweling, with six to eight layers between the athlete's skin and the pack (Fig. 5–9).

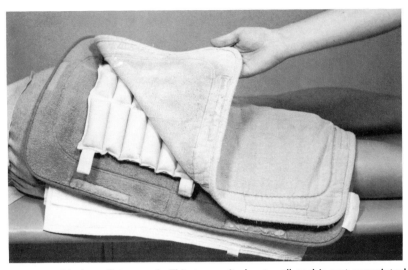

FIGURE 5–9 Hydrocollator pack. This transmits heat well and is not associated with a high incidence of overheating or skin burns.

APPLICATION The packs can be molded to irregular surfaces and held in place by small weights or loosely applied elastic wraps. The athlete should never lie on top of a pack, because this could squeeze water out into the protective layers of toweling, possibly causing a skin burn.[29, 39] Packs are usually applied for 20 minutes; they must be reimmersed in the water bath for at least 30 minutes before reuse.[39]

ADVANTAGES AND DISADVANTAGES Hot packs are convenient to use and are not particularly expensive. They usually provide good transmission of heat and are not associated with a high incidence of overheating or skin burns. They are difficult to apply to curved surfaces, however, because of their stiffness, which often prevents total surface contact. Athletes should not lie on top of the hydrocollator pack, and those who are in pain may not be able to tolerate the weight of the pack and toweling as it is placed onto the body part to be heated. Position modifications to allow hot pack placement are common.

Whirlpools

Whirlpool tanks can be of extremity, lowboy, or Hubbard size. They are commonly used to clean open wounds and prior to exercises for the relief of pain and stiffness (Fig. 5–10). If wound healing is the purpose of the treatment, various antibacterial agents can be added to the whirlpool; the most common additives are povidone-iodine (Betadine) and 5% bleach (Dakin's) solutions. Whirlpools are especially useful in the treatment of the athlete who has just resumed activity following casting or prolonged immobilization and whose primary problem is restricted range of motion. The heat diminishes joint and tissue stiffness while the body part is moved and stretched.

APPLICATION Water for the tank is usually at a temperature between 36.5 and 40° C (98 to 104°F) and can be agitated by turbines, which mix air and water. The body part is submerged and can be actively moved during the treatment. The usual length of treatment is 20 minutes.

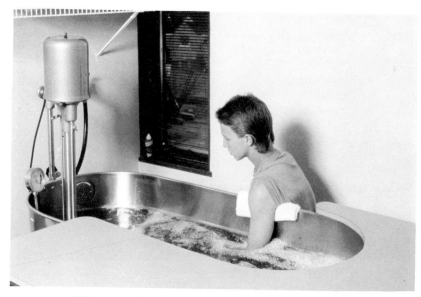

FIGURE 5–10   Whirlpool bath. This is ideal for wound cleaning. The warmth of the water and buffeting of the agitator help relieve pain. (Photo courtesy of *Sports Medicine Update,* Birmingham, AL.)

ADVANTAGES AND DISADVANTAGES   As a tool in the rehabilitation of athletes, whirlpools have several advantages for both the acute and long-term phases of care. Whirlpools are ideal for cleaning large, open wounds that might have grass, soil, or surface particles embedded in them. The water cleans the wounds mechanically and introduces anti-bacterial agents into the tissues. Both the warmth of the water and the buffeting of the agitator relieve pain according to the gate theory of pain modulation.

Warm whirlpools should not be used when edema is present. The heat of the water causes vasodilation, and creates an outward fluid filtration; when combined with the dependent position of the body part or extremity, this brings about a definite increase in edema. Active movement of the body part during the whirlpool treatment facilitates venous and lymphatic return, which helps to reduce the edema formed but does not eliminate it altogether.

Contrast Baths

Contrast baths are a special form of therapeutic heat and cold that can be applied to distal extremities. They are frequently used in the treatment of ligament and joint capsule sprains as well as stasis edema because of the vigorous hyperemia they elicit. Also, they can be used in patients with peripheral vascular disease to improve circulation in the contralateral extremity by consensual vasodilation and to improve range of motion in arthritic joints.

APPLICATION   Two tubs are used, one containing warm water (approximately 38 to 44°C or 100 to 111° F) and one containing cold water (approximately 10 to 18°C or 50 to 66° F). The extremity is initially submerged in the warm bath for 10 minutes. It is then alternated between the cold bath for 1 minute and the warm bath for 4 minutes, ending in the warm bath. The cycle is repeated four times, with the total treatment time usually being 30 minutes.

ADVANTAGES AND DISADVANTAGES   Judging by the skin color changes seen in those treated with contrast baths, they do elicit a vigorous hyperemia, which is not a common feature of superficial heating agents, but studies reporting this physiologic effect are scarce. The cold cycle can be uncomfortable for the athlete and may create a problem of compliance.

Paraffin Baths

Paraffin baths are liquid mixtures of paraffin wax and mineral oil. Body parts are either dipped into the bath or painted with the mixture. Use of this modality is usually followed by stretching exercises in the treatment of painful, arthritic joints, because the heat diminishes pain and joint stiffness. When applied to joints covered by subcutaneous soft tissue, paraffin baths produce only mild heating but, when applied to the joints of the hands, wrist, foot, or ankle, internal temperatures approach 45° C (113° F). Thus, for these joints, paraffin baths are considered to be a deep heating modality.

APPLICATION   A commercially available mixture of paraffin wax and mineral oil is heated in a thermostatically controlled bath to temperatures ranging from 47.8 to 54.5° C (117 to 130° F).[39] The athlete's hand or foot is dipped into the bath (Fig. 5–11), or, if a larger joint is to be

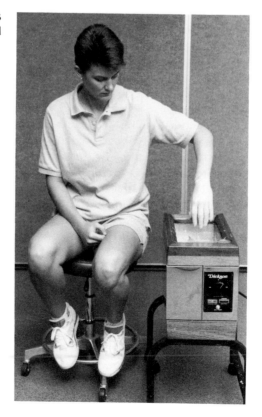

FIGURE 5–11   Paraffin bath. This is effective for heating small joints.

treated, the paraffin is painted onto the body. The skin must be cleaned thoroughly and all jewelry removed prior to application. Treatment of the hand or foot can be accomplished by repeatedly dipping the body part into the bath, gradually producing a thick layer of paraffin. The paraffin-coated body part is wrapped in plastic and five or six layers of toweling for 20 minutes. A more vigorous heating can be obtained if the body part is dipped several times to form a protective layer and then immersed for 20 minutes.[29] Paraffin is contraindicated if the athlete has an open wound.

ADVANTAGES AND DISADVANTAGES   Paraffin baths are effective for heating small joints of the upper and lower extremities. Coupled with range-of-motion stretching, this can be an excellent method for regaining mobility. Because significant heating and vigorous vasodilation occur, however, the clinician should expect edema formation. If edema is a problem prior to treatment, this modality should not be used.

Fluidotherapy

Fluidotherapy treatments consist of warm air (37.8 to 48.9° C or 99 to 119° F) blown through fine glass beads or, more commonly, cellulose particles.[20] The air–particle mixture is housed in containers. Fluidotherapy tanks come in various sizes, allowing treatment of all body parts. Nylon mesh sleeves are attached to the body part being treated and help prevent escape of the particles.

APPLICATION   The machine must be warmed up and should be turned on in advance (exact times are given in the instruction manual). The athlete places the body part to be treated into the tank, with the nylon sleeve securely fastened. The athlete can easily move the body part within the tank—the concentration of particles and size of the tank allow active movement. The skin should be cleaned thoroughly prior to treatment, and any open wound should be protected with a plastic dressing to prevent particles from being embedded in the wound or contaminated.

ADVANTAGES AND DISADVANTAGES   According to the gate theory of pain control, the combination of heat, movement of the body part, and mechanical stimulation of the skin (bombardment by the particles) should result in a potent pain reliever. Because this modality relieves pain and allows the athlete to move during treatment, it is an outstanding method for regaining mobility lost to restricted range of motion. As with a paraffin bath, vigorous heating of the hands and feet occurs, so an athlete who still has significant edema in an extremity should avoid use of this modality.

Deep Heating Modalities

Physiologic Effects

In contrast to the superficial healing agents, deep heating modalities can produce much higher temperatures in tissues and therefore a more vigorous response. Deep heating agents typically raise temperatures at a fairly rapid rate, elevate tissue temperatures close to tolerance levels

(45° C or 113° F), and maintain peak temperatures for a relatively long period.[29] Neither superficial nor deep heating agents transmit their energy into the body through conduction, but act on specific tissues through sound waves and electromagnetic energy to bring about tissue heating.

Specific Modalities and Their Application

Shortwave Diathermy

Shortwave diathermy machines create high-frequency alternating currents that produce a magnetic field when applied to electrical wires. A more intense magnetic field is created if the coils are formed into a solenoid shape. Diathermy machines available for clinical use operate at a frequency of 27.12 MHz. Application of a high-frequency alternating current to electrical wires yields electromagnetic waves composed of transverse electrical and magnetic fields.[39] Although both capacitance and inductance electrodes are capable of delivering both types of fields concurrently, they each favor delivery of one type over the other.[39] Capacitance electrodes build up electrical charges on two plates separated in space. Because of the separation of opposite charges, a strong electrical field develops between the two plates. In an electrical field, tissues that are poor conductors (e.g., fat and skin) act to resist current flow and thus can be overheated by the diathermy wave.[12]

Inductance electrodes create a magnetic field that envelops the body part. The electromagnetic wave affects biologic tissues differently, depending on their fluid content and consequent electrical conductivity. In a magnetic field, tissues with a high fluid content (e.g., skeletal muscle and fluid-filled cavities) absorb more of the electromagnetic wave and are heated to a greater extent (Fig. 5–12).[12] Fat tissue does not produce as great a resistance in magnetic fields as in an electric field and thus is not heated as much.[12]

THERAPEUTIC ACTIONS   The chief therapeutic action of shortwave diathermy is derived from its ability to elevate temperatures in deep tissues, specifically skeletal muscle and joints. Whatever type of electrode is used, shortwave diathermy has been shown to bring skeletal muscle tissue at depths of 2 to 3 cm to therapeutic levels of temperature (40 to 50° C, or 104 to 122° F). As tissue temperatures increase, vasodilation occurs, bringing large amounts of relatively cool blood in an attempt to reduce temperatures back to homeostatic levels.[31] As before, increased blood flow provides tissues with greater than usual quantities of oxygen and nutrients; combined with an increased rate of chemical reaction, this speeds healing of stretched or torn tissues. This increased blood flow also aids in the resolution of inflammatory infiltrates and exudates.[39] As with other heating modalities, joint stiffness decreases and both pain and muscle spasm are relieved.[39]

Knowledge of its physiologic effects helps provide indications for using shortwave diathermy. Of all the therapeutic modalities currently available, shortwave diathermy is probably the most effective for heating skeletal muscle.[26] Thus, if an increased rate of healing or resolution of inflammatory by-products of skeletal muscle is desired, shortwave

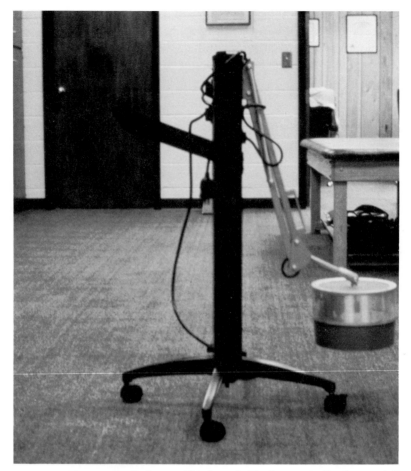

FIGURE 5—12   Shortwave diathermy. This is probably the most effective modality for heating skeletal muscle.

diathermy is recommended. It is also excellent for relieving muscle spasms that encompass a large area.

There are many contraindications to the use of shortwave diathermy. As Dowling[12] has noted, shortwave diathermy has all the contraindications common to heating modalities: tissue not adequately perfused with blood, pregnancy, cancer, infections, inflammation of any tissue, edema, and effusion. This modality, however, has additional contraindications that are not usually considered. These include the presence of any metal in the field, whether internal (surgical implants), worn by the individual (jewelry, watches), or environmental (stools, tables).[12] Shortwave diathermy interferes with the usual function of devices such as pacemakers and urinary simulators so any one with such a device should avoid the area where shortwave diathermy treatments are being given.[12] Shortwave diathermy is contraindicated on bony prominences and in any fluid-filled cavity, so application to the eyes, testes, or brain is not recommended. Finally, because the clinician must rely on the subjective report from the athlete to determine adequate or excessive dosage, this modality is not recommended for individuals with anesthetic skin.

APPLICATION   When using capacitance electrodes, physical contact between the plate surface and the athlete's body is prevented by interposing layers of towels or air spaces. Inductance electrodes have coils or wire placed close together, with electric currents running through them. They can be wrapped around the body part or housed in a drum. A layer of towels 1 to 2 cm thick must separate the wrapped coil from the skin. For both forms of electrodes at least one layer of toweling must be placed over the athlete's skin to absorb perspiration, which, because of its high water content, is selectively heated and could cause a skin burn. Care must be taken to prevent the wires from touching each other, the athlete, or furniture to avoid burns. Dosage is determined by report of the athlete. A warm, toasty feeling that is not excessively hot should be described. Usual treatment length is 20 minutes.

ADVANTAGES AND DISADVANTAGES   As noted previously, shortwave diathermy is probably the most effective modality for heating skeletal muscle.[26] Because heating is accomplished without physical contact between the modality and skin, it can also be used even if the skin is abraded, as long as significant edema is not present. The inconvenience of diathermy is its primary disadvantage. The equipment is large, bulky, and difficult to maneuver and set up. The area must be cleared of all metal, and anyone possessing a pacemaker must be at least 4.5 m (15 feet) away.[39]

Ultrasound

Therapeutic ultrasound is a deep heating modality that produces a sound wave of 0.8 to 1.0 MHz. The sound wave is produced by applying a high-frequency, alternating electrical current to a natural quartz or synthetic crystal. This converts the electrical current to a mechanical vibration,[34] a reversal of the piezoelectric effect. In piezoelectricity, compression and elongation of a neutral crystal alter its configuration (Fig. 5–13). This relative change in the mechanical orientation of the crystal produces a dipole. When the process is repeated rapidly, the dipole alternates its charges and an alternating current to

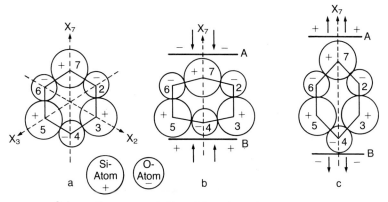

FIGURE 5–13   Schematic representation of the piezoelectric effect. (From Licht, S. (1965): Therapeutic Heat and Cold, 2nd ed., p. 331, © 1965, the Williams & Wilkins Co., Baltimore.)

the crystal causes it to distort into its compressed and elongated forms. Molecules next to the crystal are moved forward by the longitudinal compression wave created by movement of the crystal. The frequency of the compression wave is exactly equal to that of the electrical current applied to the crystal.

THERAPEUTIC ACTIONS   In the human body, ultrasound has several pronounced effects on biologic tissues. It is attenuated by certain tissues and reflected by bone. Thus, tissues lying immediately next to bone can receive an even greater dosage of ultrasound, as much as 30% more.[30] Because of the increased extensibility ultrasound produces in tissues of high collagen content, combined with the close proximity of joint capsules, tendons, and ligaments to cortical bone where they receive a more intense irradiation, it is an ideal modality for increasing mobility in those tissues with restricted range of motion. Sonation of tissues must be combined with passive stretching to gain permanent motion in tight tissues, with stretch applied during and for a time after the treatment has ended.[33] Long-duration, low-load stretching has been found to produce elongation effectively while causing the least tissue damage.[52]

In addition to increasing collagen tissue extensibility, ultrasound also increases blood flow to an area as the body attempts to cool overheated tissue. This action is thought to be useful in the resolution of inflammatory exudates and calcium deposits in bursae and tendon sheaths. Ultrasound is an accepted and recommended clinical treatment for bursitis, although research studies have failed to substantiate this.[13] Heating of tissues is thought to be responsible for the temporary increase in nerve conduction velocity seen in sonated peripheral nerves.[27]

A final effect of ultrasound is the stirring and streaming of molecules in the path of the sound wave. This nonthermal effect is believed to be partly responsible for the positive effect of ultrasound on chronic wounds and is the basis for phonophoresis. With phonophoresis, it is believed that drug molecules are propelled forward into the body. A cream emulsion containing the medication is placed on the skin and used as a coupling agent while molecules of the medicine are propelled into the body. Pharmacologic agents introduced in this fashion include hydrocortisone and lidocaine. Studies have reported that greater amounts of medication are found in tissues following phonophoresis than those found if the medication is applied topically.[39] Additionally, animal studies have reported medication introduced by phonophoresis at tissue depths of 5 to 6 cm.[39]

INDICATIONS AND CONTRAINDICATIONS   Ultrasound is the modality of choice when heating to the deepest level possible or when increased extensibility of joint, ligament, or scar tissue is desired. It has also been reported to temporarily alleviate pain, possibly by the alteration of threshold stimulation in free nerve endings.[39]

Because ultrasound causes an increase in local blood flow and enzymatic activity, it should not be applied to edematous or ischemic tissues. Similarly, joints that are hypermobile should not receive ultrasound unless any stretching movement, which would increase the preexisting hypermobility, can be controlled. Athletes with anesthetic skin or bleeding disorders also should not receive ultrasound therapy.[34] Because of the damaging effect on a fetus of increasing tissue temperature, therapeutic ultrasound is contraindicated to the pregnant uterus and should not be applied to the abdomen or low back area of a woman unless she is certain she is not pregnant. The possibility of cavitation prevents clinicians from applying ultrasound to fluid-filled cavities such as the eye, brain, and heart. Ultrasound applied directly to cardiac pacemakers can interfere with their functioning, so such individuals need to be protected from any stray sound waves.[39] Stirring effects have been implicated in increased detachment of cancer cells, with an increased possibility of metastasis, so no cancer patient should receive ultrasound except for special hyperthermic treatment of the cancer.[39] The vibrational qualities of ultrasound dictate that it should not be applied to the epiphyseal plates of children or to unhealed surgical sites, where the movement of adjacent molecules would retard or damage ongoing healing processes.

APPLICATION   In order for the sound wave to be propagated forward, it must pass through a medium that can be compressed. It cannot move through air, so a coupling agent is used to make a connection between the sound head or applicator and the athlete's skin (Fig. 5–14). The most commonly used coupling agents are commercially prepared gels, water, and mineral oil. Various studies have examined their efficacy. Commercially prepared gels have consistently been found to be the most efficient in transmitting sound waves.[3, 51] Water is less efficient, but is advocated for body surfaces too irregular to ensure transmission when using gel (e.g., hand, elbow, ankle). The body part is immersed in a water bath. Care must be taken to remove air bubbles when sonating underwater, because they interfere markedly with sound wave transmission.[51] For small areas or body parts where gel would be unpleasant, such as the face, transmission can be accomplished by a water-filled balloon (Fig. 5–15). A balloon is filled with water until all air is removed, and the neck of the balloon is placed over the sound head. A thin layer of gel is placed between the balloon and the skin.

Newer models of ultrasound units use small-diameter applicators. They have an extremely small depth of penetration because of the problem of beam divergence.[34] Customary use of ultrasound for target

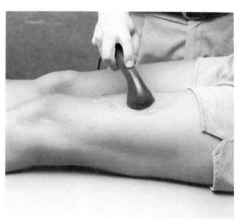

FIGURE 5–14   Ultrasound. This is effective for increasing collagen extensibility and blood flow in an area. A coupling agent such as commercial gel is required to transmit the sound waves from the applicator to the skin.

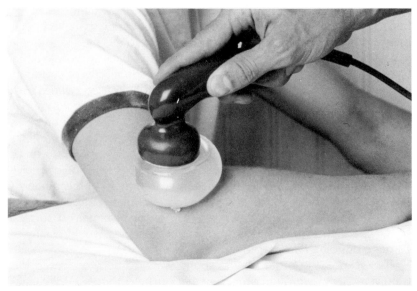

FIGURE 5–15   Ultrasound. A balloon filled with water can be used for sonation over very small areas or body parts where gel would be unpleasant or over bony prominences where good surface contact cannot be made.

tissues at a depth of 3 to 5 cm requires a sound head no smaller than 5 cm^2.[34] Usual dosages range from 0.5 to 3.0 W/cm^2 with the specific dosage for each individual being determined by the depth of the target tissue, the degree of heating desired, and the athlete's response. If an even lower level of heating or nonthermal effects are desired, the sound wave can be pulsed, although few studies have demonstrated the efficacy of this method.

Using an adequate layer of coupling medium, the clinician moves the sound head in circular, overlapping strokes. Recommended field size of sonation is a 3- to 4-inch square.[34] If tissue temperatures exceed tolerance levels, so that tissue damage is imminent, the athlete experiences periosteal pain. This is usually reported as a deep aching or soreness. The clinician should immediately reduce the intensity by 10 to 15% or expand the field size.[26] Periosteal pain should quickly subside. If it does not, the intensity should be reduced further. A note should be made for future treatment sessions about the proper dosage for each athlete.

Stationary application of ultrasound (the sound head is simply held in position over the target structure) is discouraged because of the rapid temperature rise creating "hot spots"[34] and increasing the possibility of blood clot formation.[42] To ensure temperature elevation to therapeutic levels, sonation needs to last at least 5 to 10 minutes.[32]

ADVANTAGES AND DISADVANTAGES   Ultrasound is an extremely useful clinical tool, especially when stretching tight ligaments, tendons, and capsular tissues. It effectively induces therapeutic temperatures in deep tissues to speed healing. It is relatively easy to apply and is comfortable for the athlete to experience. It is not the panacea many clinicians seem to expect, however, and successfully executes only those functions for which it is designed. It also has several potentially serious complications if applied improperly.

Considerations for Use

After a through history and physical examination have identified the target tissue, the clinician must decide which heating modality is most likely to accomplish the desired goal (e.g., increased blood flow, relief of pain, resolution of inflammatory exudates, increased extensibility of collagen tissue) without bringing about unwanted side effects. Of primary consideration is the type of heat energy that the target tissue selectively absorbs. Shortwave diathermy, especially the induction method, is selectively absorbed by skeletal muscle, whereas ultrasound is effective on connective tissues. Of equal importance is the depth of the tissue to be heated. Superficial heating agents rarely penetrate to a depth greater than 1 to 2 cm unless soft tissue covering is minimal (e.g., the hand), whereas ultrasound effectively penetrates up to 5 cm of tissue depth. Inherent in this consideration is the thickness of the subcutaneous fat layer, expecially for the superficial heating agents, which transmit their energy through conduction. For the obese athlete, superficial heating agents may require longer than usual application periods or may produce only slight temperature changes in tissue below the skin. Finally, the expected vascular response must be considered. If tissue heating is slight, the increased homeostatic blood flow to the area may prevent any change in cellular metabolic rate, nerve conduction velocity, or joint stiffness, so the goal of treatment will not be reached. If tissue heating approaches tolerance levels, however, vasodilation is vigorous. Blood flow to the area increases dramatically, the rates of chemical reactions increase, and stiffness of involved joints diminishes. The clinician should also expect an increase in edema. In a tissue whose healing is already impeded by the presence of excessive edema, this can further compromise the healing process.

THERAPEUTIC ELECTRICITY

Basic Considerations

Before going into a detailed discussion of therapeutic electricity it is necessary to review terms and mechanisms. Atoms are composed of protons, neutrons, and electrons. Protons are positively charged, electrons are negatively charged, and neutrons have no charge (neutral). Protons and neutrons are clustered in the nucleus of the atoms, with electrons orbiting around them. Protons and electrons are electrically equivalent, so that equal numbers of each produce an overall electrical neutrality of the atom. To transfer a charge from one atom to another only electrons are moved—protons are never removed from the nucleus.

Subtraction or addition of electrons to the orbit of an atom creates an electrical imbalance, so that the atom becomes electrically charged. An atom that is electrically charged is known as an ion. Ions with a deficiency of electrons—that is, more protons than electrons—are positively charged and are known as cations. Ions with an excess of electrons—that is, more electrons than protons—are negatively charged and are known as anions. Ions of similar charge repel one another, whereas ions of dissimilar charge attract each other. This force of attraction or repulsion is directly proportional to the strength of the charges on the two ions and inversely proportional to the distance between them. It causes ions to move toward or away from one another, depending on the strength and direction (attraction or repulsion) of the force. The force that causes ions to move is known as voltage. While voltage is the force that causes ions to move, the actual movement of the ions is known as current. Current can be defined as "the movement of charged particles in a conductor in response to an applied electrical force," with the applied electrical force being the voltage.[46] Current is measured in amperes, with 1 ampere (A) being equal to 1 coulomb of electrons moving past a defined point in 1 second. Current and voltage are thus proportional. High voltage (all other things being equal) produces a movement of many ions, which represents a high level of current flow.

As might be expected, however, all other things are rarely equal. The media through which ions are moving and whether these media facilitate or inhibit this movement must be considered. Media that facilitate movement are known as conductors. Biologic conductors are water, blood, and electrolyte solutions, such as perspiration. Media that inhibit movement of ions are known as resistors. Biologic resistors include skin, fat cells, and lotion.

The relationship among voltage, current, and resistance of the medium to the movement of ions is described by Ohm's law,

$$I = V/R$$

where I is current, V is voltage, and R is resistance. The law states that the current (I) induced in a conductor increases as the applied driving force is increased (V becomes larger), or as opposition to the movement of ions is decreased (R becomes smaller).

Despite the plenitude of names to the contrary, only three types of electrical current are applied to biologic tissues: direct, alternating, and pulsed (Fig. 5–16). Direct current is a continuous, one-directional flow of charged ions, and is sometimes known as galvanic current. Alternating current is a continuous, two-directional flow of charged ions, and may be referred to as faradic current. Pulsed current is a flow of ions that is periodically discontinued for a finite period of time, and the flow can be unidirectional or bidirectional.

As can be seen from Fig. 5–16, pulsed current is actually direct or alternating current that is cyclically interrupted. Pulsed currents are described by their waveforms. They can be monophasic, in which the deviation from the baseline occurs in one direction only, or biphasic, in which the deviation from the baseline occurs in two directions. The phase can be symmetric or asymmetric depending on whether the sizes of the two phases are equal. Once a specific current has been identified as direct, alternating, or pulsed, with monophasic or biphasic

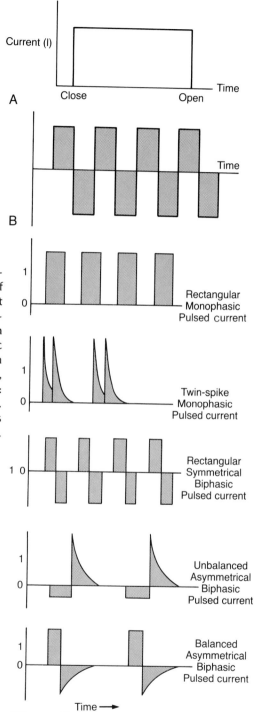

FIGURE 5-16 Graphic representation of the three types of electrical current. *A*, Direct current. *B*, Alternating current. *C*, Pulsed currents. (From Robinson, A.J. (1989): Basic concepts and terminology in electricity. *In:* Snyder-Mackler, L., and Robinson, A.J., (eds.): Clinical Electrophysiology, pp. 9,11,13, © 1989, the Williams & Wilkins Co., Baltimore. Drawing by David Lessard.)

waveforms, symmetric or asymmetric, additional terms can be used to describe the phases of a pulse and the pulses themselves (Fig. 5–17).

1. Peak amplitude: the maximum value a current can reach in a monophasic current or in either phase of a biphasic current
2. Phase duration: the amount of time during which a single phase of the current is applied
3. Pulse duration: the amount of time that passes from the begin-

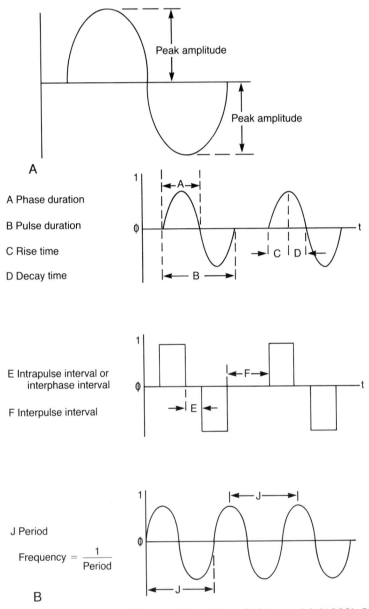

FIGURE 5–17   A, B, Electricity characteristics. (From Robinson, A.J. (1989): Basic concepts and terminology in electricity. In: Snyder-Mackler, L., and Robinson, A.J., (eds.): Clinical Electrophysiology, p. 15, © 1989, the Williams & Wilkins Co., Baltimore. Drawing by David Lessard.)

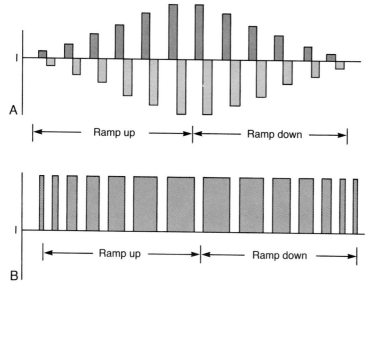

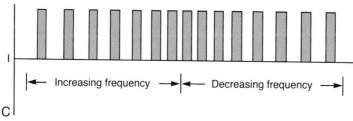

FIGURE 5–18   Methods of ramping current. *A,* Amplitude modulation. *B,* Pulse duration modulation. *C,* Frequency modulation. (From Robinson, A.J. (1989): Basic concepts and terminology in electricity. *In:* Snyder-Mackler, L., and Robinson, A.J. (eds.): Clinical Electrophysiology, p. 18, © 1989, the Williams & Wilkins Co., Baltimore. Drawing by David Lessard.)

ning to the end of a single pulse (the term "pulse width" is sometimes used to denote this)
4. Intrapulse interval: the amount of time elapsed from one phase of a pulse to the next (also described as the interphase interval)
5. Interpulse interval: the amount of time between pulses
6. Frequency: the number of pulses that occur in 1 second

Phases can also be modified so that the full strength of the current is not applied all at once or turned off abruptly. Rise time (the time during which the current of a phase increases from zero at the baseline to the peak amplitude) and decay time (time during which the current of a phase decreases from peak amplitude to zero) denote these modifications. Similarly, the current itself can be altered in this same manner through ramping (Fig. 5–18). Current can be ramped up or down by increasing or decreasing current intensity, the length of the pulse duration, or the pulse frequency.

Electrical current is passed into the body through electrodes and a conducting medium. Water or an electrolyte gel is a common conducting medium. Electrodes can be arranged in several configurations.

A monopolar arrangement (Fig. 5–19A) is a single electrode placed at a distance. The single electrode, because of its relatively smaller size, has a greater current density (amount of current/surface

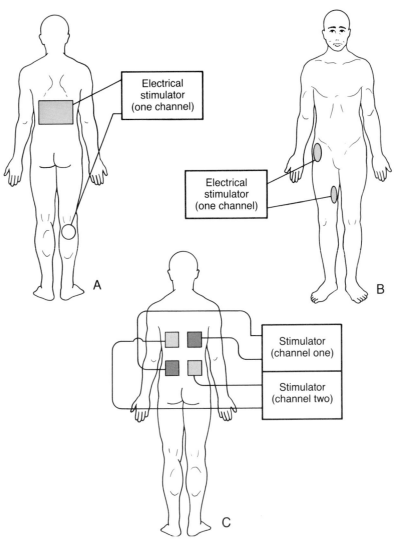

FIGURE 5–19   Electrode placement configurations in clinical electrical stimulation. A, Monopolar orientation, with a small "active" electrode over the posterior calf target region and a large "dispersive" or "indifferent" electrode in the low back region. B, Bipolar orientation, with two electrodes placed over the anterior thigh musculature target area; electrodes might not be the same size in all applications. C, Quadripolar orientation of electrodes, with two electrodes from each of two separate stimulation "channels" placed in the low back target region. (From Myklebust, B.M., and Robinson, A.J. (1989): Instrumentation. In: Snyder-Mackler, L., and Robinson, A.J. (eds.): Clinical Electrophysiology, p. 31, © 1989, the Williams & Wilkins Co., Baltimore. Drawing by David Lessard.)

area), and thus induces activity in electrically excitable tissue. Bipolar arrangements (Fig. 5–19B) involve two electrodes, both of which are placed over the target tissue; these may or may not be of equal size. If the two electrodes are of the same size, both are electrically active. Quadripolar arrangements (Fig. 5–19C) have two channels of current with at least two electrodes each.

Physiologic Effects

Generally, therapeutic electricity appears to have a role in the maintenance or gain of muscular strength, the relief of pain, increased vascularity of tissues, edema reduction, and healing of chronic wounds and nonunion fractures. Electricity is not as well understood as therapeutic cold and heat; despite many studies of the various electrical modalities, the precise mechanisms of its effects remain mostly unknown.

Muscle Strength

The research findings of studies concerning the effects of therapeutic electricity on muscle strength are confusing and controversial. Some relationships have been elucidated, however, and may lead to a greater understanding of the effects of therapeutic electricity.

For example, it is known that in healthy humans the recruitment of motor units in skeletal muscle follows a consistent and orderly pattern. When central nervous system input demands initiation of contraction in a muscle, the smallest alpha motoneurons are recruited first. As the central nervous system's demand for a greater strength of contraction continues, larger and larger motoneurons are recruited, with the largest being enlisted last. This recruitment pattern is known as the size principle, with size referring to the alpha motoneuron cell body.

Another way in which the human body can produce a greater strength of contraction is through a change in the motoneuron discharge rate, a process known as rate coding. Increasing the discharge frequency from the alpha motoneurons already firing acts to increase the tension developed by individual muscle fibers, and may fuse the twitches into a tetanic contraction. Thus, greater torque is developed by the muscle. Discharge rates developed in this way from healthy motoneurons are rarely greater than 30 pulses/second.[46]

Finally, the electrical action of skeletal muscle motor units is guided by the absolute refractory period of the motor units. The absolute refractory period for normal subjects is such that motor units can only be stimulated approximately 1000 times/second.[46] Any greater frequency of stimulation does not produce a greater strength of contraction.

A number of general guidelines in rehabilitation encourage the use of electrical stimulation to increase muscle strength and endurance. Wolf's law of functional adaptation, the specific adaptation to imposed demand (SAID) principle, and the overload method of strength training all indicate that, if a muscle contraction can be induced in some way, strength and endurance are encouraged in that muscle. Following these guidelines, the clinician should logically be led to use electrical stimula-

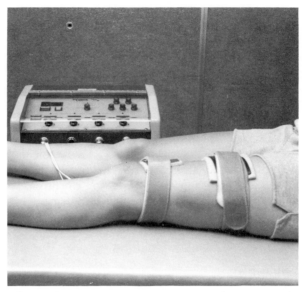

FIGURE 5-20   Electrical muscle stimulation (EMS). The efficacy of EMS for strengthening muscle is unclear, but it appears to be better than no exercise at all and is advocated for muscle re-education.

tion for maintaining and regaining muscular strength, but research studies have been frustratingly inconclusive. In an extensive literature review, DeLitto and Robinson[11] surveyed 16 well-controlled studies on the effects of neuromuscular stimulation on voluntary muscle strength of healthy individuals. They concluded that although neuromuscular electrical stimulation is a better method for improving muscle strength than no exercise at all, it is no more effective than voluntary exercise (Fig. 5-20).[11] Also, they found no advantage in using electrical stimulation and voluntary exercise together.[11]

An excellent study by Mohr and colleagues[40] has compared the quadriceps strength of healthy subjects undergoing a regimen of high-voltage galvanic stimulation and isometric exercise. They found significantly greater strength in those in the exercise group than in those in the control or electrical stimulation groups. Another earlier study by Currier and Mann[8] on muscle torque developed in healthy individuals with isometric exercise, electrical stimulation, and a combination of isometric exercise and electrical stimulation, however, found no difference among the three groups. All those in these three groups were significantly stronger than those in the no-exercise control group, but no one method was clearly shown to be an improvement over the other two.[8] Thus, those in the group receiving only electrical stimulation were as strong as those in the group who performed only isometric exercise and those who underwent the exercise and stimulation regimen.

Both studies[8, 40] appeared to have been well controlled, thorough, and appropriately analyzed, and targeted the same subjects, but reached differing conclusions. Perhaps the reason can be found in the recruitment pattern induced by the electrical stimulation. When electrically stimulated, the largest alpha motoneurons are recruited first because they have the lowest internal resistance. The smallest fibers, which have the highest internal resistance, are recruited last. Given that a system is only as strong as its weakest part, the relatively weak muscle fibers recruited by the small alpha motoneurons may limit the response. Whatever the speculated cause, it is clear that further research is needed.

For the experienced clinician these results are puzzling. Most clinicians report that electrical stimulation helps slow the formation of disuse atrophy and appears to help athletes regain strength. The studies previously outlined, however, fail to note any difference. In their exhaustive review of the literature, DeLitto and Robinson[11], examined studies involving individuals with pre-existing muscle weakness and found a noticeable trend. They concluded that some protocols of electrical stimulation, when applied to patients, yielded greater gains in strength than voluntary exercise, and that there appeared to be a direct proportion between training contraction intensity and amount of strength gained.[11] Gould and co-workers[19] have compared the functional abilities of ten postmeniscectomy patients who received neuromuscular electrical stimulation to those of ten postmeniscectomy patients who underwent the usual isometric strengthening regimen. The electrical stimulation was of sufficient intensity to elicit a strong tetanic contraction. Those in the electrically stimulated group required significantly smaller amounts of pain medication, ambulated earlier without crutches, demonstrated greater range of motion, exhibited reduced volumes of postsurgical edema, and had significantly smaller losses of muscle volume and strength.[19]

Relief of Pain

Use of various electrical modalities for pain relief was a generally accepted practice for years, long before Melzack and Wall presented their gate theory of pain modulation in 1965. Since then the number and variety of electrical modalities used to provide analgesia for the relief of all types of pain has proliferated at an astounding rate. Relief of pain has been cited as an indication for the use of high-voltage stimulators, interferential stimulators, transcutaneous electrical nerve stimulators (TENS), Medcosonolators, and low-voltage stimulators.

It is commonly thought that these devices relieve pain by two methods. Electrical stimulation of the skin and mild contraction of muscles act on receptors within tissues that transmit their message to the central nervous system, closing the "pain gate" at the spinal cord level. This process is commonly known as counter-irritation.[26] More intense stimulation, which elicits strong muscular contractions and is reported to be a painful sensation, is believed to stimulate release of endogenous opiates into the general circulation, producing a more general analgesia throughout the body.[48]

It has been suggested that the different forms and levels of stimulation are more effective for the relief of the varying types and intensities of pain that confront the average clinician. These "modes of stimulation" are usually described as sensory level, motor level, and noxious level stimulation (Table 5–2).[48]

TABLE 5–2   **COMMON STIMULATION CHARACTERISTICS OF ELECTROANALGESIA**

Mode of Stimulation	Phase Duration (μsec)	Frequency (pps, bps, or beats/sec)	Amplitude	Duration of Treatment	Duration of Analgesia	Electrode Placement
Sensory level	2–50	50–100	Perceptible tingling	20–30 min.	Little, residual posttreatment	In the area of pain
Motor level	>150	2–4	Strong, visible muscle contraction	30–45 min.	Hours	Remote, usually in the same sclerotome
Noxious level	<1 sec	1–5 or >100	Noxious; below motor threshold	Seconds to minutes	Hours	Close or remote; widely varied

Adapted from Snyder-Mackler, L. (1989): Electrical stimulation for pain modulation. *In*: Snyder-Mackler, L., and Robinson, A.J. (eds.): Clinical Electrophysiology, p. 208. © 1989, the Williams & Wilkins Co., Baltimore.

Sensory level stimulation, also known as conventional stimulation, has a relatively high frequency, low level current (just enough to produce a skin sensation of buzzing or tingling), and the pain relief provided lasts only as long as the stimulation is applied.[48] No muscular contraction should be evident, either visually or through palpation.[48] It is thought that this form of stimulation produces analgesia by interference with pain message transmission, as described by the gate theory of pain. It is the most comfortable and least frightening of all the levels of stimulation and therefore is an excellent choice for the athlete who is apprehensive about receiving electroanalgesia treatment.

By comparison, motor level or acupuncture-type stimulation has a lower frequency of stimulation and a longer pulse duration, and uses a current strong enough to elicit a regular motor response.[48] The relief obtained through this stimulation method does not immediately follow initiation of treatment but lasts for a period after stimulation ceases.[48] Thus, it is believed to relieve pain by stimulating the release of endogenous opiates.[48]

Noxious level stimulation (as may be expected from its name) is the least comfortable of all the stimulation modes. It has a relatively low frequency of stimulation and uses sufficient current to be painful to the athlete. This current can produce a muscle contraction if the electrodes are placed close enough to a motor point.[48] The usual length of treatment is relatively short, lasting only seconds to several minutes. The discomfort from this form of stimulation relates to the long phase duration, which can last up to 1 second.[48] It produces a generalized analgesia that endures long after treatment has ceased.

Although these general guidelines are widely accepted, more specific recommendations are a subject of vast controversy. In an outstanding review of studies of TENS usage for pain relief, Gersh and Wolf[17] noted extensive variation in recommendations for clinical use in regard to pulse duration, pulse frequency, current intensity, and frequency and duration of treatments, even for patients with similar diagnoses. By comparison, Jette[23] induced pain in the form of an electrically induced pinprick sensation in healthy subjects and then treated them with one of five commonly used TENS protocols: low frequency, burst frequency, hyperstimulation, high frequency with low-voltage galvanic stimulation, a high frequency with high-voltage galvanic stimulation. No significant difference was found in measured pain threshold or tolerance to pain among those receiving differing protocols. These results contrast with those of other studies, which showed definitive relief of pain with specific protocols.[17]

The most accurate conclusion may be that, although many forms of electrical stimulation produce significant reductions in pain, the research results are both confusing and contradictory. This lack of consistency, despite widespread study, was probably stated best by Mayer and Price:

> In conclusion, acupuncture and transcutaneous electrical nerve stimulation appear to be forms of counter-irritation which activite both opiate and non-opiate systems. The variable clinical outcomes observed following these treatments probably result from differential recruitment of segmen-

tal, extrasegmental, opiate, and non-opiate pain inhibitory systems, all of which are now known to be activited by these types of stimulation in animals.[36]

Increased Blood Flow

Electrical stimulation is thought to increase tissue blood flow by two mechanisms—stimulation of the autonomic nervous system causing reflexive vasodilation and as a response to the increased metabolic demands of muscles induced to contract.[49] Reflex responses brought about by stimulation of sympathetic fibers are thought to be elicited by intensities of stimulation that are low enough to avoid muscular contractions. Leandri and colleagues[28] have studied blood flow in response to TENS stimulation at current levels of 15 to 27 mA using frequencies of 3 and 100 pulses per second (pps). They found a transient increase in skin temperature, which they attributed to increases in blood flow. Following cessation of the stimulation, skin temperatures returned to resting levels within 5 minutes. The maximal increase in temperature was found to occur at the highest level of stimulation for that individual (three times the sensory threshold) at a frequency of 100 pps.[28]

Results of studies examining the changes in blood flow caused by electrical stimulation of intensities sufficient to produce a muscle contraction have varied. Animal studies have shown that significantly higher levels of blood flow occur at frequencies that cause fused muscle contraction but do not produce tetany.[49] It has been speculated that electrical stimulation must be of sufficient intensity and frequency to induce metabolic by-products, which then stimulate flow to a muscle without occluding the arterial flow as would occur in a tetanized, continuous contraction.[49] Human studies have failed to show such clear-cut results. Reports have indicated that the type of waveform or stimulator used does not appear to influence the vascular response.[50] Pulse frequency appears to affect blood flow, but these results are not consistent. Results of a study by Tracey and associates[50] have suggested a frequency of 50 pps to be most effective in increasing blood flow when intensities are sufficient to produce a 15% maximal voluntary contraction (MVC). An earlier study,[9] using the same stimulation frequency, found no significant difference between intensity levels, which produced 10 and 30% MVCs.

Edema Reduction

Electrical stimulation of sufficient intensity to produce a muscle contraction is thought to reduce edema by stimulation of muscle pump action when athletes cannot contract the muscles themselves. Other mechanisms by which tissue edema is reduced continue to be speculative. Reed[45] has noted that, in the cheek pouch tissue of golden hamsters, high-voltage stimulation using voltages of 10, 30, and 50 Volts at a frequency of 120 pps significantly reduce microvessel leakiness, with the two higher voltages being most effective. The study is provocative in its implications, but further research is indicated before any conclusions can be reached for humans.

Wound Healing

The vast majority of research regarding the use of electrical stimulation for accelerating the closure of open wounds indicates that continuous direct current is preferable to pulsed or alternating current.[49] A study by Brown and Gogia[6] followed rabbits with surgically induced wounds for 4 and 7 days. Daily high-voltage (pulsed) stimulation was applied to the experimental group's wounds. Measures of the wounds indicated that electrical stimulation may have actually hampered wound closure in the rabbits who received 7 days of stimulation.

Use of direct current is believed to speed wound healing by two mechanisms. Placement of the negative electrode over the wound has a pronounced bacteriostatic effect on both gram-positive and gram-negative organisms.[49] Additionally, application of a low level of continuous direct current is thought to mimic the "current of injury" hypothesized by Becker. Becker's 1967 investigation[4] theorized that the homeostatic electrical currents found in normal human tissue, which are usually electropositive, become reversed during an injury. The resulting change in local tissue polarity stimulates a flow of current, known as the current of injury.[4, 7, 49]

Treatment of chronic ulcers with low-intensity (200 to 800 mA) direct current for one hour twice daily has been shown to promote healing at rates 1.5 to 2.5 times faster than traditional wound treatment regimens.[7] Those in the electrical stimulation group received two 1-hour sessions of stimulation at levels of 200 to 800 mA daily; the negative electrode was placed in wet gauze, which was then packed into the wound. Those in the control group received primarily wet-to-dry dressings, with four subjects receiving daily whirlpool treatment. Wounds were measured and photographed over a 5-week period; at that time wounds for the experimental group averaged 0.5 cm^3 in size compared to wounds for the control group, which averaged 2.16 cm^3.[7]

Specific Modalities and Their Application

Transcutaneous Electrical Nerve Stimulators

Transcutaneous electrical nerve simulators (TENS) are small, hand-held electrical simulators whose energy source is a disposable or rechargeable battery. Most TENS units are small enough to be worn clipped to the athlete's belt or clothing and produce either a monophasic rectangular or asymmetric biphasic pulse (Fig. 5–21).[41]

APPLICATION   Electrodes for TENS units are typically small, about 4 to 5 cm^2, and are commercially available in various forms. More commonly used is a carbonized silicone electrode that uses a conductive gel to transmit electrical pulses to the skin and is held to the skin with adhesive tape. It is the least expensive of the TENS electrodes and, for the athlete with long-standing chronic pain, is the electrode of choice. The electrode gel can dry out, however, creating extremely high current densities ("hot spots") which can burn the athlete. Repeated application and removal of adhesive tape can create skin abrasion, and some athletes experience allergic reactions to the glue used in the adhesive. For athletes with these problems the Karaya form of electrodes is

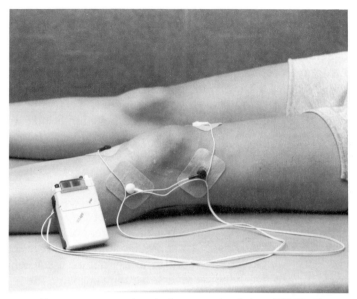

FIGURE 5–21 Transcutaneous electrical nerve stimulation (TENS). This is advocated for relief of almost all levels of pain.

available. These electrodes have a self-adhering layer of conductive polysaccharide that sticks to the skin when slightly dampened with water.[41] The thick layer of conductive polysaccharide ensures even transmission of the electrical stimulus, so current density remains constant. Because adhesive tape is not used, allergic skin reactions are not a problem.

Opinions regarding effective or optimal placement of electrodes in TENS stimulation are divided. Most clinicians appear to agree that placing electrodes around the painful area, in the relevant dermatome, or along the spinal segment of the relevant sclerotome is efficacious. Placement over acupuncture or trigger points, along peripheral nerves, or on the contralateral dermatome is also advocated.[41] Placement of electrodes over the contralateral dermatome is particularly useful in the treatment of conditions too painful to allow direct placement of an electrode, such as reflex sympathetic dystrophy or postherpetic neuralgia.[41]

Ideally, a TENS stimulator allows the clinician to modify the stimulation delivered to the patient by adjustment of the stimulation frequency, pulse duration, and intensity of the stimulating current. By adjusting these parameters, TENS units are commonly set according to the guidelines of the various modes of stimulation presented earlier (Fig. 5–22).

Conventional or high-frequency TENS units use a short-duration pulse (20 to 60 msec) combined with a 50 to 100 Hz frequency of stimulation.[41] The current is adjusted to sensory level stimulation only, delivering a slight tingling or buzzing to the athlete's skin. This form of TENS is most commonly used for those with acute or postsurgical pain[41] or as an introduction to electroanalgesia for the apprehensive athlete.[49] The relief of pain lasts only as long as the stimulus is applied, and considerable accommodation to the stimulus is thought to occur.

Therefore, frequent adjustments of the stimulus characteristics are necessary and can be performed by the athlete following instruction by the clinician. The conventional form of TENS can be used continuously, as is common in the treatment of postsurgical pain, or in a 30 to 60-minute session several times per day.[41]

The acupuncture-type TENS unit has a low frequency (1 to 4 Hz) and a long pulse duration (150 to 200 msec). The intensity is adjusted so that a strong muscular contraction is elicited.[41] This form of TENS takes longer to provide pain relief following initiation of treatment, and analgesia lasts for some time after stimulation is ended. It is believed that the acupuncture and noxious forms of TENS act to elicit the release of endogenous opiates. Usually, treatment sessions using this type of TENS units are provided daily, lasting for 20 to 30 minutes.

Use of the noxious level or brief, intense TENS unit is characterized by an extremely long pulse duration that can last up to 1 second.[49] The frequency can be low (1 to 5 Hz) or in excess of 100 Hz.[49] Current amplitude is adjusted to the greatest intensity the athlete can tolerate. This form of TENS produces a long-lasting, profound, and generalized analgesia, believed to be mediated by the endogenous opiates, which are released following brief periods of extreme discomfort.

INDICATIONS AND CONTRAINDICATIONS   TENS units are indicated for those with almost all levels of pain. They have not been found to be effective in the treatment of chronic, psychogenic, or centrally pro-

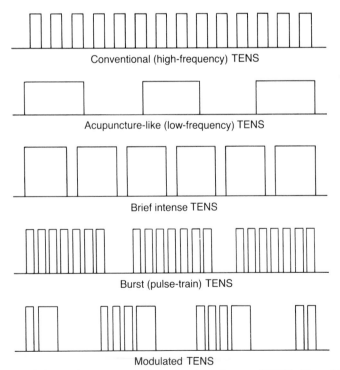

FIGURE 5–22   Schematic representation of various forms of TENS. (From Nelson, R.M., and Currier, D.P. (1987): Clinical Electrotherapy. Los Altos, CA, Appleton and Lange, p. 222.)

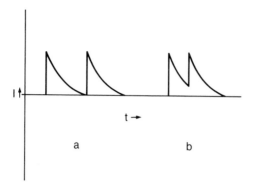

FIGURE 5–23 Schematic representation of a high-voltage pulsed galvanic waveform. (From Nelson, R.M., and Currier, D.P. (1987): Clinical Electrotherapy. Los Altos, CA, Appleton and Lange, p. 166.)

duced pain, however, but are otherwise useful in the treatment of other forms of pain, including sports injuries, peripheral nerve injuries, mild ischemic pain associated with Raynaud's phenomenon, and peripheral vascular disease.[41] They are an excellent adjunct to medication following surgery or during labor and delivery. The use of TENS units is contraindicated for the area of the carotid sinus and pharynx, low back, and pelvic regions of pregnant women, and for all individuals using a synchronized or demand form of pacemaker.

High-Voltage Galvanic Stimulation

High-voltage galvanic stimulators (HVGS) deliver a monophasic pulse with a double-peak configuration (Fig. 5–23). A twin peak is used because the duration of each individual peak does not have enough current that can be delivered to the electrical excitable tissues to ensure a response, especially if a muscle contraction is desired.[41] As can be noted in Fig. 5–23, because the pulses are monophasic the current leaves a charge in the tissues.[2]

An HVGS is a stimulator having an output greater than 100 to 150 V. For most stimulators now in use this range is usually about 300 to 500 V.[2] Their pulse duration is approximately 5 to 75 μsec/peak; with the combined duration of the two peaks lasting up to 200 μsec.[2, 41] The pulse frequency can be varied, ranging from 1 to 120 pps. They are not actually galvanic stimulators, because this would indicate use of a continuous direct current.[2] HVGSs generate a pulsatile current, but the descriptor "galvanic" has remained throughout the years and will probably continue to be used.

Because of the high voltages generated by these stimulators, pulse durations can be short and still deliver sufficient current to elicit a response in electrically excitable tissue. Therefore, these stimulators can be comfortably used by the athlete. Discomfort reported to electrical stimulation is related to pH changes occurring in the skin directly under the stimulating electrode. Currents that leave a net charge in the tissue attract high concentrations of positive or negative electrons to the area under them, an uncomfortable condition for the athlete. This is especially true of the alkaline response occurring under the cathode.[41] The short duration of current provided by HVGSs prevents a large amount of charge from accumulating under the electrodes. Pairing the short pulse duration with a long interpulse interval makes the chemical and thermal changes in the skin negligible when high-voltage stimulation is used.[2]

APPLICATION   High-voltage stimulators can be set so that current flows through both pads, first one, and then the other, or surges to peak current over a set number of pulses. These forms of current delivery are known as modes.[41] In continuous mode, a nonstop train of monophasic current is delivered to the athlete, with one electrode positive and the other negative. In reciprocating mode, one electrode is active and the other electrode is dispersive for a finite period of time. The direction of current flow then switches, so that the dispersive pad becomes the active one and the active pad becomes dispersive. This mode is particularly useful if a large muscle mass is to be stimulated, such as the thoracic or lumbar paraspinals. Surge mode allows a gradual build-up to peak current and is therefore preferred by most individuals, especially those apprehensive about or inexperienced in the use of therapeutic electrical stimulation. It is similar to the ramping mode used with TENS units (see above); each successive set of pulses is of a slightly greater amplitude than the one that preceded it, until peak current is reached.[41]

INDICATIONS AND CONTRAINDICATIONS   High-voltage pulsed stimulators are indicated for reduction of edema, stasis, and blood pooling; relief of pain; maintenance of muscle size and strength during periods of disuse; muscle re-education; and when an increase in blood flow to tissues is indicated.[41] They have also been advocated for the reduction of muscle spasm.[2] It has been suggested that the electrical stimulation reduces painful spasms through several mechanisms: fatiguing the muscle (a continuous train of pulses at a rate of 100 to 200 pps is used); relieving the pain through counter-irritation, which in turn reduces the need for protective muscle guarding (e.g., muscle spasm); and eliciting a strong muscle contraction, which then is followed by a more thorough relaxation.

Because of their extremely short pulse durations, high-voltage stimulators are not effective for stimulating denervated muscle or performing iontophoresis.[2] Like many electrical stimulators, high-voltage devices are contraindicated for people with impaired vascularity to the target tissue, pregnant women, patients with synchronous pacemakers, and those prone to seizures.[41] Regardless of past medical history, electrical stimulation should never be applied to the carotid sinus or over the heart.

Interferential Current

Interferential current is a relative newcomer to the field of physical rehabilitation, It was originally invented by Dr. Hans Nemec in the mid-1950s but has only recently gained commercial popularity. As with other electrical modalities, studies of its efficacy have yielded conflicting results.

The term "interferential" refers to the manner in which the electrical current is generated. Two independent generators and a quadripolar electrode arrangement are needed for the two currents that produce the final current acting on the tissues. These two currents operate within the mid-frequency range, 1,000 to 10,000 Hz. This takes advantage of the dramatically lower skin resistance in this frequency range. In a 100-cm^2 area of tissue, skin resistance to a current of 50 Hz is about 3,000 ohms.[10] If the frequency is increased to 4,000 Hz, this resistance decreases to approximately 40 ohms. The decrease in skin resistance therefore makes the use of this current more comfortable for the athlete.

Merely stimulating the tissues at this more comfortable frequency does not yield the desired results if muscle strengthening is the goal, because the absolute refractory period of electrically excitable biologic tissues limits current frequencies to 0.1 to 200 Hz.[10] The two currents are usually about 4000 Hz, differing from each other by about 100 to 200 Hz. For example, circuit 1 might be operating at a frequency of 4000 Hz and circuit 2 operating at 4125 Hz. The two current frequencies are known as the carrier frequencies—that is, they "carry" the current into the tissues. Because the currents are slightly out of phase with one another at some point, they summate or diminish each other to an intensity greater or lesser than either current alone. The resultant current, which is not formed until the two carrier currents meet inside the tissues, is a waveform whose intensity is constantly changing. The number of times that the intensity rises to its maximal level and drops to its minimal level is the beat frequency. Usually this frequency is the difference between the two carrier frequencies or, in the case of the example above, 125 Hz.

APPLICATION   A fairly precise knowledge of target tissue location is essential, because the final stimulating current is a synthesis of the two

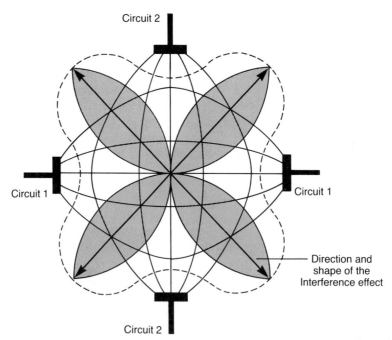

FIGURE 5–24   Current pathways and electrode placement for a static interferential field in a homogeneous medium. (From DeDomenico, G. (1988): Interferential Stimulation: A Monograph. Chattanooga, Chattanooga Corporation, p. 17.)

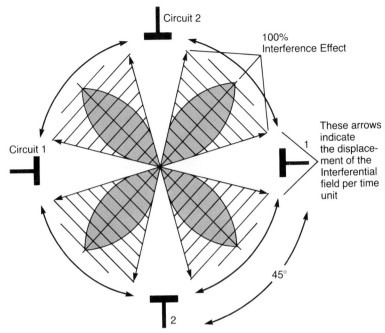

Circuit 2

100%
Interference Effect

These arrows
indicate
the displace-
ment of the
Interferential
field per time
unit

Circuit 1

45°

2

FIGURE 5–25   Current pathways and electrode placement for a dynamic interferential field. (From DeDomenico, G. (1988): Interferential Stimulation: A Monograph. Chattanooga, Chattanooga Corporation, p. 19.)

currents delivered from the four electrodes and is formed within the tissues. Typically, the two circuits are arranged to intersect each other in a diagonal pattern. The resultant interference current occurs midway between the diagonals. In a homogeneous field a cloverleaf pattern should be formed (Fig. 5–24). This type of homogeneous field in no way represents the human body with its muscle-fascial interfaces and skeletal bones. The static interferential field shown (Fig. 5–24) requires that the athlete be able to locate the painful area and perceive the stimulus to be in that area. If this cannot be done, a dynamic interferential field that moves across (scans) the area is used (Fig. 5–25). In this modification the intensities of the two circuits are unbalanced, so that the resultant interferential current moves closer to the stronger of the two circuits. If this balance is reversed the interferential current sweeps across an area of tissue to align itself more closely with the more intense circuit. Once the interferential current is arranged over the target tissue, the intensity is increased to sensory, motor, or painful response levels, depending on the type and severity of the problem being treated.[10]

Interferential current can be delivered to the skin using various electrodes or a combination of electrodes. The usual rubber electrodes can be used with a damp sponge or electrolyte gel conductor. Usually, however, interferential current is delivered using vacuum electrodes containing a damp sponge, which apply suction to the skin. The suction units, which provide the vacuum to keep the electrodes attached to the skin, may provide equal pressure to all four electrodes or allow independent modulation of different electrodes (Fig. 5–26). It has been

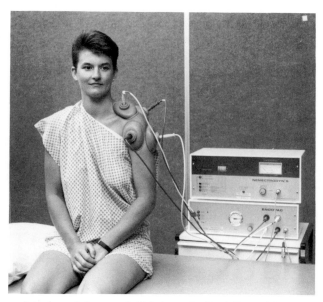

FIGURE 5–26 Interferential current. This is typically delivered by vacuum electrodes, which are ideal when attempting to provide stimulation to irregularly shaped body parts.

recommended that the amount of suction in the electrodes not exceed 0.25 atmospheres.[10] If the area being treated has significant edema, suction electrodes should not be used. Some suction electrodes allow four small electrodes to be housed in one suction cup. For a small area these single-cup or quadripolar plate electrodes can be useful. Quadripolar plate electrodes consist of four plate electrodes contained in a nonconductive panel that separates them. Because the electrical current still follows the path of least resistance and the clinician cannot adjust the distances among the four electrodes, however, care must be taken to avoid intensities that would create an edge effect and burn the athlete. Finally, plate electrodes and suction electrodes can be combined in a quadripolar arrangement.[10] The usual length of treatment is 20 to 30 minutes, with the intensity adjusted to the athlete's report.

INDICATIONS AND CONTRAINDICATIONS   Interferential current is recommended for the treatment of all types of pain because of its improved comfort of application, the strengthening of weak muscles, reduction of acute and chronic edema, relief of painful muscle spasms, improved blood flow to an area, healing of chronic wounds, and relief of abdominal organ dysfunction, specifically stress incontinence.[10] This modality is contraindicated for those with conditions usually contraindicated for electrical stimulation, such as pregnancy, cardiac pacemakers, thrombophlebitis, bleeding disorders, active cancer in the area being treated, open wounds in the area of the electrodes, or anesthetic skin, or if the individual being treated reports adverse effects. Additionally, interferential current devices should not be operated in the same area as a shortwave diathermy machine. If they must be in use at the same time it is recommended that the devices be at least 9 feet apart.[10]

Direct Current

Direct current electrical stimulation involves the uninterrupted uni-directional flow of electrons. Current flow is usually long, about 1 second, and can be modified to be surged, interrupted, or reversed.[41] Waveforms are usually monophasic with the exception of reversed direct current, which has a biphasic waveform.

Stimulation of Denervated Muscle With the advent and improved comfort of electrical stimulators using an alternating biphasic waveform or shortened pulse duration, direct current stimulators are used primarily to stimulate denervated muscle and in the process of iontophoresis. Recently small amperage direct current stimulators have been advocated for healing of chronic wounds.

APPLICATION Because of the extremely long duration of stimulus, application current intensities are relatively low, about 0.5 to 1.0 mA/cm^2.[41] Even with these low levels of current flow considerable charge accumulates in the skin and superficial tissues directly under the electrodes. The pH of the skin under the cathode gradually becomes more alkaline as positive ions are attracted to it, whereas the skin under the anode undergoes the opposite reaction. These chemical changes elicit a reflex vasodilation, presumably for the purpose of maintaining homeostatic pH. Because the alkaline reaction occurring under the cathode is considerably more harmful than the acidic reaction under the anode, it is recommended that the electrode that serves as the cathode be increased in size.[41] This reduces current density under the cathode, thus diluting the ensuing chemical changes in the tissues.

INDICATIONS AND CONTRAINDICATIONS Electrical stimulation of denervated muscle for the purpose of preventing disuse atrophy has been a traditional practice. As is true for the use of many of the electrical modalities, however, research substantiating or denying this technique is contradictory. For those athletes whose nerves are expected to regenerate within 12 to 18 months, electrical stimulation is unnecessary because human muscle tissue does not degenerate that quickly.[41] This does not imply that improvement of range of motion, friction massage to scar adhesions, and other methods of treatment are not necessary to maintain the limb, so that when the nerve finally does innervate, the limb muscles are functional. Rather, rigorous stimulation to the denervated muscles is not necessary if it is believed that the muscle can be reinnervated within 12 to 18 months following injury.

For those individuals whose nerve regeneration is not expected to occur within 24 months following injury, electrical stimulation is thought by some researchers to be a useful method of slowing or delaying irreversible fibrosis. Animal studies have found that 5 minutes of stimulation every half hour, spread out over an 8-hour day, is an optimal schedule.[41] Good results were also obtained using 30 minutes of stimulation twice daily, which was found to be almost as beneficial as 5 minutes of stimulation every half hour, and is a more feasible schedule for clinical use on humans.

After considering these factors, if the clinician decides to undertake the arduous task of instructing an individual in direct current stimulation for denervated muscles during the regeneration period, the following guidelines are recommended:

1. A portable, hand-held stimulator be rented or purchased by the individual.
2. A map of motor points be provided.
3. Stimulation should begin as soon after the injury as possible.
4. Pulse duration must be longer than 10 msec, and current intensity must be sufficient to elicit a tetanic contraction.
5. Passive range-of-motion exercises should be included in the treatment program to maintain connective tissue flexibility.
6. Volumetric or girth measurements should be performed regularly.
7. The individual must be encouraged and supported in this lengthy, time-consuming task so that treatment is performed regularly.[11, 41]

Iontophoresis   Currently, iontophoresis is the other primary clinical use of direct current. In iontophoresis, charged molecules of medication are driven into the tissues by placing them under an electrode of the same polarity. When a direct current is applied, these molecules move away from the electrode into the skin and toward the target tissues. Neither pulsed nor alternating current can be used because uniform forward movement of the molecules does not occur. Both animal and human studies on the efficacy of iontophoresis have been found to be inconclusive, with a slight edge given to those studies substantiating its effectiveness.[18] Clinically, iontophoresis appears to be an effective means of introducing various medications into a specific area of the body. Thus, the expense and the athlete's experience with systemic treatment are avoided. Iontophoresis does not require that

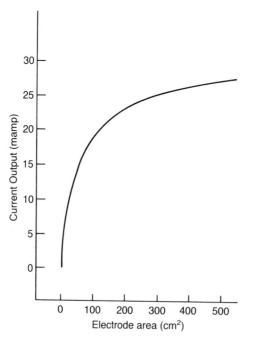

FIGURE   5–27 Recommended currents for electrodes of various sizes. (From Glick, E., and Snyder-Mackler, L. (1989): *In* Snyder-Mackler, L., and Robinson, A.J. (eds.): Clinical Electrophysiology, p. 257, © 1989, the Williams & Wilkins Co., Baltimore.)

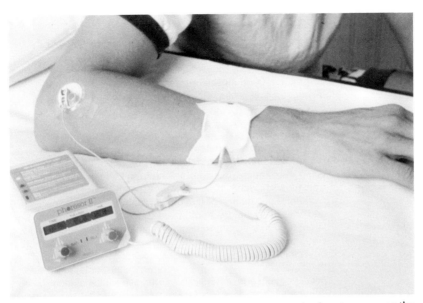

FIGURE 5–28 Commercial iontophoresor. This has several advantages over the use of the self-prepared electrodes. (Photo courtesy of *Sports Medicine Update,* Birmingham, AL.).

the medication be administered by a physician each time. Also, damage to tissue from the introduction of a needle through or into delicate structures is avoided.

APPLICATION   The amount of medication introduced into the tissues is determined by various factors: the intensity and duration of the current, skin resistance to ion movement, ionization potential of the medication or the solvent in which it is dissolved, and electrode size (Fig. 5–27).[18] Treatment sessions usually last 10 to 20 minutes at current levels of 3 to 5 mA. Electrodes can be home-made by interposing a medication-soaked gauze pad between the athlete's skin and a conducting electrode attached to a direct current generator. Commercially prepared electrodes are available and have a semipermeable membrane. The membrane contacts the skin and the drug is injected into a cavity contiguous with the membrane.

Although the electrodes are more expensive, commercially prepared iontophoresors with current regulators have several important advantages over the home-made variety. (Fig. 5–28): (1) medication introduced into the athlete's skin can be done under sterile conditions; (2) amount of medication being introduced into the tissues is known in advance, so that dosage can be controlled; and (3) the devices can turn themselves off automatically if tissue impedance becomes too high or the contact area becomes disconnected.[18] This last feature is important, because skin burns caused by the electrical current are common and can be serious. Self-monitoring by the athlete for painful sensations under the electrodes has been shown to be an unreliable method for avoiding these burns.

INDICATIONS AND CONTRAINDICATIONS   Depending on the drug used, iontophoresis is indicated for a wide variety of conditions, including bursitis, tendinitis, adhesive capsulitis, open wounds, scar tissue, cal-

TABLE 5–3 NONSTEROIDAL IONS AND RADICALS

Ion or Radical (Charge)	Features*
Magnesium (+)	From magnesium sulfate (Epsom salts), 2% aqueous solution; excellent muscle relaxant, good vasodilator, mild analgesic
Mecholyl (+)	Familiar derivative of acetylcholine, 0.25% ointment; powerful vasodilator, good muscle relaxant and analgesic; used with discogenic low back radiculopathies and sympathetic reflex dystrophy
Iodine (−)	From Iodex ointment, 4.7%; bactericidal, fair vasodilator, excellent sclerolytic agent; used successfully with adhesive capsulitis ("frozen shoulder"), scars
Salicylate (−)	From Iodex with methyl salicylate, 4.8% ointment (if desired without the iodine, can be obtained from Myoflex ointment—trolamine salicylate, 10%—or from a 2% aqueous solution of sodium salicylate powder); a general decongestant, sclerolytic, and anti-inflammatory agent; used successfully with frozen shoulders, scar tissue, warts, and other adhesive or edematous conditions
Calcium (+)	From calcium chloride, 2% aqueous solution; believed to stabilize the irritability threshold in either direction, as dictated by the physiologic needs of the tissues; effective with spasmodic conditions, tics, "snapping joints"
Chlorine (−)	From sodium chloride, 2% aqueous solution; good sclerolytic agent; useful with scar tissue, keloids, burns
Zinc (+)	From zinc oxide ointment, 20%; trace element necessary for healing; especially effective with open lesions and ulcerations
Copper (+)	From 2% aqueous solution of copper sulfate crystals; fungicide, astringent, useful with intranasal conditions (e.g., allergic rhinitis—hay fever), sinusitis, and dermatophytosis (athlete's foot)
Lidocaine (+)	From Xylocaine 5% ointment; anesthetic and analgesic, especially with acute inflammatory conditions (e.g., bursitis, tendinitis, tic douloureux, and temporomandibular joint pain
Lithium (−)	From lithium chloride or carbonate, 2% aqueous solution; effective as an exchange ion with gouty tophi and hyperuricemia†
Acetate (−)	From acetic acid, 2% aqueous solution; dramatically effective as a sclerolytic exchange ion with calcific deposits‡
Hyaluronidase (+)	From Wydase crystals in aqueous solution, as directed; for localized edema
Tap water (+/−)	Usually administered with alternating polarity, sometimes with glycopyrronium bromide in hyperhidrosis
Ringer's solution (+/−)	With alternating polarity; used for open decubitus lesions
Citrate (+)	From potassium citrate, 2% aqueous solution; reported effective in rheumatoid arthritis
Priscoline (+)	From benzazoline hydrochloride, 2% aqueous solution; reported effective with indolent ulcers
Antibiotics— Gentamycin Sulfate (+)	8 mg/ml; for suppurative ear chondritis

From Kahn, J. (1987): Non-steroid iontophoresis. Clin. Management, 7:15. Reprinted from CLINICAL MANAGEMENT with the permission of the American Physical Therapy Association.

* All solutions are 2%; ointments are also low percentage compounds. The literature and clinical reports agree that the lower the percentage, the more effective the ionic exchange and transfer. Whether this is purely a physical chemistry phenomenon or an example of the Arndt–Schultz law, which states that "the smaller the stimulant, the greater the physiological response,"[25] remains to be proven.

† The lithium ion replaces the weaker sodium ion in the insoluble sodium urate tophus, converting it to soluble lithium urate.

‡ The acetate radical replaces the carbonate radical in the insoluble calcium carbonate calcific deposit, converting it to soluble calcium acetate.

cium deposits, and hyperhidrosis.[18] Table 5–3 was developed by Kahn[25] and lists medications and their uses. Iontophoresis is contraindicated for patients with anesthetic skin or a known drug allergy. Initial sessions should be conducted with caution because allergic reactions are always possible and can be serious medical emergencies.

OTHER MODALITIES

Compression

The formation of edema following an injury is a common problem. Typically, edema is formed by a blockage or overflow of the lymphatic drainage system or by frank bleeding within the tissues. Edema collects primarily in joints of soft tissues.[44] Frank bleeding, the result of ruptured capillaries, is associated with a hematoma, whose appearance is usually delayed by several hours to days following the original trauma. Edema formation not occurring because of actual bleeding is usually caused by leakage of plasma proteins out of the capillaries into the interstitial spaces. This can happen because of actual trauma to the capillaries themselves, allowing proteins to escape, or as a response to histamine or kinin action in the inflammatory process.[16]

As the serous or lymphatic edema accumulates in tissues, the normal contour of the body part is obliterated. This condition, known as pitting edema, is graded by the length of time required to fill in a cavity made by pressing a finger or thumb into the tissue. Although edema is a common response to injury, this makes it no less harmful to the athlete. Increased internal pressure caused by excess fluid can slow or even stop nutrient exchange, thus delaying the healing process. The stasis pooling of fluid results in a toxic environment, which promotes cell death with consequent necrosis. Additionally, the excess fluid can actually stretch or tear small structures in the edematous area, initiating the inflammatory response and worsening an already bad situation.

In attempting to limit edema formation and thus minimize the damage it can cause, the clinician has several tools available. Most clinicians would probably agree that the optimal technique for dealing with edema is to prevent it from forming. Thus, following an injury in which the trainer or therapist believes edema formation to be a likely consequence, many clinicians actively take steps to avoid edema formation before it is apparent. This can be done by elevating the extremity, allowing gravity to assist lymphatic drainage. The application of a compression bandage, which increases external hydrostatic pressure and prevents fluid from moving into the interstitial spaces, is an almost universal practice and typically accompanies elevation of the limb. The bandage can be applied in a spiral wrap or figure-of-eight fashion. When these two methods were compared the figure-of-eight method was found to be more effective than the spiral wrap technique.[54]

Once edema has formed it can be reduced or controlled in several different ways. These methods act to increase external hydrostatic pressure temporarily by compressing the limb, which prevents more fluid from leaking out of the capillaries and pushes fluid out of the extracellular space into the lymphatic-venous drainage system. If the edema is not too severe or is located in the hand, wrist, foot, or ankle, centripetal massage followed by application of a compression bandage can be sufficient to reduce edema. The hands of the operator are held in a pétrissage position and stroked repetitively in a centripetal direction along the limb. The goal is to stroke or milk the fluid into a more proximal location, where a muscle mass capable of pumping the fluid back into the lymphatics exists. Alternating contractions of major muscle groups (e.g., a muscle pump) in the area of the edema is another method that moves the excess fluid along and out of the tissues.

If the edema is widespread or severe, the clinician can apply intermittent compression using a mechanical pump and sleeve that covers the entire length of the upper or lower extremity (Fig. 5–29). Pressure is applied intermittently to force fluid into the lymph vessels, with periods of relaxation to allow fluid movement within the system. There is no consensus concerning the length or ratio of on–off times between the compression and relaxation periods. Some have recommended that the time of compression exceed the time of relaxation by a factor of 2, 3, or even 4, whereas others have reversed this.[44, 47] The length of treatment varies and is determined by athlete tolerance of the procedure. In treating athletic injuries, 10- to 30-minute sessions are commonly used and seem to be effective for the types of conditions treated.[44]

APPLICATION   Prior to applying intermittent compression, both the involved and uninvolved limbs should be measured either circumferentially or volumetrically to determine the amount of edema present. If circumferential measurements are taken, the precise location of the measurement should be the same at each session and should include the joint (if one is affected). Usually the length of the involved limb is

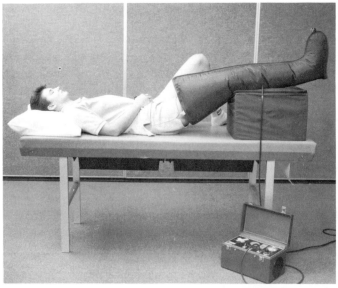

FIGURE 5–29   Intermittent compression. This is indicated for edema reduction in which pressure is applied intermittently, alternating with periods of relaxation.

divided into thirds, with measurements taken at these points.[47] Volumetric measurements are more precise and are determined by the amount of water displaced by the limb; they are also more time-consuming to perform, however, and require special equipment.

For hygienic reasons a tubular stockinette covering is placed over the skin before the compression sleeve is placed on the extremity. The athlete's limb is placed in an elevated position so that the effects of gravity can be added to those of the compression pump. The time of treatment is set according to severity and expected tolerances. In the initial treatment session, it is recommended that the pressure be set at 80 mm Hg.[47] Consequent settings can be either at this generic setting or 20 mm Hg below the athlete's systolic pressure.

At the end of a treatment session the involved extremity should be remeasured to determine the amount of edema removed from the limb, remembering to use the same location if circumferential measurements are taken. Optimally, the same person should perform the measurements. A compression bandage should be applied to the limb before upright or limb-dependent activities are resumed.

Portable units have been developed that use chemical coolants or ice water. The coolant or ice water circulates through a hand or foot sleeve, providing a cold modality in combination with compression. Although these units are convenient and provide an excellent tool for on the field treatment of the injured athlete, they are not an adequate substitute for mechanical compression units because they do not provide as much pressure.

INDICATIONS AND CONTRAINDICATIONS Mechanical compression is usually confined to the treatment of edema. It is contraindicated in conditions of congestive heart failure, pulmonary edema, thrombophlebitis, and active inflammatory or infectious processes.[47]

Friction Massage

Friction massage is a specialized form of massage that uses subcutaneous friction of tissues for various purposes. It was popularized in the late 1970s by Dr. James Cyriax and is also known as deep transverse massage or cross-fiber massage. It is not a method of massage designed to promote relaxation and can be somewhat painful for the athlete, even if properly applied.

Physiologic Effects

Friction massage has a number of effects on human tissues. Perhaps its most significant effect is on collagen fiber orientation. It is thought that friction massage causes healing collagen fibers to be laid down parallel to each other. This increases the strength of the tendon or ligament involved, allowing it to withstand greater levels of longitudinal stress. Generally, after an injury, these tissues are "rested" while adequate healing occurs. After this period the athlete is allowed to gradually resume a normal activity level. Without any stimulus to increase cross-sectional area, the ligament or tendon is usually weak when activities are resumed and the rehabilitation period prolonged. Too much early stress to the tissue can result in reinjury. Use of friction massage during the interim healing period and rehabilitation process is believed to stimulate the ligament or tendon to orient its fibers longitudinally without actually stressing the tissue.[21] Friction massage also improves the extensibility of tissues.

Friction massage is believed to be useful in destroying adhesions. Adhesions, both those that would bind the structure to those around it and those between the fibers of the structure itself, are broken apart and discouraged from re-forming.[21] This is the rationale for applying friction massage to surface scar tissue—to break down skin and subcutaneous tissue adhesions that would prevent full range of motion from being achieved.

Friction massage produces a significant hyperemia in the target tissues.[21] This is especially important in the treatment of structures experiencing tissue breakdown caused by overuse or poor vascular perfusion. The combination of stimulus with proper collagen fiber orientation and strengthening with improved circulation may be sufficient to allow an athlete to maintain a high level of activity long after that which would have been possible without treatment.

APPLICATION   The athlete is positioned comfortably, with the limb supported. If the purpose of the massage is to break up adhesions between the target tissue and adjacent structures, the target tissue is placed on slight stretch. To break up adhesions between a surface scar and subcutaneous tissues, a light to moderate pressure (sufficient to stretch the scar without damaging or blistering the skin) is applied along the length of the scar. The scar is stretched along its length with one finger or thumb, with tension being maintained until the second finger or thumb can be drawn up the scar. This process is repeated for several minutes. Greater pressure can be applied as some of the tenderness diminishes. Athletes should be instructed in the performance of this procedure at home on a daily to twice-daily basis. Pressure is never applied across or perpendicular to the scar because this can widen it, a cosmetically undesirable outcome.

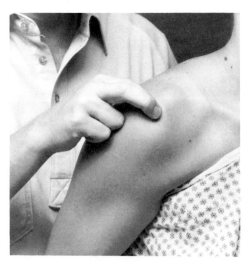

FIGURE 5–30 Deep friction massage to the supraspinatus tendon.

If the purpose is to treat an underlying structure, the athlete is again positioned comfortably, this time with the target tissue slack (Fig. 5–30). The therapist or trainer places himself so that his fingers are perpendicular to the target structure and in a comfortable position. It is recommended that the therapist be seated.[21] Only one or two fingertips are used, and the others maintain positioning of the athlete. No oil or lotion is applied to the skin. The clinician applies enough pressure to the skin so that it moves with the fingers. The clinician rubs across the structure slowly in a controlled fashion. Only light pressure is applied initially, and the pressure is deepened as treatment progresses. Excursion of the movement is small, no massage is applied to any of the surrounding tissues, and there should be no tension on the skin, which might cause a blister.

The athlete generally reports some tenderness in the first 1 to 2 minutes of treatment, which should disappear. Pressure of the massage can then be increased. Greater pressure should not be applied, however, if tenderness has not diminished significantly or disappeared altogether. This may indicate that the initial pressure was too great. If the pressure has not vanished after 4 minutes or has actually increased, treatment should be discontinued.[21]

The length of treatment is 5 to 6 minutes for the initial session and is gradually increased in 3-minute increments to 12 to 15 minutes per session.[21] Treatment session are usually done twice to three times weekly, with most problems resolving within 2 to 3 weeks.

The stress that this technique may place on the joints of the therapist's or trainer's treatment fingers may be a problem. This can be reduced by stabilizing the affected joint with the opposite hand.[21]

INDICATIONS AND CONTRAINDICATIONS Friction massage is ideal for overuse conditions of tissues that are poorly perfused or have diminished energy-attenuating properties. Thus, conditions such as rotator cuff tendinitis, tennis and golfer's elbows, DeQuervain's tendinitis, plantar fasciitis, and mild or chronic sprains of wrist, ankle, and surface ligaments of the knee are ideal for treatment with friction massage. Additionally, any surface scar that might prevent full range of motion from occurring can also benefit from treatment by friction massage. This technique is contraindicated for an individual with anesthetic skin who cannot report tenderness accurately or in the presence of acute inflammatory or infectious conditions.

The therapist or trainer treating an injured athlete has a wide variety of tools available. Most of these are effective, if applied appropriately, and can be even more useful if combined with others that reinforce their actions. For example, an athlete with a sprained ankle is expected to develop pain, edema, possible joint instability, and loss of function. These symptoms can be treated with ice packs and an assistive ambulatory device but would probably respond better if the ice were combined with elevation, compression bandaging, and possibly electrical stimulation, and the joint protected from hypermobility by a removable brace. Home use might include ice packs and the use of a TENS unit at night.

Although it seems reasonable to use these modalities in combination and with other therapeutic techniques, the problem of overtreatment can develop from this strategy. The experienced clinician must determine, in each *individual* case, where the proper use of techniques and modalities ends and overtreatment begins. A worse problem is the unfortunate practice of treating the athlete with a combination of modalities that may actually act against each other. This so-called "shotgun" strategy, used when the clinician does not know where to start treatment, at the least, has no benefits to the athlete or clinician and may even serve to retard healing. Using this method only confuses the issue and delays healing.

The judicious, timely, and thoughtful use of various modalities requires time and energy on the part of the clinician, two factors frequently in short supply in busy training rooms and clinics. Practicing a logical strategy in developing each athlete's treatment program, however, with frequent reappraisal, cannot fail to reward the clinician willing to make this effort.

References

1. Abramson, D.I., Bell, Y., Tuck, S., *et al.* (1961): Changes in blood flow, oxygen uptake and tissue temperatures produced by therapeutic physical agents. Am. J. Phys. Med., 405:5–13.
2. Alon, G. (1984): High Voltage Stimulation: A Monograph. Chattanooga, TN, Chattanooga Corporation.
3. Balmaseda, M.T., Fatehi, M.T., Koozekanani, S.H., and Lee, A.L. (1986): Ultrasound therapy: A comparative study of different coupling media. Arch. Phys. Med. Rehabil., 67:147–150.
4. Becker, R.O. (1967): The electrical control of growth processes. Med. Times, 95: 657–669.
5. Bierman, W.S., and Friedlander, M.(1940): The penetrative effect of cold. Arch. Phys. Ther., 21:585–592.
6. Brown, M., and Gogia, P.P. (1987): Effect of high-voltage stimulation on cutaneous wound healing in rabbits. Phys. Ther., 67:662–669.
7. Carley, P.J., and Wainapel, S.F. (1985): Electrotherapy for acceleration of wound healing: Low intensity direct current. Arch. Phys. Med. Rehabil., 66:443–446.
8. Currier, D.P., and Mann, R. (1983): Muscular strength development by electrical stimulation in healthy individuals. Phys. Ther., 63:915–921.
9. Currier, D.P., Pettrilli, C.R., and Threlkeld, A.J. (1986): Effect of graded electrical stimulation on blood flow to healthy muscle. Phys.Ther., 66:937–943.
10. DeDomenico, G. (1988): Interferential Stimulation: A Monograph. Chattanooga, TN, Chattanooga Corporation.
11. DeLitto, A., and Robinson, A.J. (1989): Electrical stimulation of muscle: Techniques and applications. *In:* Snyder-Mackler, L., and Robinson, A.J.,(eds.): Clin. Electrophysiology. Baltimore, Williams & Wilkins, pp. 97–138.
12. Dowling, J.C. (1987): Shortwave diathermy. Sports Med. Update, 3:7–8.
13. Downing, D.S., and Weinstein, A. (1986): Ultrasound therapy for subacromial bursitis. Phys. Ther., 66:194–199.
14. Drez, D., Faust, D.C., and Evans, J.P. (1981): Cryotherapy and nerve palsy. Am. J. Sports Med., 9:256–257.
15. Fox, R.H. (1961): Local cooling in man. Br. Med. Bull., 17:14–18.
16. Ganong, W. (1977): Review of Medical Physiology. Los Altos, CA, Lange.
17. Gersh, M.R., and Wolf, S.L. (1985): Applications of transcutaneous electrical nerve stimulation in the management of patients with pain. Phys. Ther., 65:314–336.
18. Glick, E., and Snyder-Mackler, L. (1989): Iontophoresis. *In:* Snyder-Mackler, L., and Robinson, A.J. (eds.): Clinical Electrophysiology. Baltimore, Williams & Wilkins, pp. 247–259.

19. Gould, N., Donnermeyer, D., Gammon, G.G., *et al.* (1983): Transcutaneous muscle stimulation to retard disuse atrophy after open meniscectomy. Clin. Orthop. Rel. Res., 178:190–197.

20. Henley, E.J. (1982): Fluidotherapy: Clinical Applications and Techniques. Sugarland, TX, Henley International.

21. Hertling, D., and Kessler, R.M. (1990): Management of Common Musculoskeletal Disorders, 2nd ed. Philadelphia, J.B. Lippincott.

22. Hocutt, J.E., Jaffe, R., Rylander, C.R., and Beebe, J.K. (1982): Cryotherapy in ankle sprains. Am. J. Sports Med., 10:316–319.

23. Jette, D.U. (1986): Effect of different forms of transcutaneous electrical nerve stimulation on experimental pain. Phys. Ther., 66:187–193.

24. Johnson, D.J., and Leider, F.E. (1977): Influence of cold bath on maximal handgrip strength. Percept. Mot. Skills, 44:323–326.

25. Kahn, J. (1987): Non-steroid iontophoresis. Clin. Management, 7:14–15.

26. Kessler, R.M., and Hertling, D. (1983): Management of Common Musculoskeletal Disorders. Philadelphia, Harper & Row.

27. Kramer, J.F. (1985): Effect of therapeutic ultrasound intensity on subcutaneous tissue temperature and ulnar nerve conduction velocity. Am. J. Phys. Med., 64:1–9.

28. Leandri, M., Brunetti. O., and Parodi, C.I. (1986): Telethermographic findings after transcutaneous electrical nerve stimulation. Phys. Ther., 66:210–213.

29. Lehmann, J.F. (1982): Therapeutic Heat and Cold, 3rd ed. Baltimore, Williams & Wilkins.

30. Lehmann, J.F., DeLateur, B.J., and Silverman, D.R. (1966): Selective heating effects of ultrasound in human beings. Arch. Phys. Med. Rehabil., 66:331–339.

31. Lehmann, J.F., DeLateur, B.J., and Stonebridge, J.B. (1969): Selective muscle heating by shortwave diathermy with a helical coil. Arch. Phys. Med. Rehabil., 50:117–123.

32. Lehmann, J.F., DeLateur, B.J., Stonebridge, J.B., and Warren, C.G.(1967): Therapeutic temperature distribution produced by ultrasound as modified by dosage and volume of tissue exposed. Arch. Phys. Med. Rehabil., 48:662–666.

33. Lehmann, J.F., Masock, A.J., Warren, C.G., and Koblanski, J.N.(1970): Effect of temperature on tendon extensibility. Arch. Phys. Med. Rehabil., 51:481–487.

34. Licht, S. (1965): Therapeutic Heat and Cold, 2nd ed. Baltimore, Waverly Press.

35. Lowdon, B.J., and Moore, R.J. (1975): Determinants and nature of intramuscular temperature changes during cold therapy. Am. J. Phys. Med., 54:223–233.

36. Mayer, D.J., and Price D.D. (1989): Neurobiology of pain. *In:* Snyder-Mackler, L., and Robinson, A.J., (eds.): Clinical Electrophysiology. Baltimore, Williams & Wilkins, pp. 141–201.

37. McMaster, W.C., and Liddle, S. (1980): Cryotherapy influence on edema. Clin. Orthop. Rel. Res., 150:283–287.

38. McMaster, W.C., Liddle, S., and Waugh, T.R. (1978): Laboratory evaluation of various cold therapy modalities. Am. J. Sports Med., 6:291–294.

39. Michlovitz, S. (1986): Thermal Agents in Rehabilitation. Philadelphia, F.A. Davis.

40. Mohr, T., Carlson, B., Sulentic, C., and Landry, R. (1985): Comparison of isometric exercise and high volt galvanic stimulation on quadriceps femoris muscle strength. Phys. Ther., 65:606–612.

41. Nelson, R.M., and Currier, D.P. (1987): Clinical Electrotherapy. Los Altos, CA, Appleton and Lange.

42. Oakley, E.M. (1978): Dangers and contraindications of therapeutic ultrasound. Physiotherapy, 64:173–174.

43. Oliver, R.A., Johnson, D.J., Wheelhouse, W.W., and Griffin, P.P. (1979): Isometric muscle contraction response during recovery from reduced intramuscular temperature. Arch. Phys. Med. Rehabil., 60:126–129.

44. Prentice, W.E. (1986): Therapeutic Modalities in Sports Medicine. St. Louis, Times Mirror/Mosby.

45. Reed, B.V. (1988): Effect of high voltage pulsed electrical stimulation on microvascular permeability to plasma proteins. Phys. Ther., 68:491–495.

46. Robinson, A.J. (1989): Basic concepts and terminology in electricity and physiology of muscle and nerve. *In:* Snyder-Mackler, L., and Robinson, A.J., (eds.): Clinical Electrophysiology. Baltimore, Williams & Wilkins, pp. 3–19, 61–94.

47. Sculley, R.M., and Barnes, M.R. (1989): Physical Therapy. Philadelphia, J.B. Lippincott.

48. Snyder-Mackler, L. (1989): Electrical stimulation for pain modulation. *In:* Snyder-Mackler, L., and Robinson, A.J. (eds.): Clinical Electrophysiology. Baltimore, Williams & Wilkins, pp. 205–227.

49. Snyder-Mackler, L. (1989): Electrical stimulation for tissue repair. *In:* Snyder-Mackler, L., and Robinson, A. J. (eds.): Clinical Electrophysiology. Baltimore, Williams & Wilkins, pp. 231–244.

50. Tracey, J.E., Currier, D.P., and Threlkeld, A.J. (1988): Comparison of selected pulse frequencies from two different electrical stimulators on blood flow in healthy subjects. Phys. Ther., 68:1526–1532.

51. Warren, C.G., Koblanski, J.N., and Sigelmann, R.A. (1976): Ultrasound coupling media: Their relative transmissivity. Arch. Phys. Med. Rehabil., 57:218–222.

52. Warren, C.G., Lehmann, J.F., and Koblanski, J.N. (1976): Heat and stretch procedures: An evaluation using rat tail tendon. Arch. Phys. Med. Rehabil., 57:122–126.

53. Wessman, H.C., and Kottke, F.J. (1967): The effect of indirect heating on peripheral blood flow, pulse rate, blood pressure, and temperature. Arch. Phys. Med. Rehabil. 48:567–576.

54. Whitmore, J.J., Burt, M.M., Fowler, R.S., *et al.* (1972): Bandaging the lower extremity to control swelling: Figure-8 versus spiral technique. Arch. Phys. Med. Rehabil., 53:487–490.

55. Wright, V., and Johns, R.J. (1960): Physical factors concerned with the stiffness of normal and diseased joints. Bull. Johns Hopkins Hosp., 106:215–231.

56. Zankel, H.T. (1966). Effect of physical agents on motor conduction velocity of the ulnar nerve. Arch. Phys. Med. Rehabil., 47:787–792.

CHAPTER 6

◆

Range of Motion and Flexibility

Karen Middleton, A.T., C., P.T.

Range of motion is a joint's available amount of movement, whereas flexibility is the ability of soft tissue structures, such as muscle, tendon, and connective tissue, to elongate through the available range of joint motion. Whether undergoing therapeutic stretching during postinjury rehabilitation or in a routine flexibility program, connective tissue is the most important physical focus of range-of-motion exercises. Connective tissue involved in the body's reparative process after trauma or surgery often limits normal joint motion. Understanding the biophysical factors of connective tissue is important in determining optimal ways of increasing range of motion. Histologic evidence has shown that fibrosis can occur within 4 days of the onset of immobility.[22] Pathologic connective tissue conditions of scarring, adhesions, and fibrotic contractures must be addressed therapeutically.[11, 21] Similarly, when a normal relaxed muscle is physically stretched, most of the resistance to the stretch is a result of the muscle sheath and connective tissue framework.[22]

BIOPHYSICAL CONSIDERATIONS OF STRETCHING

Connective tissue is composed of collagen and other fibers within a ground substance, a protein polysaccharide compound (see Chap. 2). Connective tissue has viscoelastic properties, defined as two components of stretch, which allow elongation of the tissue.[4, 7, 12, 21, 22] The viscous component allows for a plastic stretch, which results in a permanent tissue elongation after the load is removed. Conversely, the elastic component allows for an elastic stretch, a temporary elongation, and the connective tissue returns to its previous length once the stress is removed. Range-of-motion exercise techniques should primarily be designed to produce plastic deformation.

The amount and duration of the applied force and the tissue

temperature when performing the stretch are the principal factors affecting how much elastic or plastic stretch occurs with connective tissue stretching. Elastic stretch is enhanced by high-force, short-duration stretching, whereas plastic stretch is favored by low-force, long-duration stretching. Numerous studies have noted the effectiveness of prolonged stretching at low to moderate tension levels.[1, 2, 4, 5, 11–13, 16, 21, 23, 24, 31, 32]

Research has shown that temperature has a significant influence on the mechanical behavior of connective tissue under tensile stretch.[3, 7, 15, 20, 21, 32, 33] Treatment procedures were evaluated for the residual length increase and the damage produced. It was concluded that higher therapeutic temperatures at low loads produce the greatest elongation with the least damage. Increased connective tissue temperature increases extensibility. The use of ultrasound prior to joint mobilization has proved effective in elevating deep tissue temperature and extensibility.[14] Greater plastic stretch results if the tissue is allowed to cool before releasing tension.[12] Examples of clinical application of these considerations include the following:

1. Muscular activity demands an increased blood flow to muscle, resulting in increased intramuscular temperature; therefore, stretching should not be performed at the beginning of a warm-up because tissue temperature is low. Cold muscles and tendons are less "stretchable" and thus more vulnerable to injury.

2. It is advantageous to stretch immediately after a rehabilitative exercise session and then to apply ice to the involved part while stretching is continued (e.g., "cryostretching" of the hamstrings).

Limited joint range of motion caused by soft tissue restriction often inhibits the initiation or completion of the rehabilitative process. Conservative treatment of contractures only meets with moderate success, and overly aggressive stretching may result in undesired adverse effects. In rehabilitative treatment of contractures there is often a fine line of "pushing hard enough, but not pushing too much." Optimal passive stretching is achieved only when voluntary and reflex muscle resistance is eliminated. Ballistic stretching is not a favorable method because as the muscles stretch rapidly the intrafusal muscle spindles may be activated and cause a reflex protective muscle contraction, which is a contradictory aim of increased muscle flexibility.[30] Forceful ballistic stretching can also result in microtrauma of muscle fibers.

Passive Stretching and Active-Assisted Techniques

Various passive and active-assisted techniques augment manual passive stretching. Methods of achieving the desired outcome are often limited only by an individual's creativity and improvisational skills. Once the soft tissue restriction has been assessed, the clinician should analyze appropriate and effective ways of carrying out the treatment and rehabilitation plan. Several methods of stretching can be used.

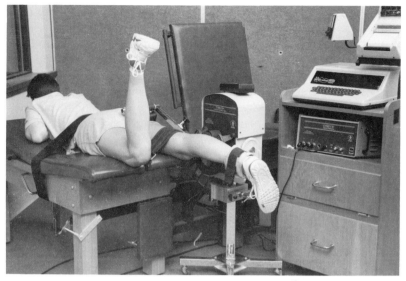

FIGURE 6–1 Prolonged stretching of knee in the prone position.

Spray and Stretch This technique has been described in detail by Travell and Simons.[28] Fluori-Methane* spraying of taut muscle fibers and desensitizing palpable myofascial trigger points facilitates stretching of the muscle to its full length. Passive stretch remains the central component.

Prolonged Weighted Stretch The rationale of a prolonged duration, low-load stretch has been discussed. Figure 6–1 illustrates a

_____

* Gebauer Chemical Co., Cleveland, OH.

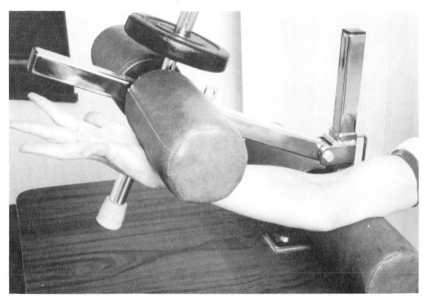

FIGURE 6–2 Weighted elbow stretch. (Courtesy of Sports Medicine Update, Birmingham, AL, Health South Rehabilitation Corporation.)

method of prolonged weighted stretching for the knee using the Cybex as a support and stabilizer. With the athlete in a prone position, a weight is attached to the ankle to aid in decreasing any extension limitations present. Figure 6–2 shows a weighted stretch of the forearm in the treatment of elbow ankylosis.

Assistive Devices   These aid in gaining and maintaining end range of motion. Assistive devices include pulleys, extremity traction,[15, 21] T bars or wands, and continuous passive range-of-motion units.[4] Pulleys are commonly used for those with joint restriction of the shoulder and knee (Figs. 6–3 and 6–4). Wands, T bars, sport sticks, or other similar sports apparatus may be used for individual assistive stretching of the upper extremity.

Continuous passive motion units are often a valuable mechanical device that can benefit various joints. They can provide constant movement of the joint(s) after surgical repair. A passive mode can be used on other equipment, such as the Biodex and Lido isokinetic units, to allow a controlled passive range of motion with a pause to provide a stretch at the end range of motion (Fig. 6–5).

Walk-Away Casts   These are effective in providing a progressive high-tension, prolonged stretch of ankylosed knees. A cylinder cast is applied to the athlete's knee from midthigh to ankle in as much passive extension as can be obtained. Foam pads are placed on the posterior

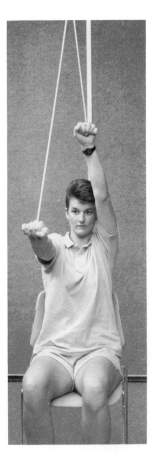

FIGURE 6–3   Active-assisted range of motion of the shoulder.

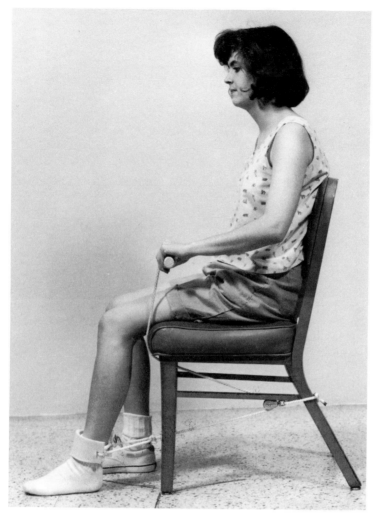

FIGURE 6–4 Active-assisted range of motion of the knee with the use of pulleys.

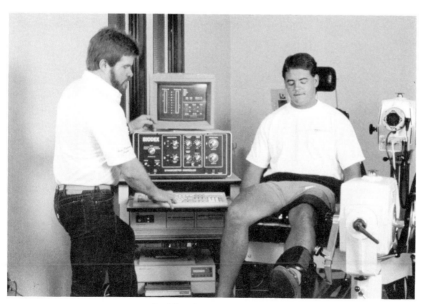

FIGURE 6–5 Isokinetic setup in a passive mode.

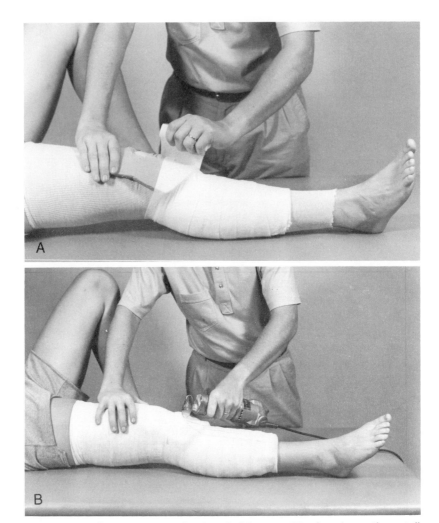

FIGURE 6–6   Walk-away cast application. *A,* A foam pad is placed over the patella to decrease pressure. *B,* A large front opening is cut from the infrapatellar area, parallel to the medial and lateral malleoli.

thigh, patella (with a doughnut hole cut to relieve patella pressure), and at the distal aspect of the calf. With frequent cast applications, one must note excessive pressure areas, which can result in skin breakdown and blisters. After cast drying, a large front opening is cut from the infrapatellar area, parallel to the medial and lateral malleoli; this part of the cast is removed. Subsequently, the posterior cast (calf area) is packed with padding and progressed as tolerated, allowing for increased pressure. This stretch is facilitated by active quadriceps contraction to gain increased knee extension as the athlete "walks away" from the cast (Figs. 6–6 and 6–7).

Dynasplints   These adjustable dynamic splints can produce low-intensity, prolonged duration force. They are composed of two stain-

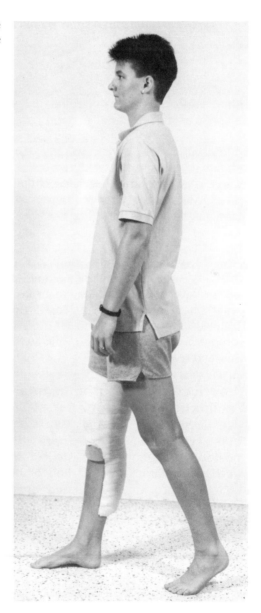

FIGURE 6–7   Dynamic use of the walk-away cast as the athlete "walks away" from the cast.

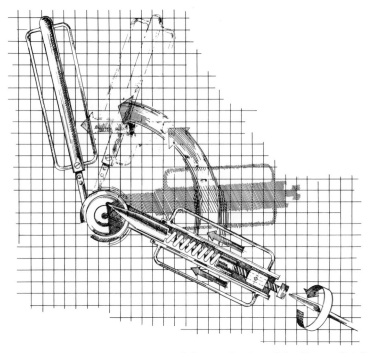

FIGURE 6–8   Schematic representation of the mechanics of the Dynasplint. The force can be gradually increased to offer prolonged and progressively higher loads to contracted tissues. (Courtesy of Dynasplint Systems, Baltimore, MD.)

less steel medial and lateral struts and a compression coil spring. Mechanically, the Dynasplint* has a three-point pressure system.[4, 5] This offers a lower progressive load that can be self-adjusted and graduated as orthotic tolerance time increases (Fig. 6–8). The Dynasplint is also relatively easy to apply and take off after the initial adjustment as compared to the higher-load walk-away cast, which should be cut off daily and reapplied (Fig. 6–9).

Proprioceptive Neuromuscular Facilitation Techniques

Proprioceptive neuromuscular facilitation (PNF) can be defined as a method of "promoting or hastening the response of neuromuscular mechanisms through stimulation of the proprioceptors."[10, 29] PNF stretching techniques are based on reduction of sensory activity through spinal relaxes to bring about relaxation of the muscle to be stretched. Sherrington's principle of reciprocal innervation demonstrates relaxation of the muscle being stretched (agonist) through voluntary concentric contraction of its opposite (antagonist).[9, 10, 19, 27] Research has been done specifically to determine effective techniques

---

* Dynasplint Systems, Baltimore, MD.

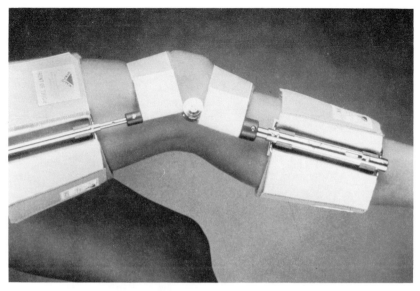

FIGURE 6–9   Knee Dynasplint. This is used for low-intensity, prolonged stretching of contracted tissues. (Courtesy of Dynasplint Systems, Baltimore, MD.)

for range-of-motion exercises. Several studies[19, 27, 30, 34] have found greater increases in flexibility when using the PNF technique as compared to static or dynamic stretching techniques.

Contract-Relax Technique   The contract-relax technique[10, 25, 26, 29] achieves increased range of motion in the agonist pattern by using consecutive isotonic contractions of the antagonists. The body part to be stretched is moved passively into the agonist pattern until range-of-motion limitation is felt. At this point, the athlete contracts isotonically into the antagonistic pattern against strong manual resistance. When the clinician realizes that relaxation has occurred, the body part is again moved passively into as much range of motion as possible until limitation is again felt. The procedure is repeated several times, followed by the athlete moving actively through the obtained range (Figs. 6–10 and 6–11).

Hold-Relax Technique   Hold/relax[10, 25, 26] is a PNF technique used to increase joint range of motion and is based on an isometric contraction of the shortened muscle performed against maximal resistance. This technique is performed in the same sequence as contract-relax, but, because no motion is allowed on isometric contraction, this is the method of choice when joint restriction is accompanied by muscle spasm and pain. The intensity of each contraction is gradually increased with each successive repetition.

Slow Reversal Hold-Relax Technique   The slow reversal hold-relax[10, 25, 29] technique uses reciprocal innervation, as does the hold-relax technique. The reciprocal innervation of the slow reversal hold-relax technique is repeated several times. The body part is moved into the agonistic pattern to the point of pain-free limitation and is then returned passively to the starting position several times before iso-

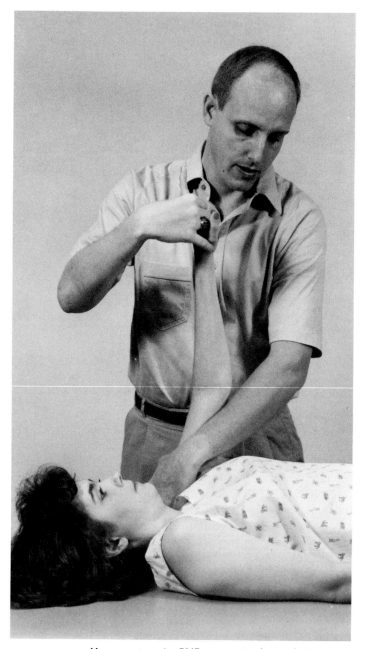

FIGURE 6–10   Upper extremity PNF contract-relax technique.

metric contraction is performed, relaxation obtained, and passive stretch achieved.

Joint Mobilization Techniques

Manual (hands-on) joint mobilization techniques are a form of passive range of motion. The proper use of mobilization helps facilitate healing, reduce disability, relieve pain, and restore full range of motion. When

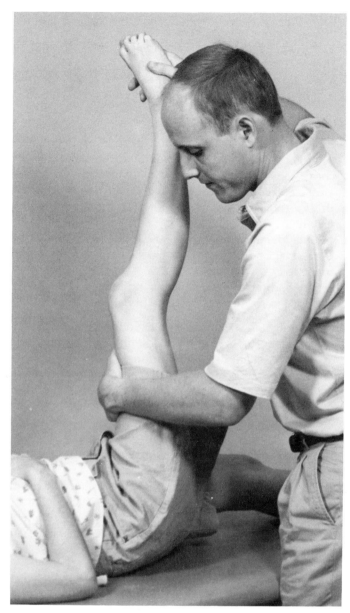

FIGURE 6–11   Lower extremity PNF.

restriction of a joint is assessed on passive movement, determination should be made as to whether restriction is in a capsular or noncapsular pattern. Capsular patterns or restrictions indicate loss of mobility of the entire joint capsule from fibrosis, effusion, or inflammation. Differentiation can be made by noting the "end-feel" at the extremes of movement. The following end-feels may be normal or pathologic:[7]

1. Capsular end-feel: firm feeling, as when forcing the shoulder into full external rotation; when felt in conjunction with a capsular pattern of restriction, indicates capsular fibrosis

2. Bony end-feel: abrupt feeling, as when moving the elbow into

full extension; when felt in conjunction with joint restriction, may indicate bony changes

3. Soft tissue approximation end-feel: as when flexing the normal knee or elbow
4. Muscular end-feel: "rubbery feel"; similar to that felt on tension of tight hamstrings when testing flexibility

Pathologic end-feels include the following:

1. Adhesions and scarring: sudden sharp arrest in one direction
2. Muscle spasm end-feel: "rebound end-feel"; usually accompanies pain felt at the end of restriction
3. Loose end-feel: ligamentous laxity, such as a hypermobile joint
4. Boggy end-feel: soft, mushy end-feel associated with joint effusion
5. Internal derangement end-feel: pronounced, springy end-feel; may result from a mechanical block, such as a loose body or torn meniscus
6. Empty end-feel: no resistance to motion felt, but movement has stopped because of complaints of pain

Manual stretching techniques are used in cases of capsular tightness; therefore, the goal is to apply an intermittent stretch to an aspect of the capsule. Mechanical effects include "stretching out" capsular restrictions and breaking adhesions, distracting impacted tissue, providing movement needed for normal cartilage, and maintaining lubrication and fiber distance for an orderly disposition of new collagen fibrils.[7] True contraindications of mobilization are hypermobility and inflammation; relative contraindications include conditions requiring special precautions, such as excessive pain, hypermobility in associated joints, unhealed fractures, bone disease, and malignancy.[8]

Systems of grading immobilization have been described by Maitland,[17] Kaltenborn,[6] and Wright and Johns.[35] Maitland has outlined four grades of oscillations, the first two used primarily for treating joints limited by pain and the last two used primarily as stretching maneuvers (Table 6–1). The neurophysiologic effects of providing oscillations include firing dynamic mechanoreceptors to decrease muscle tension and stimulation of fast-conducting fibers to block small pain-conducting fibers.[7] Kaltenborn has described three grades of joint play or oscillations, the first used for the relief of pain and the last grade of traction or glide used to stretch the joint capsule.[6] A gradual increase in the amplitude of movement progressed to a prolonged stretch with superimposed rhythmic oscillations is safe and effective and discourages pain and muscle spasm.

Fundamentals of mobilization include the following guidelines:[8]

1. Remove jewelry and rings.
2. The athlete and clinician should be relaxed.
3. Always examine the contralateral side.
4. Use a loose-packed joint position.
5. Provide stabilization.
6. Avoid causing pain, which leads to muscle spasm.
7. Apply smooth, regular movements.

TABLE 6–1   MAITLAND'S GRADES OF MOVEMENT

Grade	Description
I	Small-amplitude movement at the beginning of the accessory range
II	Large-amplitude movement within the available range but not to either limit
III	Large-amplitude movement beginning and extending up to the end of the accessory range
IV	Small-amplitude movement at the end of the accessory range
V	A manipulation (a high-velocity thrust)

Modified from Wallace, Lynn A., Mangine, Robert E., and Malone, Terry R.: The Knee. In Gould, James A., III, editor: Orthopaedic and Sports Physical Therapy, ed. 2, St. Louis, 1990, The C.V. Mosby Co., p. 340. Reproduced by permission.

The loose-packed position is the resting position in which the joint capsule and ligaments are most lax and the volume of intracapsular space is at its greatest. This is the optimal position for applying therapeutic distraction and mobilization.[6–8, 17, 18]

APPLICATION

Upper Extremity

Shoulder

Distraction with Oscillations; Progressive Anterior, Posterior, and Inferior Glides

POSITION   The athlete is supine, with the arm resting at the side.

PROCEDURE   The scapula may be stabilized with a small towel roll at the posterior aspect and the hand held at the inferior aspect of the glenoid.

MOVEMENT   The humerus is moved distally along its long axis for distraction, with small articulation movements performed. The head of the humerus can be mobilized in anterior, posterior, and inferior glides. As the athlete relaxes, the arm can be gradually moved toward abduction (Fig. 6–12).

Inferior Glide Moving Toward Flexion

POSITION   The athlete is supine, with the humerus flexed to 60 to 100° and the elbow flexed.

PROCEDURE   The proximal humerus is contacted with both hands and the clinician's fingers interlaced.

MOVEMENT   The clinician pulls inferiorly with the trunk to produce a movement of combined flexion of the humerus in an inferior glide. As the athlete relaxes, the arm is gradually moved toward greater ranges of flexion (Fig. 6–13).

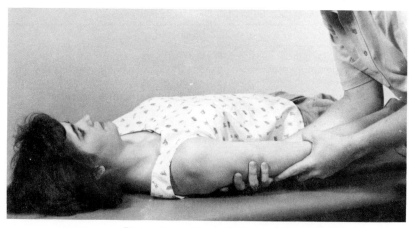

FIGURE 6–12 Distraction with oscillations of the shoulder.

Distraction and Glides of the Acromioclavicular Joint

POSITION   The athlete is in the seated position.

PROCEDURE   One of the clinician's hands stabilizes the clavicle or scapula at the acromion process.

MOVEMENT   The clavicle is either moved on the acromion process or the thumb of the hand is placed posteriorly on the clavicle and pushed anteriorly (Fig. 6–14).

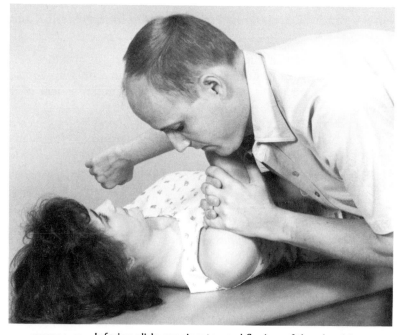

FIGURE 6–13   Inferior glide moving toward flexion of the shoulder.

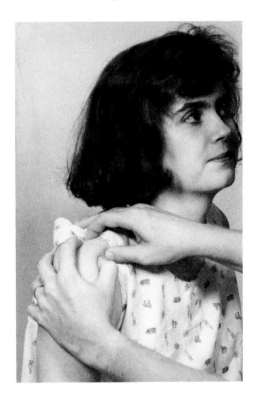

FIGURE 6–14 Distraction and glide of the acromioclavicular joint.

Elbow

Joint Distraction and Flexion

POSITION   The athlete is supine, with the arm by the side, elbow flexed, and forearm supinated.

PROCEDURE   Contact is made high on the proximal forearm.

MOVEMENT   The elbow is moved inferiorly, resulting in joint distraction. As the athlete relaxes, the elbow can be progressively flexed.

Joint Distraction Moving Toward Extension

POSITION   The athlete is supine, with the arm by the side, elbow bent, and forearm in neutral position.

PROCEDURE   The distal humerus is contacted.

MOVEMENT   Distraction results from a distal pull and slight supination. The elbow may be gradually extended as movement increases (Fig. 6–15).

Anterior and Posterior Glides of the Radioulnar Joint

POSITION   The athlete is supine, sitting, or standing.

PROCEDURE   The clinician uses one hand to hold the radius and the other one to hold the ulna.

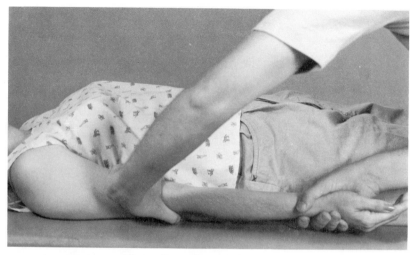

FIGURE 6–15   Elbow distraction moving toward extension.

MOVEMENT   The ulna is stabilized and the radius moved in anterior and posterior positions at the proximal, middle, and distal forearm (Fig. 6–16).

Wrist

Radiocarpal Joint Distraction

POSITION   The athlete is sitting.

PROCEDURE   The clinician places the hands at the radiocarpal joint.

MOVEMENT   The clinician pulls along the long axis of the extremity, moving the carpals distally (Fig. 6–17).

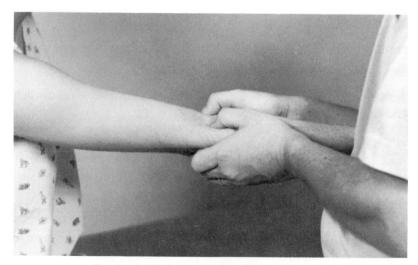

FIGURE 6–16   Proximal anterior-posterior glides of the radioulnar joint.

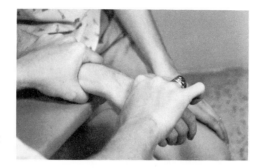

FIGURE 6–17   Radiocarpal joint distraction.

General Mobilization—Dorsal and Volar Glides

POSITION   The athlete's forearm is resting over the edge of the table and may be supported over a small towel roll.

PROCEDURE   The clinician uses one hand to stabilize the distal forearm and the other to grasp the radiocarpal joint.

MOVEMENT   The carpals are moved into dorsal and volar glides, perpendicular to the long axis of the extremity (Fig. 6–18).

Thumb and Fingers

Distraction of the Carpometacarpal Joint

POSITION   The athlete is sitting, with the forearm and hand in a resting position on the table.

PROCEDURE   The clinician uses one hand to stabilize the distal bone and the other to grasp the proximal bone.

MOVEMENT   The clinician applies long axis distraction to separate the joint surfaces. As the athlete relaxes, the ulnar, dorsal, and volar glides may be progressed.

Interphalangeal Joint Distraction of the Fingers

POSITION   The athlete is sitting, with the forearm and hand in a resting position on the table.

PROCEDURE   The proximal and distal bones are stabilized.

MOVEMENT   Long axis distraction is applied to separate the joint

FIGURE 6–18   Dorsal and volar glides of the radiocarpal joint.

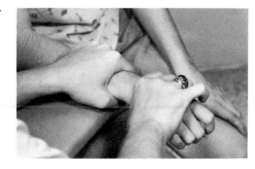

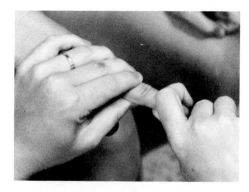

FIGURE 6–19 Distraction of the interphalangeal joint.

surfaces. As movement increases, oblique force may be applied by the clinician's thumb against the proximal end of the bone to be moved. A volar glide may be progressed to increase flexion, a dorsal glide to increase extension (Fig. 6–19).

Lower Extremity

Hip Joint

General Distraction

POSITION   The athlete is supine, with the hip in a resting position and the knee extended. Support may need to be provided with a belt for stabilization at the hip.

PROCEDURE   The clinician grasps the ankle proximally and the femur distally.

MOVEMENT   Long axis distraction is applied by pulling the leg and leaning backward with the trunk. As the athlete relaxes, this may be performed through various degrees of abduction (Fig. 6–20).

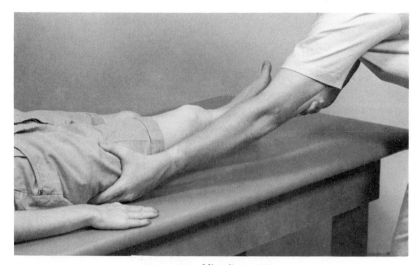

FIGURE 6–20   Hip distraction.

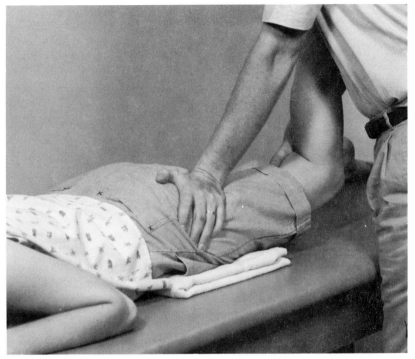

FIGURE 6-21   Anterior glide of the hip.

Anterior Glide to Increase Hip Extension and External Rotation

POSITION   The athlete is prone, with the knee bent to 90°.

PROCEDURE   Toweling may be placed under the anterior aspect of the pelvis while the clinician contacts the posterior aspect of the proximal femur with one hand and the other hand supports the knee.

MOVEMENT   Anterior glide is applied to the proximal femur. The support hand at the knee may glide the leg into increased extension (Fig. 6-21).

Knee

Patellofemoral Superior and Inferior Glides

POSITION   The athlete is supine, with the knee slightly flexed.

PROCEDURE   The patella is grasped between the thumb and fingers.

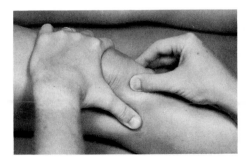

FIGURE 6-22   Superior glide of the patella.

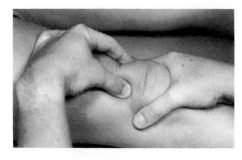

FIGURE 6–23 Inferior glide of the patella.

MOVEMENT   The patella is mobilized proximally and distally to increase patellar mobility (Figs. 6–22 and 6–23).

Patellar Medial and Lateral Glides

POSITION   The athlete is supine, with the knee slightly flexed.

PROCEDURE   The clinician grasps the patella with the thumbs and the fingers of both hands.

MOVEMENT   The patella is forced medially and laterally between the clinician's thumbs and fingers to increase patellar mobility (Figs. 6–24 and 6–25).

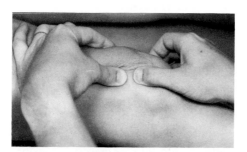

FIGURE 6–24 Medial glide of the patella.

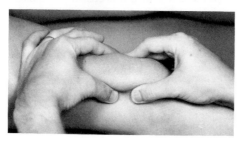

FIGURE 6–25 Lateral glide of the patella.

Anterior and Posterior Glides

POSITION   The athlete is supine, with the knee bent, and the foot resting on the table.

PROCEDURE   The procedure is the same as that for performing an anterior-posterior drawer test.

MOVEMENT   The proximal tibia is grasped and mobilized either anteriorly to encourage extension or posteriorly to increase flexion on the femur.

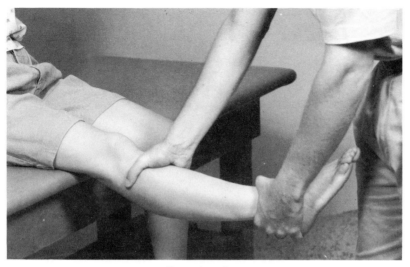

FIGURE 6-26   Posterior glide of the knee.

Posterior Glide in Alternate Position

POSITION   The athlete is seated, with the knee flexed over the edge of the table in a resting position.

PROCEDURE   The clinician stands on the medial side of the athlete's leg, holding the distal leg with one hand and placing the palm of the other hand on the proximal aspect of the tibia.

MOVEMENT   Extending the clinician's elbow and providing a body weight force into the tibia results in gliding of the tibia posteriorly (Fig. 6-26).

Ankle

General Joint Distraction

POSITION   The athlete is supine with the ankle in a resting position (range between plantar flexion and dorsiflexion).

PROCEDURE   The fingers of both of the clinician's hands are placed over the dorsum of the athlete's foot.

MOVEMENT   The clinician applies a distal force along the long axis of the leg distally.

Subtalar Distraction with Posterior-Medial-Lateral Glides

POSITION   The athlete is supine with the leg supported and the heel over the edge of the support.

PROCEDURE   The clinician's hand grasps the forefoot or calcaneus from the posterior aspect of the foot and the other hand stabilizes the tibia.

MOVEMENT   A posterior glide can be provided to increase dorsiflexion by mobilizing the talus posteriorly with respect to the tibia. Medial glides can be progressed to increase extension or lateral glides to increase inversion by providing force with the fingers on the lateral side

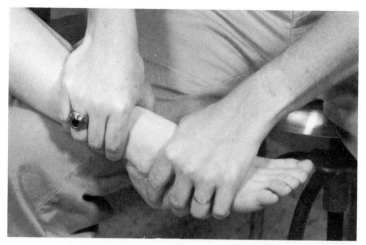

FIGURE 6-27   Subtalar distraction with posterior, medial, and lateral glides.

of the foot in a medial direction, or with the thumbs on the medial side in a lateral direction. (Fig. 6–27).

Subtalar Anterior Glide

POSITION   The athlete is prone, with the foot over the edge of table.

PROCEDURE   The clinician places one hand around the distal tibia for stabilization while the web space of the other hand is placed on the posterior aspect of the talus and calcaneus.

MOVEMENT   The calcaneus is distracted and forced in the anterior direction, providing an anterior glide of the talus (Fig. 6–28).

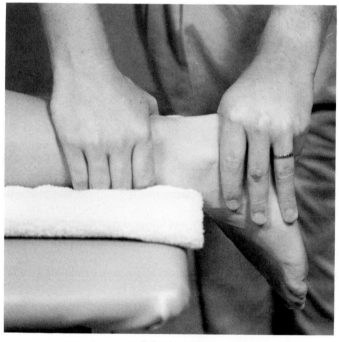

FIGURE 6-28   Subtalar anterior glide.

References

1. Becker, A.H. (1979): Traction for knee flexion contractures. Phys. Ther., 59:114.
2. Bohannon, R.W., Chavis, D., Larkin, P., et al. (1985): Effectiveness of repeated prolonged loading for increasing flexion in knees demonstrating post-operative stiffness: A clinical report. Phys. Ther., 65:494–496.
3. Henricson, A.S., Fredrikisson, K., Persson, I., et al. (1984): The effect of heat and stretching on the range of hip motion. J. Orthop. Sports Phys. Ther., 6:110–115.
4. Hepburn, G.R. (1987): Case studies: Contracture and stiff joint management with Dynasplint. J. Orthop. Sports Phys. Ther., 8:498–504.
5. Hepburn, G.R., and Crivelli, K.J. (1984): Use of elbow Dynasplint for reduction of elbow flexion contractures: A case study. J. Orthop. Sports Phys. Ther., 5:269–274.
6. Kaltenborn, F.M. (1980): Mobilization of the Extremity Joints, Examination and Basic Treatment Techniques. Oslo, Olaf Norlis Bokhand.
7. Kessler, R.N., and Hertling, D. (1983): Management of Common Musculoskeletal Disorders. Philadelphia, Harper & Row.
8. Kisner, C., and Colby, L.A. (1985): Therapeutic Exercises, Foundations and Techniques. Philadelphia, F.A. Davis.
9. Knortz, K., and Rongel., C. (1985): Flexibility techniques. Natl. Strength Conditioning Assoc. J., 7:50–54.
10. Knott, M., and Voss, D.E. (1968): Proprioceptive Neuromuscular Facilitation, 2nd ed. New York, Harper & Row.
11. Kottke, F.J. (1982): Therapeutic exercise to maintain mobility. In: Kottke, F.J., Stillwell, G.K., and Lehmann, J.E. (eds.): Krusen's Handbook of Physical Medicine and Rehabilitation, 3rd ed. Philadelphia, W.B. Saunders, pp. 389–402.
12. Kottke, F.J., Pauley, D.L., and Ptak, K.A. (1966): The rationale for prolonged stretching for correction of shortening of connective tissue. Arch. Phys. Med. Rehabil., 47:345–352.
13. LaBan, N.M. (1962): Collagen tissue: Implications of its response to stress in vitro. Arch. Phys. Med. Rehabil., 43:461–466.
14. Lehmann, J.F., DeLateur, B.J., and Silverman, D.R. (1966): Selective heating effects of ultrasound in human beings. Arch. Phys. Med. Rehabil., 47:331–339.
15. Lehmann, J.F., Masock, A.J., Warren, C.G., and Koblanski, J.N. (1970): Effect of therapeutic temperatures on tendon extensibility. Arch. Phys. Med. Rehabil., 51:481–487.
16. Light, K.E., Nuzik, S., Personius, W., and Barstrom, A. (1984): Low load prolonged stretch versus high load restretch treating knee contractures. Phys. Ther., 64:330–333.
17. Maitland, G.D. (1977): Peripheral Manipulation, 2nd ed. Boston, Butterworth.
18. Mennell, J. (1964): Joint Pain. Boston, Little, Brown & Company.
19. Moore, M.A., and Hutton, R.S. (1980): Electromyographic investigation of muscle stretching technique. Med. Sci. Sports Exerc., 12:322–329.
20. Prentice, W.E., Jr. (1982): An electromyographic analysis of the effectiveness of heat, cold and stretching for inducing relaxation in injured muscle. J. Orthop. Sports Phys. Ther., 3:133–140.
21. Sapega, A.A., Quedenfeld, T.C., Moyer, R.A., and Butler, R.A. (1981): Biophysical factors in range of motion exercise. Physician Sportsmed., 9:57–64.
22. Stap, L.J., and Wodfin, P.M. (1986): Continuous passive motion in the treatment of knee flexion contracture. Phys. Ther., 66:1720–1722.
23. Starring, D.T., Grossman, M.R., Nicholson, G.G., and Lemons, J. (1988): Comparison of cyclic and sustained passive stretching using a mechanism device to increase resting length of hamstring muscles. Phys. Ther., 68:314–320.
24. Stromberg, D., and Wiederhielm, C.A. (1969): Viscoelastic description of a collagenous tissue in simple elongation. J. Appl. Physiol., 26:857–862.
25. Sullivan, P.E., Markos, P.D., and Minor, M.A. (1982): An Integrated Approach to Therapeutic Exercise. Reston, VA, Reston Publishing.
26. Sullivan, P.E., and Markos, P.D. (1987): Clinical Procedures in Therapeutic Exercise. Norwalk, CT, Appleton & Lange.
27. Tanijawa, M.D. (1972): Comparison of the whole-relaxed procedure in passive immobilization on increasing muscle length. Phys. Ther., 52:725–735.
28. Travell, J.G., and Simons, D.G. (1983): Myofascial pain and dysfunction. The Trigger Point Manual. Baltimore, Williams & Wilkins.

29. Voss, D.E., Ionta, M.K., and Myers, B.J. (1985): Proprioceptive Neuromuscular Facilitation: Patterns and Techniques, 3rd ed. Philadelphia, Harper & Row.
30. Wallin, D., Ekblon, B., Grahn, R., and Nordenborg, T. (1985): Improvement of muscle flexibility. Am. J. Sports Med., 13:263–268.
31. Warren, C.G., Lehmann, J.F., and Koblanski, J.N. (1971): Elongation of rat tail tendon: Effect of load and temperature. Arch. Phys. Med. Rehabil., 52:465–474.
32. Warren, C.G., Lehmann, J.F., and Koblanski, J.N. (1976): Heat and stress procedures: An evaluation using rat tail tendon. Arch. Phys. Med. Rehabil., 57:122–126.
33. Wiktorsson-Moller, M., Oberg, B., Ekstrand, J., and Gillquist, J. (1988): Effects of warming up, massage, and stretching and range of motion for muscle strength in the lower extremity. Am. J. Sports Med., 11:249–252.
34. Williford, H.N., and Smith, J.F. (1985): A comparison of proprioceptive neuromuscular facilitation and static stretching techniques. Am. Correct. Ther. J., 39:30–33.
35. Wright, V., and Johns, R.J. (1962): Relative importance of various tissues in joint stiffness. J. Appl. Physiol., 17:824–828.

CHAPTER 7

◆

Introduction to Rehabilitation

Gary L. Harrelson, M.S., A.T., C.

Rehabilitation, or reconditioning, is a dynamic program of prescribed exercise for preventing or reversing the deleterious effects of inactivity while returning individuals to their former level of competition.[33] Athletic rehabilitation combines exercise and therapeutic modalities to restore athletes to their supernormal level of activity. It is unlike conventional rehabilitation, in which complete return of function may not be possible, and the ultimate goal of treatment is below the patient's level of prior activity. Athletic rehabilitation not only includes complete restoration of unrestricted performance, but strives for a level of conditioning above that which the athlete had prior to injury. It must take into account muscular strength, power, flexibility, and endurance, as well as balance, proprioception, timing, and cardiovascular performance.[33] Each rehabilitation program must be individualized to meet the special needs of each athlete.

Athletic rehabilitation primarily encompasses the restoration of traumatized musculoskeletal structures. Rarely is an injury so mild that some form of rehabilitation is not necessary, and, as a rule, the more serious an injury, the more prolonged and necessary the rehabilitation.[1] The effectiveness of rehabilitation in the recovery period, either postinjury or postsurgical, usually determines the degree and success of future athletic competition.[1] Hughston[24] has stated that rehabilitation accounts for 50% of a successful result following injury or surgery. Moreover, injuries sustained during athletic participation are usually produced by circumstances inherent to the respective athletic performance; therefore, the athlete can be exposed to recurrent identical trauma, making reinjury likely.[30] Figure 7–1 illustrates the body's response to injury and the result of inadequate rehabilitation.

In any injury sequence, specific physiologic effects occur in response to trauma (see Chap. 2). It is the clinician's role to reduce the severity of these physiologic effects, speed up healing time, and return the athlete to competition as soon as possible without compromising

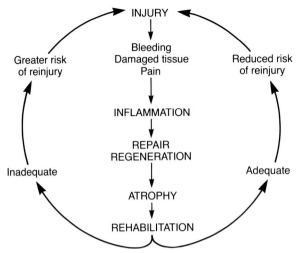

FIGURE 7–1   The body's response to injury and the role of rehabilitation. (From Welch, B. (1986): The injury cycle. Sports Med. Update, 1:1.)

the athlete's well-being. The goals of any rehabilitation program, in conjunction with the use of specific modalities, include the following:

1. Decrease pain
2. Decrease inflammatory response to trauma
3. Return full, pain-free, active range of motion
4. Decrease effusion
5. Return full muscular strength, power, and endurance
6. Regain full asymptomatic functional activities at the preinjury level

Swelling, pain, and spasm can inhibit early institution of a rehabilitation program. The use of various modalities (e.g., cryotherapy, thermotherapy, electrical stimulation) can help control and reduce effusion, pain, spasm, and inflammation, allowing the athlete to begin early range-of-motion and strengthening exercises. The modality itself, however, is never considered the *cure* for most athletic injuries. Only through therapeutic exercise can the injured body part(s) be returned to the preinjury level. If a rehabilitation program is not instituted in conjunction with modalities, the injury cycle is likely to continue as a result of reinjury to the same body part that was susceptible because of the initial injury.

Early exercise is essential to rehabilitation. Athletes can improve their physical condition daily about 1%, whereas they lose from 3 to 7% daily if totally inactive; therefore, the longer an athlete is inactive, the longer it takes to complete the rehabilitation program.[9, 23] The proper use of exercise can expedite the healing process, and the lack of exercise during the early stages of rehabilitation may result in permanent disability. Caution must be observed, however, because exercise that is too vigorous can also result in permanent disability. Some limitations may be required to protect a surgical repair or allow an injury to heal properly. Thus, excessive stress to the traumatized area may not allow for reapproximation of tissues and can result in additional injury or disfigurement. Optimal conditions for healing depend on a fine balance between protection from stress and return toward normal function at the earliest possible time.

Each rehabilitation program must be individualized—there is no "cookbook" rehabilitation program for every injury that can be used for every athlete. Procedures should be shaped to meet the athlete's needs, rather than the athlete fitted into a treatment procedure.[29] Athletes must be treated individually and instructed in their own personal rehabilitation program, with concentration on each athlete's deficiencies.

The general goals of rehabilitation have already been mentioned. Before the rehabilitation program begins, the clinician and athlete should develop a set of short- and long-term goals based on the athlete's injury and/or surgical procedure. The use of pre-established rehabilitation protocols as guidelines for advancement of the athlete through the rehabilitation program can be valuable. Protocols should be based firmly on principles derived from research on healing time and joint kinematics. Goals can be outlined in relationship to range of motion, weight-bearing, and progressive resistance exercise (PRE) weight progression. Rehabilitation protocols are only guidelines, however, and individuals tolerate pain differently and heal at varying rates. The athlete's rehabilitation advancement should be based on the clinician's daily assessment of subjective reports and objective findings. Advancement from one rehabilitation phase to another should not occur until the athlete has achieved the goals outlined in the current phase.

REHABILITATION CONCEPTS

Healing Constraints

The most important factor to consider in designing a rehabilitation program is the consideration of physiologic healing restraints. Wounds in muscle and skin tissue are usually closed securely within 5 to 8 days. Tendons and ligaments may take 3 to 5 weeks to achieve sufficient strength to allow movement without damage to the scar tissue.[11] The rate of healing in bone is highly variable, more than that of other body tissues. The healing time in bone may be estimated by considering the patient's age, site and type of injury, and blood supply to the area.

Physiologic healing is affected by the age, health, and nutritional status of the athlete, as well as by the magnitude of the pathology. The structured rehabilitation program must be based on consideration of the physiologic healing restraints. For example, in postoperative rehabilitation of an athlete with an ulnar collateral ligament repair, the primary consideration is protection of the surgical repair during the healing process. A brace that provides protective (limited) motion and support accomplishes this goal. Therapeutic exercise and modalities may be used concurrently, as appropriate, always recognizing the primary concern of protecting the surgical repair.

Management of Pain and Swelling

Pain and swelling are major factors in the initiation of a therapeutic exercise program and are usually the first signs of injury. Pain varies according to the nature of the injury and the athlete's individual pain tolerance threshold. In treating pain, it is first necessary to classify pain as acute or chronic. Pain is a symptom that helps in evaluating an injury and in determining the course of treatment. Acute pain is typically short-term and is associated with an injury or surgery. It is often a protective response by the body, warning that something is wrong and inducing a cycle of muscle spasm and protective guarding. Chronic pain is present for a long period, frequently recurs, and often serves no purpose. It may exist long after the original injury has healed as a result of such factors as altered biomechanics or learned habits of guarding. In the person with chronic pain, the pain may actually become a dysfunction in itself.[32]

It is important to know the underlying cause of pain (e.g., acute trauma, inflammation) because this has a direct bearing on the approach to pain management. Numerous therapeutic modalities can be used to control or manage pain. It is necessary for the clinician to understand the principles and applications of specific therapeutic choice(s) for pain management (see Chap. 5).

The control of existing swelling and prevention of further effusion are critical in the rehabilitation process. Swelling can compress sensory nerve endings and contribute to pain. In the acute injury state, ice, compression, and elevation should be used. Ice promotes local vasoconstriction, helping to control hemorrhage and edema. Application of external pressure to the injury site helps control the amount of swelling. Compression wraps should be applied in a distal to proximal direction, with a decreasing pressure gradient. Tubi-Grip* or a stockinette is excellent for compression and can be applied and removed easily by the athlete. Elevation assists the lymphatic system in moving any extracellular tissue fluid away from the injury site.

Various modalities may be used in the management of swelling. The use of intermittent compression units such as the CryoTemp† in conjunction with elevation aids greatly in edema reduction. Electric muscle stimulation (EMS) can be used to create a muscle-pumping effect, facilitating removal of excess fluid. This can be further enhanced by voluntary isometric muscle contractions, as tolerated. Once the acute stage has subsided, contrast therapy may be implemented to create a pumping action within the capillary system. The pumping action created by alternating treatments of thermotherapy and cryotherapy helps facilitate excess fluid removal. Also, centripetal massage in conjunction with extremity elevation assists the lymphatic system in dissipating swelling.

Therapeutic exercise itself helps diminish swelling, which is an advantage of early motion. Pain and swelling can often cause transitory

---

* Available from Sepro, Montgomeryville, PA.
† Available from Jobst, Toledo, OH.

paralysis of a body part. For example, in the knee, swelling can result in "quad shutdown" (inability to tighten the quadriceps muscle independently) through neural inhibition.[16] Along with the use of EMS for muscle re-education, as the pain and effusion decrease, the athlete's ability to recruit and control the quadriceps muscle improves.

Circumferential measurements taken on a regular basis, using anatomic landmarks as reference points, provide objective data regarding the effectiveness of treatments to manage swelling. Once swelling has been controlled, the athlete may continue to use ice and compression postrehabilitation as a prophylactic measure to prevent further swelling and inflammation.

Assessment

Whether the athlete is postinjury or postsurgery, the body part must be evaluated as to its current ability and limitations. For postsurgical patients, the clinician must stay within the physician's guidelines for limitations. Parameters such as effusion, circumference, strength (if possible), and range of motion should be measured and documented to determine progress. Short- and long-term goals should be stated and noted in the athlete's progress chart as they are achieved.

Types of Exercises

As defined earlier, therapeutic exercise involves bodily movements prescribed to restore or favorably alter specific functions in an individual following injury. Exercise movements may be active or passive. Active exercise is purposeful voluntary motion that is performed by the injured athlete, with or without resistance and with or without the aid of gravity. Active exercise may be assistive, where the clinician helps the athlete perform the movement, or resistive, which can be static or dynamic. Static training refers to contraction against a fixed resistance. Dynamic refers to moving the resistance through a range of motion. Two types of muscle contractions exist with dynamic training: (1) concentric, which is a shortening of muscle fibers that results in a decrease of the joint angle where the muscle inserts, also known as positive work; and (2) eccentric, which occurs when the muscle resists its own lengthening so that the joint angle increases during the contraction, also known as negative work.[33] During maximal effort twice as much force is generated eccentrically than concentrically; therefore, concentric exercise may begin earlier than eccentric exercise.

Static exercise (isometrics) is performed without restricting movement or changing the joint angle (Fig. 7–2). The muscle being used maintains a fixed length, with the tension generated equal to the resistance encountered. Isometric contractions are exertional where the velocity is zero.[33] It is the least effective method of building strength. Isometric contractions can increase the circumference and strength of the muscles exercised, but the strength increase is related to the joint angle at which the isometric contraction is achieved. In the early phases

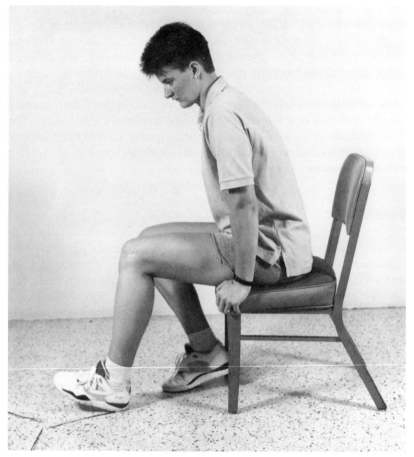

FIGURE 7–2 Isometric cocontractions of the quadriceps and hamstrings. This is an example of an isometric exercise in which the velocity is zero and the muscle maintains a fixed length.

of rehabilitation this may be the only type of exercise permitted and is preferable to no exercise at all.

Dynamic exercise can be of several types: (1) isotonic, in which the fixed weight is moved through a range of motion (e.g., ankle weights); (2) variable resistance, in which resistance varies in a fixed ratio through a full range of motion (e.g., Nautilus* and Eagle* equipment); and (3) isokinetic—accommodating variable resistance in which the speed of motion is fixed and the resistance varies to accommodate the force input (e.g., Cybex* and Biodex† equipment and manual resistance).

Isotonic exercise causes actual muscle length to change, causing or resisting a change in joint angle. In pure isotonic exercise, resistance remains constant while velocity is inversely proportional to the load. This type of exercise is readily available in the form of ankle weights, free weights, and weight machines (Fig. 7–3). Additionally, both eccentric and concentric contractions can be achieved. Some inherent disadvan-

---

* Nautilus available from Nautilus, DeLand, FL, and Eagle available from Cybex, Ronkonkoma, NY.

† Available from Biodex, Shirley, NY.

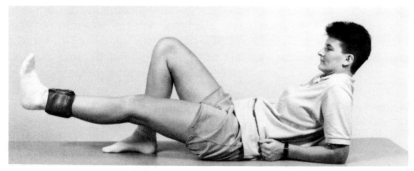

FIGURE 7–3 Traditional straight leg raises. This is an example of an isotonic exercise in which the resistance remains constant and the velocity is inversely proportional to the load.

tages, however, include the following: (1) the weight is fixed and does not adjust to strength differences in various ranges of motion; and (2) with speed work, the weight is propelled so that the strength required diminishes in the extremes of motion.[40]

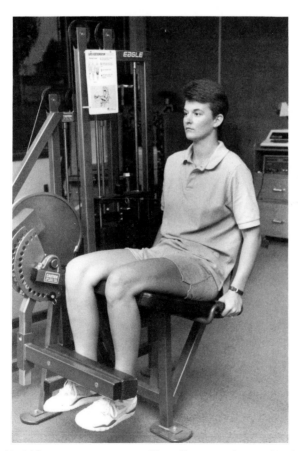

FIGURE 7–4 Variable resistance exercise. This offers an isokinetic-like feel through a cam but, because the angular velocity is not controlled, it cannot provide isokinetic resistance.

In variable resistance exercise, the resistance varies through the range of motion to match the difference in strength through this range.[40] With these types of machines the axis of rotation of the weight generates an isokinetic-like feel to the motion, but because angular velocity is not controlled, this equipment cannot provide isokinetic resistance (Fig. 7–4).

Isokinetic exercise or accommodating variable resistance is performed at a set speed, with resistance matching the input of force at that speed.[40] As the input changes, the resistance changes to match the input, but the speed remains constant.[40] The application of one's own muscular resistance is met with a proportional amount of resistance through full agonist (muscle that causes the joint motion) and then antagonist (opposing muscle group—works in cooperation with the agonist, but has the opposite motion) range of motion (Fig. 7–5).

Manual progressive resistance exercise is a variation of accommodating variable resistance.[40] The clinician provides the resistance with this mode of exercise and can modify the resistance and speed during the exercise as the athlete's fatigue is recognized. This exercise mode is applicable during early rehabilitation phases and can produce patterns that cannot be duplicated on machines, not unlike proprioceptive neuromuscular facilitation (PNF) techniques.

Passive exercises are performed for the injured athlete by the clinician or by a mechanical appliance (e.g., a continuous passive motion (CPM) machine; also, some isokinetic units provide a passive mo-

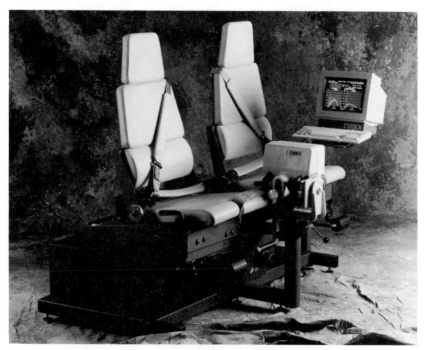

FIGURE 7–5   The Cybex 350 Extremity System is an example of an accommodating variable resistance piece of equipment. The resistance changes to match the input, but the speed remains constant. (Photo Courtesy of Cybex, a division of Lumex, Inc. Photographer, Darrell Peterson.)

TABLE 7–1   **COMPARISON OF STRENGTH EXERCISES**

Parameter	Type of Exercise			
	ISOMETRIC	ISOTONIC	ISOKINETIC	VARIABLE RESISTANCE
Resistance	Accommodating at one angle	Constant	Accommodating through range of motion	Fixed ratio through range of motion
Velocity (speed)	Zero	Variable	Constant	Variable
Reciprocal contraction	None	None	Yes	None
Eccentric contraction	None	Yes	None	Yes
Safeness	Excellent	Poor	Excellent	Poor
Specificity to sport	Low	Medium	Very high	Medium
Motivation	Low	High	Medium	High

Modified from Arnheim, D.J. (1989): Modern Principles of Athletic Training. St. Louis, C. V. Mosby, p. 86.

tion setting). Passive exercise is carried out by the application of some external force, with minimal participation of muscle action by the injured athlete. It may be forced or nonforced. Nonforced exercises are those used to help maintain normal joint motion, which are usually kept within a painless range of motion. Conversely, forced passive exercises generally produce movement beyond the limits of free range of motion and are associated with some discomfort to the individual.

Finally, plyometrics, which are drills or exercises aimed at linking strength and speed of movement to produce an explosive-reactive type of movement, can be employed.[43] Plyometrics was initially used in off-season strength training programs, and only recently has it become part of therapeutic rehabilitation. Plyometrics is based on maximizing the myotactic or stretch reflex—by means of an eccentric contraction, the muscle is fully stretched immediately preceding the concentric contraction.[2] The greater the stretch placed on the muscle from its resting length immediately before the concentric contraction, the greater the load the muscle can lift or overcome.

Plyometrics was originally used to describe box jumps or depth jumps, but its use has evolved to include hops and bounds that can be used to increase the athlete's speed, power, and skill of movement. Plyometrics can be implemented in the late stages of rehabilitation and can mimic a sports-specific skill. Plyometrics should be used judiciously, however, because it can cause overuse injuries. Two to three times weekly in conjunction with functional activities is a reasonable schedule. Absolute contraindications for plyometrics include acute surgical cases, gross instability, pain, and athletes not previously in a weight program. Although traditionally considered a lower extremity exercise, upper extremity plyometrics can be instituted with the use of a medicine ball or surgical tubing (Figs. 7–6 and 7–7).

Kinematic Chain

The term "kinematic" chain was introduced by Reuleaux[37] in 1875 to refer to a mechanical system of links in engineering. The term was

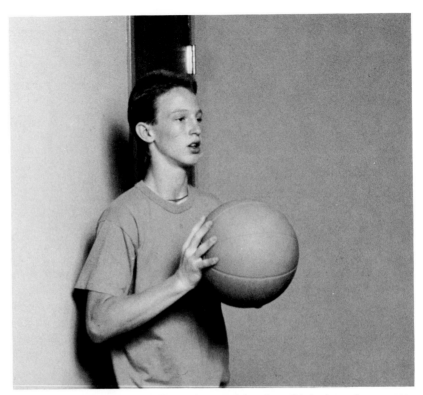

FIGURE 7–6 The medicine ball can be used by the athlete in various upper extremity plyometric exercises, such as the chest pass demonstrated here. The athlete catches the ball out in front of the body and decelerates the force of the ball before it hits the chest, initiating the stretch reflex. The athlete then explodes forward with the arms to pass the ball back.

FIGURE 7–7 Use of surgical tubing for plyometrics. By placing the connective tissue on stretch the athlete moves the extremity as fast as possible through the range of motion.

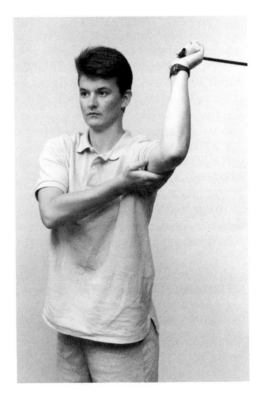

subsequently applied to biomechanics.[7] In engineering, a kinematic chain is usually a closed system of links joined together so that if any one is moved on a fixed link, all the other links move in a predictable pattern.[20, 34] In 1955, Dempster,[12] a kinesiologist, was the first to apply this concept to those problems involving kinetic and kinematic movements of the human body.[20] The kinematic chain in the human body is a combination of successively arranged joints that constitutes a complex motor unit.[7, 41] The kinetic chain concept allows the action of the total lower or upper extremity to be viewed in a functional relationship.[19]

The human kinematic chain can be an open or closed system. An open kinematic chain is characterized by the distal segment terminating freely in space. For example, waving of the hand is an open kinetic chain in which the shoulder, elbow, and wrist joints are successively involved. In a closed kinematic chain the distal segment of the joint is fixed and meets with considerable external resistance, which prohibits or restrains its free motion. Eventually the external resistance may be overcome and the peripheral portion of the joint may move against this resistance—for example, pushing a cart or lifting a load.[41] The closed link system is common to machines, whereas an open link system is more common in the human body.[7, 31]

The closed kinematic chain is exemplified by the erect weight-bearing, standing position. With few exceptions, however, the system of skeletal links in the human body is generally not composed of closed chains but of open ones, because the peripheral extremity ends can move freely.[20, 34] The lower extremity is considered an open kinetic chain when the foot is off the ground and is considered a closed kinetic chain when the foot is in contact with a supporting surface.[19] The significant difference between open and closed systems is that a closed kinetic chain is an encapsulated system that prohibits the function of one portion of the system (e.g., the foot) to the exclusion of the remaining parts (e.g., the knee and hip).[19] Forces, if abnormal, cannot be dispersed but must be absorbed into other tissues in the closed kinetic chain.

The spatial relationships among the foot, ankle, knee, thigh, and hip in the overall recovery of the athlete are often overlooked when developing a rehabilitation program. During the rehabilitation process, not only should the traumatized area be addressed, but also the joint(s) and/or areas proximal and distal to the traumatized region must be considered. For example, during the throwing mechanism of a baseball pitcher, the trunk, shoulder, elbow, and wrist in the upper extremity work as a kinematic chain to throw the baseball (the lower extremity is also involved).

Athletic activities are composed of two types of skills: (1) closed skills, in which the environment is predictable and the performer is free to execute a skill without having to make quick decisions (e.g., archery and bowling); and (2) open skills, in which the environment is constantly and perhaps unpredictably changing, so that the performer cannot effectively plan a response (e.g., football player returning a punt, tennis player responding to a serve). Both types of skills are encountered in athletic activities, but open skills require a greater dynamic reaction that requires feedback through the full kinetic chain to make an unplanned

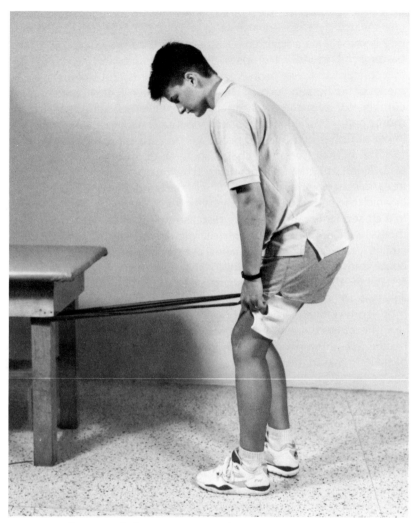

FIGURE 7–8 The use of Thera-Band to perform a closed chain terminal knee extension is excellent, particularly in patellofemoral problems, because the shear forces across the patellofemoral joint are lower when compared with those of the traditional open chain terminal knee extension.

response. Thus, the initial implementation of functional activities in a controlled setting, with gradual return to sports-specific skills at one-half, three-fourths, and then full speed to redevelop the spatial relationships in the kinematic chain, is paramount. Many rehabilitation specialists advocate closed kinetic chain exercises, because this type of program stresses functional progression without exerting potentially dangerous, open chain, high-torque–producing activities with forced coupling mechanisms.[8] Because the shear forces with closed chain exercises are reduced, these exercises are generally safer for the athlete to perform (Fig. 7–8). They can also be performed at varying rates of speed and adjusted to mimic the athlete's skill patterns.

Progressive Resistance Exercise

Before beginning active resistance exercises, the athlete's range of motion must be assessed. Range of motion can be limited by pain swelling, spasm, shortening of soft tissues, or a mechanical block. Many athletes develop loose bodies, bone spurs (osteophytes), or shortening of connective tissue, which results in a partial loss of their range of motion but may not be a hindrance early in the condition's onset. Most mechanical blocks eventually cause pain and have to be surgically corrected.

If active range of motion (AROM) is within normal limits (WNL) when compared bilaterally, the athlete may begin active resistive exercise. If full AROM is not WNL, however, active assistive range of motion (AAROM) or passive range of motion (PROM) is indicated to help regain full, pain-free AROM. The clinician must be careful with the use of PROM because of the possibility of further injury or damage to a surgical repair or healing process.

It is not a prerequisite that full, pain-free AROM be attained before beginning active resistive exercise. The athlete may begin isometric, manual resistance or active resistive exercise in a limited range of motion as long as the healing process is not jeopardized. Initiation of manual resistance and progressive resistance exercise (PRE) is determined by the extent and nature of the injury. Athletes with chronic conditions may begin PRE on the first day of rehabilitation, whereas those with acute injuries may require several weeks or longer before beginning PRE because of pain, effusion, and biologic healing. The athlete may not be able to tolerate active movement or weight in the early stages after injury or surgery.

Progressive resistance exercise is used to increase muscular strength and endurance in an orderly and progressive manner. This method permits an overload to be applied to the musculature and allows for the adaptation of bones, ligaments, tendons, and muscles so that the imposed overload is not applied too quickly and further damage incurred. This philosophy is based on the specific adaptation to imposed demands (SAID) principle. [42] This implies that the body responds to a given demand with a specific and predictable adaptation.[44] Stated another way, "specific adaptation requires that a specific demand be imposed."[28] Therefore, if strength is to be developed in a particular muscle group, those muscles must be contracted repeatedly against resistance.

When using the PRE concept in therapeutic rehabilitation the clinician must remember that it is an orderly progression and the athlete should show improvement each day, whether this involves an increase in repetitions or an increase in weight. The theory behind therapeutic rehabilitation is to apply an overload to increase muscular strength while at the same time maintaining the integrity of the surgical repair and/or not impeding the healing process. Therapeutic rehabilitation should be based on the concept of low weight and high repetition. This not only builds muscular strength and endurance but helps retard and reverse the atrophy process, while hopefully negating some potential setbacks if exercise is too aggressive.

DeLorme[13] first introduced the concept of progressive resistance exercise in 1945. The rationale of using PRE is that it creates a condition in which an individual muscle(s) must work to full capacity against an ever-increasing resistance.[21] The ever-increasing intramuscular tension, caused by an ever-increasing resistance, produces an increase in muscle strength. Gardiner[18] has reported that it is essential for the resistance to be increased as the muscle strength improves, and she further stated that "An increase in resistance which is too rapid results in overloading, preventing contraction, and may damage the muscle; conversely, underloading will not increase strength."

DeLorme's[13] initial concept of PRE was based on the amount of weight that could be carried through a full range of motion for 10 repetitions. This 10-repetition maximum (10 RM) was determined once a week, and a set of exercises of that value (10 RM) was repeated seven to ten times during each exercise session. This corresponds to 70 to 100 repetitions. On the last day of each exercise week, the maximum weight for only 1 repetition (1 RM) was determined, and the 10 RM was established from this 1 RM for the following week. DeLorme[13] has referred to this as "heavy resistance exercise" because the weights used were great when compared with those used in previous strengthening methods and an all-out effort was necessary to complete them. This mode of PRE, however, is generally not applicable to athletes in the early postoperative stages. Subjects involved in DeLorme's[13] research were usually not diseased but had lost strength from disuse. The weight lifted in DeLorme's program does not take into account healing restraints in the early postoperative phases.

DeLorme and Williams[14] revised this original work in 1948. In their revised method, 20 to 30 repetitions were used in place of the 70 to 100 previously recommended. This permitted exercise with even heavier loads and thus resulted in a more rapid gain in strength and muscle volume. In the new regimen the first 1 or 2 sets of repetitions were considered as warm-ups for the 10 RM exercises. Their revised program can be outlined as follows:

First set of 10 repetitions—use one-half 10 RM
Second set of 10 repetitions—use three-fourths 10 RM
Third set of 10 repetitions—use full 10 RM

Still, DeLorme's PRE program was skewed toward the low-repetition, high-weight concept.

There have been numerous modifications of the DeLorme[13, 14] PRE program.[23, 27, 38, 45] Knight's[27] technique of daily adjustable progressive resistance exercise (DAPRE) uses the basic principle of PRE to a greater degree than older programs. According to Knight,[27] the DAPRE technique allows for individual differences at the rate at which a person regains strength in the muscle and provides an objective method for increasing resistance in accordance with strength increases. The key to the program is that athletes perform as many full repetitions as they can in the third and fourth sets.[27] The number of repetitions performed in the third and fourth sets is then used to determine the amount of weight that is added to the working weight or sometimes removed from the working weight for the fourth set and the first set of the next

TABLE 7–2   **THE DAPRE TECHNIQUE**

Set	Portion of Working Weight Used	Number of Repetitions
1	Half	10
2	Three-fourths	6
3*	Full	Maximum
4†	Adjusted	Maximum

From Knight, K. (1985): Guidelines for rehabilitation of sports injuries. Clin. Sports Med., 4:413.

* The number of repetitions performed during the third set is used to determine the adjusted working weight for the fourth set according to the guidelines in Table 7–3.

† The number of repetitions performed during the fourth set is used to determine the adjusted working weight for the next day according to the guidelines in Table 7–3.

session. The working weight is estimated for the initial reconditioning session. A good estimate would result in 5 to 7 repetitions during the third set. More repetitions are performed if the estimate is low, and fewer are performed if it is too high.

During the first and second sets, the athlete performs 10 repetitions against half of the estimated working weight and 6 repetitions against three-quarters of the working weight (Tables 7–2 and 7–3). These sets act to warm up and educate the muscles and neuromuscular structures involved.

Emphasis during the third and fourth sets is on performing the greatest number of full repetitions possible. The full working weight is used on the third set, and the athlete performs as many repetitions as possible. The number of full repetitions performed in the third set is used to determine the adjusted working weight for the fourth set, and the number performed is used to determine the working weight for the next day.

TABLE 7–3   **GENERAL GUIDELINES FOR ADJUSTMENT OF WORKING WEIGHT**

Number of Repetitions Performed During Set	Adjustment of Working Weight for	
	FOURTH SET*	NEXT DAY†
0–2	Decrease by 5–10 lb and perform the set over	
3–4	Decrease by 0–5 lb	Keep the same
5–7	Keep the same	Increase by 5–10 lb
8–12	Increase by 5–10 lb	Increase by 5–15 lb
13–. . . .	Increase by 10–15 lb	Increase by 10–20 lb

From Knight, K.L. (1985): Guidelines for rehabilitation of sports injuries. Clin. Sports Med., 4:414.

* The number of repetitions performed during the third set is used to determine the adjusted working weight for the fourth set according to the guidelines in Table 7–2.

† The number of repetitions performed during the fourth set is used to determine the adjusted working weight for the next day according to the guidelines in Table 7–2.

The DAPRE guidelines are based on the concept that if the working weight is ideal, the athlete can perform 6 repetitions when told to perform as many as possible.[4] If the athlete can perform more than 6 repetitions, the weight is too light. Conversely, if the athlete cannot perform 6 repetitions, the weight is too heavy. The number of repetitions also helps determine the amount of weight added during the adjustment.

Athletes exercise daily, except Sundays, until the working weight of the injured limb is equal to or within 5 pounds of that of the uninjured limb. Emphasis is then shifted from strength development to strength maintenance and to the development of muscular endurance. The athlete should perform the exercise slowly and deliberately, avoiding jerky or explosive contractions. There should be a pause at the extremes of motion. The athlete should be in control of the weight at all times.

For those with injuries of insidious onset and early postoperative rehabilitation, however, high-repetition, low-weight exercise has proved to be the best regimen.[6] Potentially, exercise involving high weight or intensity could cause a breakdown of the supporting structures and only exacerbate the condition. Use of smaller weights and submaximal intensities provides a therapeutic effect that stimulates blood flow and diminishes tissue breakdown. To obtain the strengthening and endurance effect, higher repetitions must be used.[5, 6]

The PRE program outlined here can be carried out early in rehabilitation using the low-weight, high-repetition concept (Table 7–4). Early rehabilitation begins with an AROM of 2 or 3 sets of 10 repetitions (or 20 or 30 repetitions) and progressing to 5 sets of 10 repetitions (5×10, or 50 repetitions), as tolerated. The athlete must do 20, 30, 40, or 50 of the prescribed exercises. It is not necessary for the number of repetitions to be divisible by 10. The repetitions can be split in half or all performed consecutively, with no rest between repetitions. If the repetitions can be performed consecutively, the athlete's program should be upgraded by 10 repetitions the next day. The athlete should exercise 2 or 3 times per day. The prescribed repetitions and weight performed in the morning should be repeated in the afternoon, even if the athlete fits the criteria for advancement. This technique allows the body and injured area to adjust to the demands placed on it.

When 5×10 is reached and the athlete can perform 50 repetitions without stopping, 1 pound may be added and the repetitions reduced to 3×10, or 30, and the athlete once again advanced to 5×10, or 50.

TABLE 7–4   **PRE SCHEDULE FOR INITIAL REHABILITATION STAGES**

Week	SUNDAY	MONDAY	TUESDAY	Day WEDNESDAY	THURSDAY	FRIDAY	SATURDAY
1			Surgery	30 rep	40 rep	50 rep	30×—1 lb
2	40×—1 lb	50×—1 lb	30×—2 lb	40×—2 lb	50×—2 lb	30×—3 lb	40×—3 lb
3	50×—3 lb	30×—4 lb	40×—4 lb	50×—4 lb	30×—5 lb	40×—5 lb	50×—5 lb
.	etc.						
.							
.							
.							

At 50 repetitions, the cycle repeats, with the athlete adding another pound and reducing the repetitions to 30. Usually the athlete may progress through this low weight, high repetition regimen as tolerable, with emphasis placed on proper lifting technique.

All exercises should be performed smoothly, with a pause at the terminal position. The athlete must also concentrate on lowering the weight (eccentric) in a controlled fashion. In the later stages of rehabilitation, DeLorme's, Knight's, or any other type of PRE schedule may be used.

Some pain and discomfort are to be expected initially with the rehabilitation program. Moreover, the severity of the symptoms of many chronic injuries may slightly increase before abating. Soreness after initiation of the rehabilitation program is common, and cryotherapy application postexercise helps decrease the soreness, pain, and inflammation and helps control potential swelling. Prophylactic cryotherapy is recommended for at least 4 to 6 weeks after surgery and in the early, pre-exercise stages of rehabilitation following surgery. Residual pain (pain the next day) should be avoided. Residual pain generally indicates that the treatment is proceeding too quickly and should be reduced.

Prehab

Patient education plays an integral role in the rehabilitation program. By explaining the surgical procedure and the methods and rationales for protecting a surgical repair, patient compliance with orthotic devices and treatment may be enhanced.

"Prehab" is a term that refers to exercises and patient education before surgery. Ideally, particularly in the deconditioned athlete or individual, the initiation of a therapeutic exercise program 4 to 6 weeks prior to surgical intervention is preferable. This is thought to result in a decrease in morbidity and loss of muscular strength and endurance postoperatively, because the individual is beginning at a higher level of conditioning. Generally, the exercises focus on regaining range of motion and on therapeutic exercise that does not result in exacerbation of symptoms or further damage to the injured area. Usually the prehab concept can be used when a surgical procedure is not immediately mandated (e.g., chronic conditions). If the injury proves to have progressed too far for conservative treatment, the conservative exercise program now becomes the preoperative exercise program.

Fortunately, a long period of prehab is usually not necessary for the conditioned athlete. In these individuals prehab may consist of only a short session to educate the athlete about the initial rehabilitation program and what is expected of the athlete in the early phases of rehabilitation, gait training, baseline measurements (consisting of circumferential measurements, range of motion, and muscular strength tests, if indicated and tolerated by the athlete), and the fitting of any orthotic appliances that are to be used in the early postoperative phases. The athlete should also be informed about the surgical procedure to be performed, the prognosis following surgery, any potential complications, and precautions and limitations following surgery (e.g., limitation of the last 15 to 40° of elbow extension following ulnar nerve transposition). Finally, the importance of rehabilitation, its function, and its approximate duration should also be discussed.

Following surgery, the exact findings and surgical procedure as well as the prognosis and any rehabilitation program changes should once again be discussed with the athlete. It is also recommended that at this time the subjects that were discussed before surgery be reiterated so that the athlete has a clear understanding of them.

The preoperative and postoperative education of the athlete is often taken for granted, and the surgical procedure, extent of damage, prognosis, and rehabilitation course are often not discussed with the athlete. It is important that athletes be able to be involved in goal-setting and have input into their rehabilitation program, and to understand the consequences of noncompliance with rehabilitation and early rehabilitation restrictions.

Crutch Training

The correct fitting of crutches and patient education in crutch use are often a neglected part of rehabilitation. Correct crutch fitting and instruction are imperative in preventing accidents, reducing frustrations, and increasing crutch compliance, when necessary. It is often assumed that the athlete knows how to ambulate both on flat surfaces and stairs using crutches, but usually this is not the case. Ideally, in surgical lower extremity patients, in whom the potential for crutch use is the greatest, crutch training before surgery is encouraged. This results in a lower level

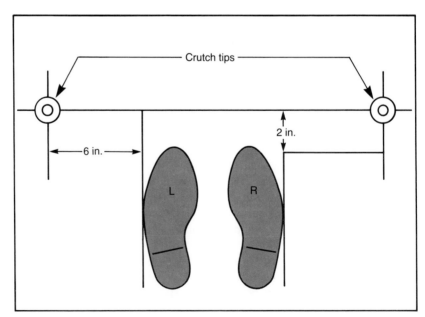

FIGURE 7–9 Schematic representation of properly adjusted axillary crutches. (From Flood, D.K. (1983): Proper fitting and use of crutches. Physician Sportsmed., 11:75.)

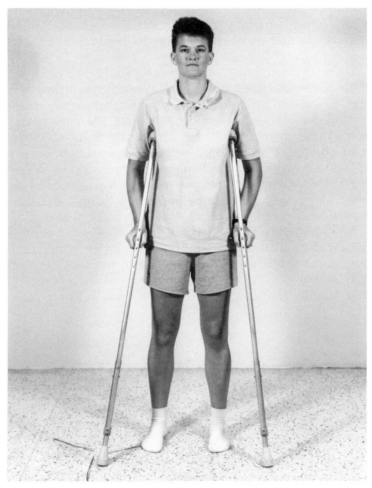

FIGURE 7–10   Correct posture for crutch adjustment.

of patient apprehension, less pain, and a lower chance of damage to repaired tissues or additional injury from a fall.

Improper crutch adjustment can cause early fatigue, axillary nerve injury, frustration, or a fall.[17] Moreover, properly adjusted crutches can help maintain good posture and strengthen the trunk, shoulders, and arms. Athletes who have not been properly instructed in crutch use tend to rest their body weight on the axillary pads. This maneuver should be avoided because it can result in temporary or permanent numbness in the hands or arms resulting from pressure on the axillary and radial nerves and blood vessels, a condition usually referred to as "crutch palsy."

Crutch adjustment consists of the following:[17] (1) adjustment with the athlete standing in good posture; (2) determination of crutch length by having the athlete stand with the feet close together and the rubber crutch tips 6 inches from the outer margin of each sole and 2 inches in front of the shoes; (3) a space of approximately two finger widths from the top of the crutch pad to the axillary skin fold; and (4) adjustment of the hand grips to allow 25 to 30° of elbow flexion with the wrist straight (Figs. 7–9 and 7–10).

Crutches are used to transfer body weight through the palms onto the hand grips. The arms may be almost fully extended at the elbow, and the axillary pads of the crutches are squeezed between the rib cage and upper arms while bearing weight.

There are five commonly used crutch gaits: (1) two-point alternate gait; (2) three-point gait; (3) four-point alternate gait; (4) swing-to gait; and (5) swing-through gait.[17] In most athletic arenas the three-point and swing-through gait is the most often used. The three-point gait is indicated when one extremity can support the body weight and the injured extremity is to be touch-down or partial weight-bearing (Fig. 7–11). Just enough pressure is placed on the crutches to eliminate limping. The athlete can gradually increase the amount of weight-bearing by decreasing the force transferred through the arms. The athlete wants to mimic a normal gait as closely as possible.

A swing-through gait is used when the athlete is to be nonweight-bearing and weight is completely removed from the injured extremity. This technique should not be used longer than necessary because it can affect kinesthetic input to the lower extremity. It can also cause hip and knee tightness.[3] In the swing-through gait, body weight is totally sup-

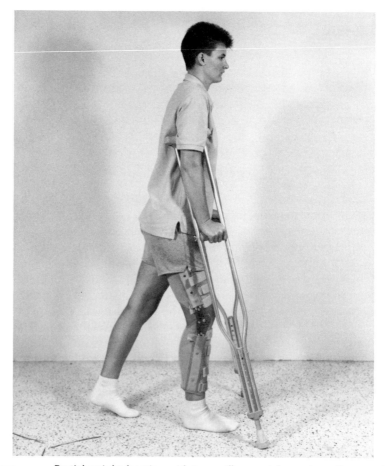

FIGURE 7–11   Partial weight-bearing with two axillary crutches using a three-point gait.

ported by the uninjured extremity while both crutches are placed 12 to 24 inches in front of the feet. Weight is then transferred to the crutches as the body is lifted and swung through to a point 12 to 24 inches in front of the crutches.[3]

Negotiating stairs with crutches presents a different problem for the injured athlete. When instructing the athlete to maneuver on stairs it is a good idea to stand close to the athlete and hold on to his or her waist belt or to use an orthopedic safety belt. This allows the clinician to be in a better position to prevent or control a fall and helps the athlete maintain balance. In ascending stairs, the supportive limb is moved up to the first step while the body weight is supported on the crutch hand grips. The body weight is then transferred to the supportive limb and the crutches in the affected limb are moved up the same step. This sequence is carefully repeated as the athlete ascends the stairs.

When descending stairs on crutches, the affected limb is placed on a lower step while the unaffected extremity, supporting the body weight, is on the upper step. Crutch placement on the lower step is critical for balance. The crutches must be placed toward the back of the step for greatest stability. After the body weight has been transferred from the unaffected extremity to the crutch hand grips, the unaffected limb is carefully brought down to the same step as the crutches and the affected extremity.

When a handrail is available it should be used instead of one of the crutches because it is safer and more stable than crutches under both arms. The sequence of moving from one step to the next using the handrail is similar to the sequence followed when using crutches bilaterally. The athlete grips the handrail and applies a downward force with one hand while applying a downward force to the crutch grip with the other.[17] The extra crutch should be carried next to the crutch in use.

APPLICATION OF EXERCISE

Rehabilitation must prepare the athlete to return to competition as soon as possible without sacrificing healing time and predisposing the athlete to reinjury or to injury to another body part as a result of the initial trauma. Intensity, duration, frequency, specificity, rhythm, and progression of the program are all related to the functional capability that is developed.

Intensity

The goal of the rehabilitation program is to overload not overwhelm.[15] Muscle and connective tissue must be subjected to a load greater than that of the usual stresses of daily activity if hypertrophy is to occur. Attempting to push too fast can result in reactive inflammatory changes.[15]

After the program is underway, an increase in exercise intensity (higher weight, lower repetition) may increase the rate of strength gain. In the initial exercise regimen the high-weight, low-repetition concept is not applicable because of the greater stresses it places on the connective tissues, but it may be used later in the program. Exercise intensity varies according to injury.

Duration

Duration of the rehabilitation program is an estimate of how long it will take to return the athlete to activity at 100%. It can vary from only a few days after a contusion to months following ligamentous injuries. Duration also encompasses the amount of time the athlete is to be performing the rehabilitation program daily. Initially this time is longer, until pain, effusion, and soreness are alleviated.

Frequency

Frequency refers to how many times the rehabilitation program should be performed. Initially, Dickinson and Bennett[15] reported that exercise performed twice daily yields a greater improvement than exercise once daily in the early phases of rehabilitation. Houglum[23] described a natural rate of progress for individuals in a rehabilitation program. In the initial phase there is a relatively rapid improvement in strength, followed by a second phase, in which there is slowing or tapering of the improvement rate, and a third (final) phase, consisting of a progression toward a plateau state in which minimal or no improvement occurs in strength (Fig. 7–12). When the athlete is in the first phase of the rehabilitation development progression, an exercise routine can be implemented twice daily.[23] With the use of this concept the athlete should be monitored, and a reduction in exercise may be needed periodically. As the athlete improves and comes closer to the final goal, a once-daily exercise program should be sufficient. This usually corresponds to a change in the PRE schedule toward higher weight, lower repetitions and advancement toward functional activities. The reduction in routine should be instituted for two reasons: (1) it helps minimize the athlete's chances

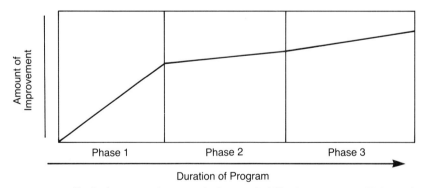

FIGURE 7–12   Typical progression rate during a rehabilitation program. (Adapted from Houglum, P. (1977): The modality of therapeutic exercise: Objectives and principles. Athletic Training, 12:43.)

of becoming bored and discontented with the program and (2) no reports have noted that exercising isotonically during the third phase more than once a day produces any significant physical benefits.[23] When the athlete returns to participation he or she can advance to a once- or twice-weekly program for maintenance. It is important that the athlete continue a rehabilitation maintenance program during the season, particularly if the regular weight room regimen does not strengthen the appropriate muscles (e.g., rotator cuff).

Specificity

There is a specific response to the type of exercise performed. An exercise program must be tailored to meet the specific needs of the individual. Obviously, the activity requirements for a homemaker are not the same as those for a football lineman, nor are the activity requirements for a football lineman the same as for a sprinter. For example, exercises that mimic the throwing motion are ideal for the baseball pitcher but are not applicable for the football lineman. Activities or exercises that simulate part of the athlete's activity are ideal for this aspect of rehabilitation.

Furthermore, the type of exercise is important. Athletes who are trained only with constant resistance (isotonic) exercise perform better with this type of testing.[40] Conversely, athletes trained with accommodating variable resistance show significant increases in strength when assessed by variable resistance procedures, but these changes diminish when assessed with constant resistant procedures.[40]

Costill and colleagues[10] evaluated the effects of training programs on postoperative knee patients. The patients in their study trained using isotonic knee extension and tested normal within 6 weeks of training. When their ability to perform other single-leg activities (e.g., leg press) was assessed, however, the maximal functional strength of the operative knee was below normal. Also, when asked to perform rapid exercises, the patients showed even poorer ability. Based on these results, Costill and associates[10] postulated that patients should be trained using various activities, and that exercise should require tension development through a full range of motion. Therefore, a rehabilitation program should consist of exercise performed at both slow and fast speeds coupled with functional training in the later stages.[40]

Rhythm

Rhythm refers to the rate at which the exercise is performed. The exercises should be performed in a slow and deliberate manner, with emphasis placed on concentric (raising weight) and eccentric (lowering weight) contractions. The athlete should pause at the end of the exercise and should exercise through the full range of motion that is allowed, avoiding jerky movements. For example, when performing a straight leg raise, the athlete should raise the leg slowly, pause, lower it slowly, relax the quad, and repeat. In addition, the larger muscle groups should be exercised first, proceeding to the smaller muscle groups. This is done because it is difficult to reach the required condition of momentary muscular exhaustion in a large muscle if a smaller muscle group that serves as a link between resistance and the large muscle group has been previously exhausted.

In the late stages of rehabilitation the exercise speed should be varied. Traditional PRE exercises are performed at about 60°/sec, which is not functional when attempting to return athletes to their sport. For example, a pitcher's throwing arm travels at approximately 7000°/sec. The continuation of a PRE program as the only tool in restoring this athlete back to function does not prepare him or her for the great demands placed on the throwing arm when returning to competition. As Costill and associates[10] have noted, it is important to vary the type and speed of the exercise. Surgical tubing can be used to implement a high-speed regimen to produce a concentric or eccentric synergist pattern, and isokinetic units at the highest speeds on the spectrum can also be used.

Progression

Progression within the rehabilitation program is of the utmost importance. There should be some type of objective improvement each day, whether this is an increase in repetitions or an increase in the amount of weight lifted. Only if the athlete has complaints of increased or residual pain should the program be maintained at the current level or possibly decreased. Muscles must be continually overloaded in order for strength to be developed. If the athlete continues to improve with repetitions or weights, he or she is getting stronger. As noted by Houglum,[23] progression is quicker at the beginning of the rehabilitation program and slows down as the athlete enters the second and third phases of rehabilitation.

In addition, there is an orderly progression from initial range-of-motion exercises to isometric, isotonic, isokinetic, and functional activities. Each phase precedes another, with some overlap in exercise types. Exercises should progress from a low-intensity to high-intensity level, with ever-increasing demands placed on the athlete as the healing process allows.

PHASES OF REHABILITATION

Knight[28] has outlined eight phases of rehabilitation to serve as a guideline for the development of the total rehabilitation sequence.

Intact Joints and Muscles

Surgery and immobilization or protected immobilization is generally necessary after the repair of ligaments, tendons, and muscles to allow for healing of the repaired structures or for the reapproximation of tissues (in conservative cases). As previously discussed, there are many deleterious effects of immobilization, and this period should be as brief as possible (see Chap. 2).

Pain-Free Articulations

Therapeutic modalities and exercise are all techniques used to decrease pain. Unfortunately, however, orthopedic surgery is painful. Pain must be monitored throughout the rehabilitation course. Although some pain is to be expected, excessive pain induced by an activity that is too strenuous or complex should result in the athlete regressing to a lesser activity and/or weight. Of further concern is residual pain, which occurs the day after the activity occurred and indicates that the previous day's activity was too strenuous; thus, the current day's activity must be adjusted accordingly. Activities that result in pain during rehabilitation hinder the rehabilitation process and induce neural inhibition.[27]

Joint Flexibility

Decreased joint flexibility results from muscle spasm, pain, and/or neural inhibition secondary to acute injury, or it may result from connective tissue adhesions and contractures secondary to surgery or immobilization. Therapeutic exercise is essential in improving flexibility and can be facilitated by thermotherapy and/or cryotherapy applications. Cryotherapy is generally more effective in relieving muscular conditions, whereas thermotherapy is preferred when connective tissue is involved.[39] If immobilization is necessary, protective or limited motion helps maintain joint flexibility. After immobilization, such techniques as cryostretch, proprioceptive neuromuscular facilitation (PNF), stationary bicycle, electrical muscle stimulation and, in severe cases, Dynasplint application can help increase the range of motion.

Muscular Strength

If the involved musculature is to gain strength and endurance, some type of PRE exercise must be performed on a regular basis. The various types of PRE exercise regimens have already been discussed.

In the early stages, if mobilization is necessary, the contralateral limb may be exercised, resulting in a crossover training effect.[22] Once the strength, power, endurance, and time-to-peak torque of the injured side are 85 to 95% of those of the contralateral side, the athlete's rehabilitation program can be changed to a maintenance program. Strength can usually be maintained with one or two workouts at near-maximum resistance weekly.

Muscular Endurance

Muscular endurance can be gained through the use of a stationary bicycle, running, aquatic therapy, and other types of rehabilitation regimens including the StairMaster, Nordic Track, and Slide Board. High-speed isokinetic and surgical tubing exercise to fatigue also produce an increase in muscle endurance and can be modified to exercise sports-specific skill patterns.

Muscular Speed

Muscular speed can be developed by participation in team drills at half-speed, three-fourths speed, and finally full speed. Also, isokinetic work helps facilitate a gain in muscular speed.

Integrated and coordinated movements can be developed only by the practice of sports-specific skill patterns. This phase is developed along with muscular speed by using increasingly complex team drills. The low-weight, high-repetition PRE regimen early in rehabilitation also confers some endurance benefits.

Neuromuscular Re-education

Although not directly outlined in the eight phases of rehabilitation, neuromuscular re-education is important in the total rehabilitation of the athlete but is often neglected. Neuromuscular re-education primarily involves the development of proprioception, which is vital in the rehabilitation of weight-bearing joints because of the importance of mechanoreceptors in providing kinesiologic input to the nervous system.[26] All injuries result in some type of damage to the joint mechanoreceptors. The more severe an injury, the greater the mechanoreceptor damage. In addition, immobilization and nonweight-bearing (NWB) result in further deterioration of proprioception in the lower extremity. Conversely, normal function usually returns more quickly in the athlete who is allowed to continue with activities that permit near-normal function but do not interfere with the normal healing process. Proprioceptive exercises can be instituted early in the rehabilitation program and are generally closed chain types of activities.

Cardiovascular Endurance

As the athlete returns to the activity, this helps develop cardiovascular endurance. Other sports-specific conditioning drills should be instituted, gradually at first and than increasing in difficulty. Cardiovascular deconditioning should be considered early in the rehabilitation program to prevent as much deconditioning as possible. This can be addressed by having the athlete perform deep-water pool exercises, stationary bicycling, or upper body ergometer, as tolerated by the athlete and as healing restraints allow.

FUNCTIONAL PROGRESSION

Determining whether an athlete has been successfully rehabilitated or may safely return to competition can be difficult. As an aid to rehabilitation, functional progressions (e.g., a plan or a progressively more difficult sequence of exercises) can help the clinician determine the status of injured athletes and prepare the athlete for competition. Clinical techniques, however sophisticated, cannot predict the complex interaction of a rehabilitated joint in response to the imposed demands of competition. Functional progressions help the clinician and physician determine an athlete's status at any time throughout the rehabilitation process. Kegerreis[25] has outlined the role of functional progression, and their concepts are presented here.

Implementation of functional progressions must be based on the following:[25, 26] (1) knowing the athlete's limitations and the inherent demands of the athlete's sport and (2) allowing enough time for maturation of collagen tissue because there is a greater risk of injury during functional levels of activity.

The basis of any rehabilitation effort remains whether the athlete can perform effectively and safely. Noyes and colleagues[36] have labeled this concept "functional stability." "Functional stability is provided by (1) passive restraints of the ligaments, (2) joint geometry, (3) active restraints generated by the muscles, and (4) joint compressive forces that occur with activity and force the joint together." They concluded that "laxity tests alone do not provide a reliable prediction of functional stability.[36] Rehabilitation should be directed toward improving strength and endurance and perhaps primarily increasing neuromuscular coordination and agility. The use of functional activities also helps the apprehensive athlete to acclimatize gradually to the inherent demands of the sport. Because each successive stage builds on preceding stages, this ensures the return of physical prowess and instills confidence in the athlete in regard to the ability to complete required tasks.[25, 26]

Just as in the PRE concept, functional progressions are based on the SAID principle. This attempts to adapt athletes to the demands that may be placed on them during athletic performance. The intensity, duration, and frequency of the activity are all related to the functional capability that is developed.

Initial considerations for implementation of a functional progression program revolve around the physical parameters of the patient's intended activity. This involves an analysis of the demands of specific athletic endeavors, which are assessed for difficulty and complexity of response. The tasks are then placed on a continuum of difficulty with respect to the athlete's status. Overlaps occasionally occur as a particular task is accomplished but remains in the athlete's program for solidification as the next task is begun. Care should be taken to ensure the blending of task progressions with specific restrictions concerning the nature of the pathology.

Kegerreis and co-workers[26] have outlined a functional progression for a second-degree medial collateral ligament sprain involving a football halfback:

Protective immobilization
Range-of-motion exercises
Strengthening exercises
Progressive weight-bearing
Proprioceptive activities
Functional strengthening
Walk–jog sequence
Hop–jump sequence
Sprinting sequence
Cutting sequence
Agility drills
Specific activities
Return to sport

Typical advancement follows a progression of half- to three-quarters speed activity, increasing gradually until full speed is reached. The athlete may be performing four or five tasks in a functional progression at one time. Conceivably, the athlete can be performing one task at half-speed while performing a less demanding skill at full speed.

Functional activities may begin as soon as 2 to 3 days postinjury or as late as 6 to 8 months after injury, as with some knee surgeries. Functional activities should be performed in conjunction with the rehabilitation program and not as a substitute for it. The athlete must ultimately be able to perform each activity asymptomatically. Functional tasks that result in apparent swelling or pain, particularly residual pain, or immediate instability or athlete anxiety should be curtailed in favor of a less aggressive activity. Prophylactic icing is encouraged post-exercise.

It is common for the athlete to have occasional setbacks requiring regression to a former functional task. Tasks are considered completed when they are performed at competitive speeds with adequate repetitions without residual pain, edema, and loss of range of motion. Skills are introduced at half-normal speed and increased in intensity and frequency until functional levels have been reached. A common occurrence is that the physician permits the athlete to engage in unlimited physical activity prior to completion of the attainment of functional skills.[25] Communication is important between the clinician and physician with regard to the current functional status of the athlete.

Clinical isokinetic data can be used to determine the athlete's strength, power, and endurance but do not indicate performance when the athlete returns to competition. Functional activities progressed along an increasing continuum of difficulty can provide the clinician and physician with some idea of functional performance when athletes return to their respective sport.

SUMMARY

Rehabilitation or reconditioning is a dynamic method or program of prescribed exercise to prevent or reverse the deleterious effects of inactivity while returning an athlete to the former level of competition. Athletic rehabilitation requires the athlete to return to a performance level equal to or higher than that of the preinjury state. The goals of rehabilitation in conjunction with the use of therapeutic modalities include decreasing pain, inflammation, and effusion; return of full, pain-free, active range of motion; return of full muscular strength, power, and endurance; and asymptomatic return to full functional activities. Early exercise is essential to restoring athletes to their former conditioning level as soon as possible, but a fine balance must be achieved between early mobilization and that which is too aggressive, which can setback the rehabilitation process.

In designing a rehabilitation program, the clinician must consider the arthrokinematics and tissues that have been traumatized or surgically repaired. In addition, harmful stimuli can result in pain, swelling, and inflammation. The initial phases of rehabilitation should mainly be concerned with reducing these responses to injury. Once these reactions have been controlled the athlete may proceed with early range-of-motion and active exercises.

There are two types of exercise: dynamic and static. Static exercise consists of isometrics. Dynamic exercise is composed of isotonic, accommodating resistance, and variable resistance (isokinetic) exercises. Concentric and eccentric muscle contractions can also be incurred with these types of exercises.

Exercises can also be classified as constituting an open or closed kinematic chain. The human body functions both as an open and closed system. The system is considered open when extremity ends are not meeting resistance and are free in space. The system is closed when the distal segment of a joint is fixed and meets with some external resistance, which prohibits or restrains its free motion. The closed system functions as a link system, with each body part being affected by its proximal and distal segments. During the rehabilitation process, closed chain exercises may be favored over open chain exercises, because they stress functional progression without exerting open chain, high-torque–producing effects.

The concept of progressive resistive exercise was first introduced by DeLorme,[13, 14] who proposed a high-weight, low-repetition regimen. Knight[27] followed with the concept of the DAPRE technique. Early rehabilitation should consist of a low-weight, high-repetition regimen allowing the body time to adjust to the demands placed on it.

"Prehab" is a term that refers to exercises and patient education before surgery. The prehab session may be as short as 1 day before surgery or as long as 4 to 6 weeks preceding it. This time should be used to educate the athlete concerning the injury, surgical technique, prognosis, and rehabilitation after surgery. If surgery is not immediately mandated, the 4 to 6 weeks of exercise help in increasing muscle strength and endurance, particularly in the deconditioned athlete. The athlete should also be instructed in gait training during the prehab session.

Intensity, duration, frequency, specificity, rhythm, and progression are all important factors that must be addressed when designing a rehabilitation program. It is important to restore muscular strength, power, and endurance, and cardiovascular endurance; and to provide neuromuscular education during the reconditioning phases.

Finally, the athlete should be tested in regard to functional ability before returning to participation. This was traditionally done with objective testing equipment that provided no information about how the athlete would perform functionally on the field. The rehabilitation program should include functional activities that athletes may incur in their sports, advancing in difficulty from easy to difficult. If athletes perform well on objective measurement and functional activity tests, with no pain or effusion, and can perform functional activities at full speed, they may return to participation.

References

1. Allman, F.L. (1985): Rehabilitative exercises in sports medicine. Instr. Course Lect., 34:389–392.
2. Arnheim, D. (1989): Modern Principles of Athletic Training. St. Louis, C.V. Mosby, p. 86.
3. Aten, D. (1980): Crutches: Essential in caring for lower extremity injuries. Phys. Sportsmed., 8:121.
4. Berger, R.A. (1962): Optimal repetitions for the development of strength. Res. Q., 33:334–338.
5. Berger, R.A. (1982): Applied Exercise Physiology. Philadelphia, Lea & Febiger, p. 267.
6. Blackburn, T.A. (1987): Rehabilitation of the shoulder and elbow after arthroscopy. Clin. Sports Med., 6:587–588.
7. Brunnstrom, S. (1972): Clinical Kinesiology, 3rd ed. Philadelphia, F.A. Davis.
8. Caillouet, H. (1989): Knee rehabilitation following anterior cruciate ligament injury. Sports Med. Update, 4:15–17.
9. Cooper, D.L., and Fair, J. (1976): Reconditioning following athletic injuries. Physician Sportsmed., 4(9):125.
10. Costill, D.L., Fink, W.J., and Habansky, A.J. (1971): Muscle rehabilitation after knee surgery. Physician Sportsmed., 5:71–77.
11. Cummings, G.S., Crutchfield, C.A., and Branes, M.R. (1983): Soft tissue changes in contractures. In: Orthopedic Physical Therapy Series, Vol. I. Atlanta, Stokesville Publishing.
12. Dempster, W.T. (1955): Space requirements for the seated operator. Wright-Patterson Air Force Base, OH, Wright Air Development Center, WADC Technical Report 55159.
13. DeLorme, T.L. (1945): Restoration of muscle power by heavy resistance exercise. J. Bone Joint Surg., 27:645–667.
14. DeLorme, T.L., and Williams, A.L. (1948): Techniques of progressive resistance exercise. Arch. Phys. Med., 29:263.
15. Dickinson, A., and Bennett, K. (1985): Therapeutic exercise. Clin. Sports Med., 4:417–429.
16. Fahere, H., Rentsch, H.U., Gerber, N.J., et al. (1988): Knee effusion and reflex inhibition of the quadriceps. J. Bone Joint Surg. [Br.] 70:635–638.
17. Flood, D.K. (1983): Proper fitting and use of crutches. Physician Sportsmed., 11:75–78.
18. Gardiner, M.D. (1975): The Principles of Exercise Therapy. London, G. Belt and Sons.
19. Gould, J., and Davies, G. (1985): Orthopaedic and Sports Physical Therapy. St. Louis, C.V. Mosby, pp. 348–349.
20. Gowitzke, B.A., and Morris, M. (1988): Scientific Basis of Human Movement, 3rd ed. Baltimore, Williams & Wilkins.
21. Helebrand, F.A. (1951): Physiological bases of progressive resistance exercise. In: DeLorme, T.L., and Watkins, A.L. (eds.): Progressive Resistance Exercise. New York, Appleton-Century-Crofts, pp. 8–16.
22. Hellebrandt, F.A., Parish, A.M., and Houtz, S.J. (1947): Cross-education. Arch. Phys. Med., 28:76.

23. Houglum, P. (1977): The modality of therapeutic exercise: Objectives and principles. Athletic Training, 12:42–45.
24. Hughston, J.C. (1980): Knee surgery—a philosphy. Am. Phys. Ther., 60:1611–1614.
25. Kegerreis, S. (1983): The construction and implementation of functional progressions as a component of athletic rehabilitation. J. Orthop. Sports Phys. Ther., 5:14–19.
26. Kegerreis, S., Malone, T., and McCaroll, J. (1984): Functional progressions: An aid to athletic rehabilitation. Physician Sportsmed., 12:67–71.
27. Knight, K.L. (1979): Rehabilitating chondromalacia patellae. Physician Sportsmed., 7:147–148.
28. Knight, K. (1985): Guidelines for rehabilitation of sports injuries. Clin. Sports Med., 4:405–416.
29. Kraus, H. (1956): Principles and Practice of Therapeutic Exercise. Springfield, IL, Charles C. Thomas.
30. Kraus, H. (1959): Evaluation and treatment of muscle function in athletic injury. Am. J. Surg., 98:353–362.
31. Lehmkunl, L.D., and Smith, L.K. (1983): Brunnstroms's Clinical Kinesiology. Philadelphia, F.A. Davis.
32. Mannheimer, J.S., and Lampe, G.N. (1984): Clinical Transcutaneous Electrical Nerve Stimulation. Philadelphia, F.A. Davis.
33. Marino, M. (1986): Current concepts of rehabilitation in sports medicine: Research and clinical interrelationship. In: Nicholas, J.A., and Hershman, E.D. (eds.): The Lower Extremity in Sports Medicine, St. Louis, C.V. Mosby, pp. 126–128.
34. Norkin, C., and Levangie, P. (1983): Joint Structure and Function: A Comprehensive Analysis. Philadelphia, F.A. Davis.
35. Noyes, F.R., Grood, E.S., Butler, D.L., and Malek, M. (1980): Clinical laxity tests and functional stability of the knee: Biomechanical concepts. Clin. Orthop. Rel. Res., 146:84–89.
36. Noyes, F.R., Grood, E.S., Butler, D.L., et al. (1980): Knee ligament tests. Phys. Ther., 60:1578–1581.
37. Reuleaux, F. (1875): Theoretische Kinematic: Grundig einer Theorie des Maschinenwessens. Braunschweig, I.F. Vieweg und Sohn. (Translated by Kennedy, A.B.W. (1876): The Kinematic Theory of Machinery: Outline of a Theory of Machines. London, Macmillan.)
38. Schram, D.A., and Bennett, R.L. (1951): Underwater resistance exercise. Arch. Phys. Med., 32:222.
39. Sapega, A., Quedenfeld, T.C., Moyer, R.A., and Butler, R. (1981): Biological factors of range of motion exercises. Physician Sportsmed., 9:57–65.
40. Steadman, J.R. (1979): Rehabilitation of athletic injuries. Am. J. Sports Med., 7:147–149.
41. Steindler, A. (1970): Kinesiology of the Human Body Under Normal and Pathological Conditions. Springfield, IL, Charles C Thomas.
42. Wallis, E.L., and Logan, G.A. (1964): Figure Improvement and Body Composition Through Exercise. Englewood Cliffs, NJ, Prentice-Hall.
43. Wilk, K.E. (1990): Plyometrics for the upper extremity. Presented at the 1990 Advances on Shoulder and Knee Symposium. Cincinnati, OH, Cincinnati Sportsmedicine and Deaconess Hospital, April.
44. Wilmore, J.H. (1976): Athletic Training and Physical Fitness. Boston, Allyn & Bacon.
45. Zinovieff, A.N. (1951): Heavy-resistance exercise, the "Oxford technique." Br. J. Phys. Med., 14:129–132.

CHAPTER 8

◆

Lower Leg, Ankle, and Foot Rehabilitation

Ed Mulligan, P.T., A.T.C., S.C.S.

The lower leg, ankle, and foot consist of 26 bones, all working as one unit to propel the body. The foot has three components: rearfoot, midfoot, and forefoot. The rearfoot and midfoot are composed of the tarsal bones. The rearfoot also contains the subtalar joints, with the talus resting on top of the calcaneus. The midfoot is composed of the navicular and cuboid and articulates with the talus and calcaneus at the transverse tarsal joint. The three cuneiform bones are located within the midfoot. Five tarsal and fourteen phalangeal bones comprise the forefoot structure. The shape of the joint, orientation of its axis, supporting ligaments, and subtle accessory motions at the joint surface are important determinants of normal biomechanical behavior. The treatment of pathologic hypomobility or hypermobility is predicated on a thorough understanding of these principles and their functional intimacy.

ARTHROKINEMATICS

Tibiofibular Joint

The tibiofibular joint provides accessory motion to allow greater freedom of movement in the ankle. Fusion or hypomobility of this joint can restrict or impair ankle function. During ankle plantar flexion, the fibula slides caudally at the superior and inferior tibiofibular joint, while the lateral malleolus rotates medially to cause an approximation of the two malleoli. With dorsiflexion, the opposite accessory motions occur to provide a slight spread of the malleoli and accommodate the wider portion of the anterior talus. Accessory motion of the tibiofibular joint also occurs with supination (calcaneal inversion) and pronation (calcaneal eversion). The head of the fibula slides distally and posteriorly with supination and proximally and anteriorly during pronation.[20]

197

Talocrural Joint

The talocrural articulation is a synovial joint with a structurally strong mortice and supporting collateral ligaments. The concave surface of the mortice is made up of the distal tibial plafond and the tibial (medial) and fibular (lateral) malleoli. Within the mortice sits the convex surface of the talar dome. The joint derives ligamentous support from the deltoid ligament medially and the anterior talofibular, calcaneofibular, and posterior talofibular ligaments laterally.

The lateral malleolus is positioned distally and posteriorly relative to the medial malleolus, causing the axis of motion for the ankle joint to run from posterolateral inferior to anteromedial superior (Fig. 8–1). This oblique orientation allows triplanar motion. Sagittal plane plantar flexion and dorsiflexion make up the prime movement of the joint and are coupled with adduction and abduction, respectively. Because the axis is nearly parallel to the transverse plane, inversion and eversion are negligible components of motion. Available range of motion is typically defined as approximately 20° of dorsiflexion and 50° degrees of plantar flexion.[1]

A small amount of talocrural physiologic accessory motion also accompanies plantar flexion and dorsiflexion.[22] As the foot plantar flexes, the body of the talus slides anteriorly. Conversely, as the foot dorsiflexes, the direction of talar slide is posterior. Maximal stability to angular and torsional stresses occurs in the closed pack position of maximal dorsiflexion, where the talus has slid posteriorly and wedged within the mortice.

Subtalar Joint

The talocalcaneal joint provides the triplanar motions of pronation and supination. The joint is supported by the medial and lateral collateral,

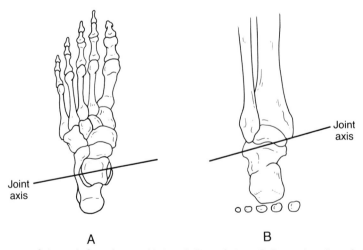

A   B

FIGURE 8–1   Joint axis for talocrural joint. *A*, Dorsal view. *B*, Posterior view. Axis of orientation runs from posterolateral inferior to anteromedial superior.

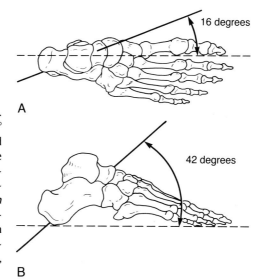

FIGURE 8–2 Subtalar joint axis. *A,* Lies approximately 16° from the sagittal plane, and *B,* 42° from the transverse plane. Reproduced by permission from Mann, Roger A.: Biomechanics of running. *In* American Academy of Orthopaedic Surgeons: Symposium on the Foot and Leg in Running Sports. St. Louis, 1982, The C.V. Mosby Co.)

the interosseous talocalcaneal, and the posterior and lateral talocalcaneal ligaments.

The joint axis runs from dorsal, medial, and distal to plantar, lateral, and proximal. It is oriented approximately 16° from the sagittal and 42° from the transverse plane (Fig. 8–2). Because of this axis of orientation, the joint provides the triplanar motions of pronation and supination. The pronation components of motion in an open kinetic chain are calcaneal dorsiflexion, abduction, and eversion. Conversely, open kinetic chain supination consists of calcaneal plantar flexion, adduction, and inversion. Functionally, however, the subtalar joint operates in a closed kinetic chain manner. Closed kinetic chain motion occurs when the distal segment is fixed and the proximal segment becomes mobile, as when the foot is in contact with the ground. The distal or terminal joints meet with considerable resistance, which prohibits or restrains free motion. During the weight-bearing portion of the stance phase gait, friction and ground reaction forces prevent the abduction–adduction and plantar flexion–dorsiflexion elements of open kinetic chain subtalar motion. To counteract these forces, the talus functions to maintain the transverse and sagittal plane motions of supination and pronation.[26] Thus, in closed kinetic chain motion, subtalar joint pronation consists of talar plantar flexion–adduction and calcaneal eversion, whereas subtalar joint supination consists of talar dorsiflexion–abduction and calcaneal

TABLE 8–1   CALCANEAL AND TALAR MOTION IN OPEN AND CLOSED KINETIC CHAINS

Position of Foot	Open Chain Motion	Closed Chain Motion
Pronation	Calcaneal eversion, dorsiflexion, abduction	Calcaneal eversion; talar plantar flexion, adduction
Supination	Calcaneal inversion, plantar flexion, adduction	Calcaneal inversion; talar dorsiflexion, abduction

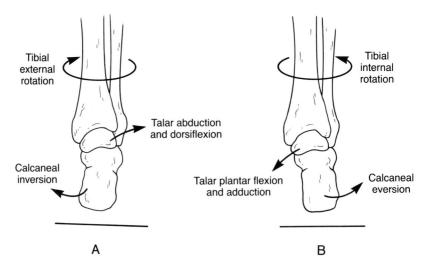

FIGURE 8–3   Closed chain subtalar motion. *A*, Supination. *B*, Pronation.

inversion (Fig. 8–3).[36] Note that calcaneal direction of movement is unaffected by open versus closed chain type of motion (Table 8–1).

The subtalar joint couples the function of the foot with the rest of the proximal kinetic chain. The prime function of the subtalar joint is to permit rotation of the leg in the transverse plane during gait. The rotation of the talus on the calcaneus allows the foot to become a

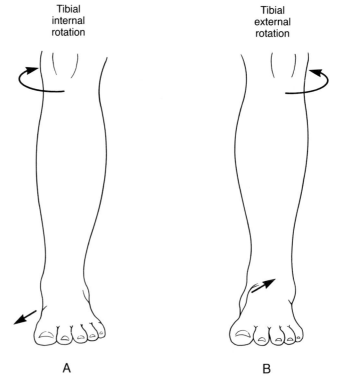

FIGURE 8–4   Relationship of the subtalar joint to the lower leg during gait. *A*, Subtalar pronation. *B*, Subtalar supination.

directional transmitter and torque converter to the kinetic chain.[29] These characteristics allow the foot to be a loose adaptor to the terrain in midstance and a rigid lever for propulsion.

Because the subtalar joint is angulated approximately 45° from the transverse plane, there is 1° of inversion−eversion for every 1° of tibial internal-external rotation. This relationship can be observed in gait. As the subtalar joint pronates, the tibial tuberosity is seen to be rotating internally (Fig. 8−4). High inclination angles (above 45°) of the subtalar joint axis cause a relative decrease in calcaneal inversion-eversion motion and an increased tibial rotation motion, leading to postural related pathologies secondary to poor absorption of ground reaction forces. The athlete with a low inclination angle (below 45°) of the subtalar joint conversely demonstrates a relative increase in calcaneal mobility, resulting in more foot-related overuse and fatigue problems secondary to the calcaneal hypermobility.[36]

The physiologic accessory motions of the subtalar joint occur in the frontal plane. The convex portion of the posterior calcaneus slides laterally during inversion (supination) and medially with eversion (pronation). From its neutral position the subtalar joint can supinate approximately twice as much as it can pronate. This motion is measured in the frontal plane of calcaneal inversion and eversion. The normal subtalar range of motion is approximately 30°. Gait requires 8 to 12° of supination and 4 to 6° of pronation.[33]

Midtarsal Joint

The midtarsal joint consists of the talonavicular and calcaneocuboid articulations. They derive their ligamentous support from the calcaneo-navicular (spring), deltoid, dorsal talonavicular, and calcaneocuboid (long and short plantar) ligaments.

The midtarsal joint has two separate axes. Functionally, these two

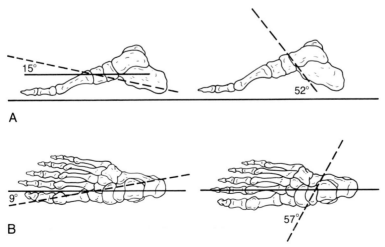

FIGURE 8−5 Axes of motion for the midtarsal joints. *A,* Longitudinal axis. *B,* Oblique axis.

axes work together to compose a triplanar motion. The two axes of the midtarsal joint are the longitudinal and the oblique. The longitudinal axis is essentially parallel to the sagittal and transverse planes, allowing only frontal plane motions of inversion and eversion, whereas the oblique axis is parallel with the frontal plane, allowing motion in the sagittal (plantar flexion–dorsiflexion) and transverse (adduction–abduction) planes (Fig. 8–5). Because the oblique axis is angulated about equally (55°) for the sagittal and transverse planes, plantar flexion–adduction and dorsiflexion–abduction are coupled equally.

From a clinical standpoint, there is no reliable method of quantifying the amount of rotation in the midtarsal joint. Midtarsal joint motion is dictated by the position of the subtalar joint. When the subtalar joint is pronated, the axes of the talocalcaneal and calcaneocuboid joints are parallel, allowing the midtarsal joint to unlock and become an adaptor with increased mobility. As the subtalar joint supinates, the midtarsal joint's motion decreases as the two axes diverge and "lock" the forefoot on the rearfoot in preparation for its rigid lever function during the propulsive phase of gait (Fig. 8–6).

The position of the midtarsal joint is dictated by ground reaction forces during the contact and midstance phases of gait and by muscular activity acting on the joint during the propulsive phase of gait.[31] The standard clinical index for determining midtarsal joint position is to compare the plantar plane position of the five metatarsal heads to the plantar plane position of the neutral rearfoot when the midtarsal joint is maximally pronated about both its axes.

Physiologic accessory motions of the midtarsal joint, which can be evaluated manually include dorsal and plantar glides of the navicular on the talus. Plantar glide accompanies supination and dorsal glide accompanies pronation.

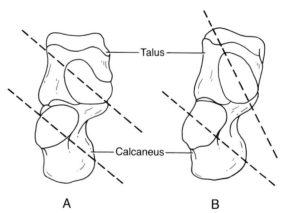

A   B

FIGURE 8–6   Axis of transverse tarsal joint. A, When calcaneus is in eversion, the conjoint axes between the talonavicular and calcaneocuboid joints are parallel to one another, so that increased motion occurs in the transverse tarsal joint. B, When the calcaneus is in inversion the axes are no longer parallel, and there is decreased motion with increased stability of the transverse tarsal joint. (Reproduced by permission from Mann, Roger A.: Biomechanics of running. In American Academy of Orthopaedic Surgeons: Symposium of the Foot and Leg in Running Sports. St. Louis, 1982, The C.V. Mosby Co.)

Tarsometatarsal, Metatarsophalangeal, and Interphalangeal Joints

The first metatarsophalangeal joint represents the articulation between the first metatarsal and the proximal phalanx of the big toe. The joint axis runs distal–lateral to proximal–medial and almost parallel to the transverse plane. Motion occurs primarily in the sagittal (plantar flexion–dorsiflexion) and frontal (inversion–eversion) planes. The axis is angulated 45° from both these planes, so for every 1° of plantar flexion there is 1° of eversion (Fig. 8–7).

First ray motion begins in the late stance phase of gait and continues late into propulsion. As with the midtarsal joint, first ray motion is controlled by the position of the subtalar joint. With the subtalar joint in pronation, the amount of first ray motion is increased. As the subtalar joint supinates, the first ray motion decreases. The normal amount of motion is 0.5 to 1 cm (thumb's width) in the plantar and dorsal directions.[31]

The clinical standard used in determining the first metatarsal's neutral position is to evaluate the first ray's position relative to the three central metatarsal heads. It should lie in the same transverse plane, neither plantar flexed nor dorsiflexed.

Minimal normal first metatarsophalangeal range of motion with the first ray stabilized is about 20 to 30° of hyperextension. Without stabilization, the first metatarsophalangeal joint should hyperextend to at least 60 to 70°.[25]

The fifth ray operates about an independent axis with the same directional orientation as the subtalar joint. The central three rays have an axis orientation parallel to the frontal and transverse planes. Consequently, there is only plantar flexion–dorsiflexion motion in the sagittal

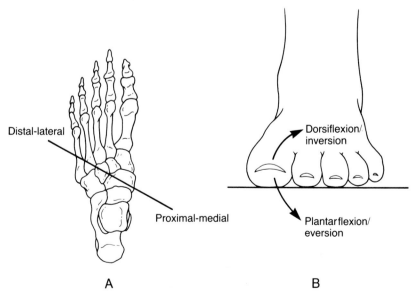

FIGURE 8–7   First ray axis and motion. *A,* First ray axis of motion, dorsal view. *B,* First ray motion.

TABLE 8–2   **LOWER LEG MUSCLE GROUPS**

Group	Muscles
Posterior superficial	Gastrocnemius, soleus, plantaris
Lateral	Peroneals
Dorsal intrinsics	Extensor hallucis brevis, extensor digitorum longus
Deep posterior	Posterior tibialis, flexor digitorum longus, flexor hallucis longus
Anterior pretibial	Anterior tibialis, extensor hallucis longus, extensor digitorum longus, peroneus tertius
Plantar intrinsics	Flexor digitorum brevis, flexor hallucis brevis, adductor and abductor hallucis, lumbricales

plane. The metatarsophalangeal joints also have an additional vertical axis, which is parallel to the frontal and sagittal planes to allow abduction and adduction of the joints.

Physiologic accessory motions of the metatarsophalangeal joints include plantar and dorsal glides. Plantar glide of the first metatarsal accompanies extension, whereas dorsal glide accompanies toe flexion.

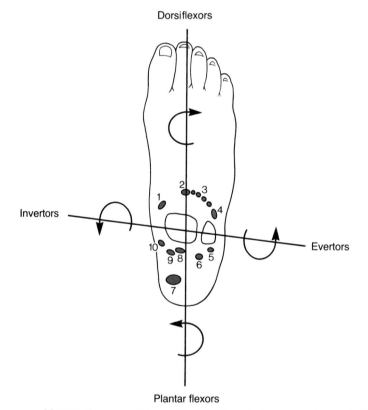

FIGURE 8–8   Motion diagram of the ankle. Tibialis anterior *(1)*, extensor hallucis longus *(2)*, extensor digitorum longus *(3)*, peroneus tertius *(4)*, peroneus brevis *(5)*, peroneus longus *(6)*, Achilles tendon *(7)*, flexor hallucis longus *(8)*, flexor digitorum longus *(9)*, tibialis posterior *(10)*. (From Magee, D.J. (1987): Orthopedic Physical Assessment. Philadelphia, W.B. Saunders.)

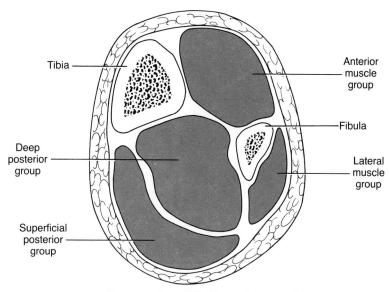

FIGURE 8–9   Cross section of the lower leg muscle groups.

MUSCULAR FUNCTION OF THE LOWER LEG, ANKLE, AND FOOT

The phasic action of the muscles of the lower leg and foot can be determined by examination of the musculotendinous unit's excursion from origin to insertion relative to the axis on which it acts (Fig. 8–8). Each muscle group has specific functions that control or provide the necessary forces to create movement. The muscles of the leg and foot can be divided into subgroups (Table 8–2; Fig. 8–9).

Posterior Superficial Muscle Group

The posterior superficial muscle group is composed of the gastrocnemius, soleus, and plantaris muscles. These muscles originate from above and below the knee joint and have a common insertion by way of the Achilles tendon on the posterior aspect of the calcaneus. In the open kinetic chain, the triceps surae provide flexion of the knee, plantar flexion of the ankle, and supination of the subtalar joint. With closed kinetic chain function, the gastrocnemius and soleus are active throughout the stance phase of gait. Initially, at heel contact, the gastrocnemius and soleus contract eccentrically to decelerate tibial internal rotation and the forward progression of the tibia over the foot. Later, during midstance and heel-off, they provide subtalar joint supination, externally rotating the tibia, and plantar flexion of the knee and ankle.

Posterior Deep Muscle Group

The posterior deep muscles of the lower leg include the posterior tibialis, flexor digitorum longus, and flexor hallucis longus. The posterior tibialis is a strong supinator and invertor of the subtalar joint that functions to control and reverse pronation during gait. It decelerates subtalar joint pronation and tibial internal rotation at heel strike, and then reverses its function to accelerate subtalar joint supination and tibial external rotation during stance. The posterior tibialis also maintains the stability of the midtarsal joint in the direction of supination around its oblique axis during the stance phase of gait.

The flexor digitorum longus functions as a supinator of the subtalar joint and flexor of the second through fifth metatarsophalangeal joints in the open kinetic chain. When the foot is in contact with the ground and the digits are stable, the flexor digitorum longus actively stabilizes the foot as a weight-bearing platform for propulsion. If the flexor digitorum longus works unopposed by the action of the intrinsic muscles, clawing of the toes results.[15]

The flexor hallucis longus has a similar function as the flexor digitorum longus in that it flexes the first metatarsophalangeal joint in the open kinetic chain. Both these long flexors help support the medial arch.

Lateral Muscle Group

The lateral muscle group includes the peroneus longus and brevis. The peroneus longus, because of its attachment to the first metatarsal and medial cuneiform on the plantar surface, functions to pronate the subtalar joint and to plantar flex and evert the first ray in the open kinetic chain. In the closed kinetic chain, the peroneus longus has many important functions. It provides support to the transverse and lateral longitudinal arches. During the latter portion of midstance and early heel-off, it actively stabilizes the first ray and everts the foot to transfer body weight from the lateral to the medial side of the foot.

The peroneus brevis is primarily an evertor in open kinetic chain motion. During gait it functions in concert with the peroneus longus. Its primary role is to stabilize the calcaneocuboid joint, allowing the peroneus longus to work efficiently over the cuboid pulley.

Anterior Muscle Group

The pretibial muscles include the anterior tibialis, extensor digitorum longus, extensor hallucis longus, and peroneus tertius. As a group they are active during the swing phase and heel contact to foot-flat phases of gait.

The anterior tibialis is primarily a dorsiflexor of the talocrural joint in open kinetic chain function. In gait, the anterior tibialis basically operates concentrically in the swing phase and eccentrically in the stance phase. At the end of toe-off, the anterior tibialis begins to contract concentrically to initiate dorsiflexion of the ankle and first ray, to assist in ground clearance at midswing, and then to supinate the foot slightly during late swing in preparation for heel contact. When the foot hits the ground, the anterior tibialis reverses its role to decelerate or control plantar flexion to foot-flat, prevent excessive pronation, and supinate the midtarsal joint's longitudinal axis. A weak anterior tibialis can lead to "foot-slap," or uncontrolled pronation in gait.

In nonweight-bearing function, the long extensors (extensor digitorum and hallucis longus) provide dorsiflexion of the ankle and extension of the toes. Because these tendons pass laterally to the subtalar joint axis, unlike the anterior tibialis, they provide a pronatory force at the joint. In fact, a prime responsibility of the long extensors is to hold the oblique axis of the midtarsal joint in a pronated position at heel strike and then assist the controlled deceleration of plantar flexion to foot-flat.

Intrinsic Muscle Group

Generally, the intrinsic muscles of the foot act together during most of the stance phase gait. Their function is to stabilize the midtarsal joint and digits while keeping the toes flat on the ground until lift-off. An unstable, pronated midtarsal joint during midstance necessitates that the intrinsics work harder and longer. This phenomenon explains the common complaint of "foot fatigue" in the athlete with a hypermobile foot.

ANTHROPOMETRIC ASSESSMENT

Anthropometric measurements of the leg, foot, and ankle provide objective evidence of effusion. Many techniques can be reliable. Volumetric displacement methods with submersion of the foot into a calibrated tank are highly reliable and easily performed. Other methods include girth assessments at selected sites using figure-eight and heel lock tape measurement techniques (Fig. 8–10A and B). Comparison to the uninvolved side is always appropriate.

Determination of Subtalar Joint, Neutral Position

To assess inversion–eversion motion of the ankle, the clinician must first identify the subtalar neutral position. This can be found through palpa-

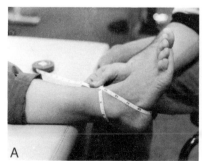 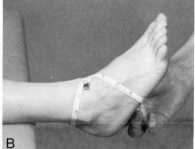

FIGURE 8–10   Ankle girth assessment. *A*, Heel lock method. *B*, Figure-eight method.

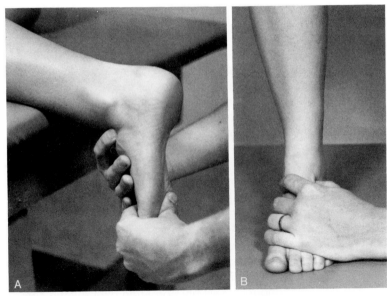

FIGURE 8–11 Subtalar neutral position. *A,* Nonweight-bearing palpation. *B,* Closed chain palpation.

tion techniques of the head of the talus as it articulates with the navicular. When the subtalar joint is pronated or supinated, the head of the talus is palpable medially or laterally. While loading the fourth and fifth metatarsal heads to pronate the forefoot to tissue resistance, the calcaneus is inverted and everted. When the subtalar joint is supinated the medial side of the talus disappears and the lateral aspect of the talus becomes prominent. The reverse is true when the subtalar is pronated. The neutral position is defined as that point where there is talonavicular congruency and neither the medial nor lateral aspects of the talus are palpable or their protrusion is symmetric. This technique can be used in a closed or open chain assessment (Fig. 8–11*A* and *B*). In a weight-

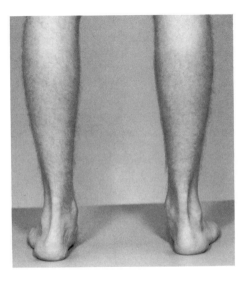

FIGURE 8–12 Pronated subtalar position with accentuated inferior curve.

bearing position, an easy visual assessment is to observe for equal concavities above and below the lateral malleolus.[31] A shallow curve superiorly and an accentuated curve inferiorly would suggest a pronated subtalar joint (Fig. 8–12).

Subtalar Range of Motion

Once the subtalar joint's neutral position has been established, calcaneal inversion–eversion range-of-motion assessment can take place. Initially, the subtalar joint's neutral position is objectively quantified through goniometric measurement. Normal is considered 2 to 3° of varus. The goniometer's arms are aligned with the longitudinal midline of the posterior calcaneus and the posterior bisection of the tibia (Fig. 8–13). Care must be taken to disregard the Achilles tendon and calcaneal fat pads, because they may produce unreliable measurements. Readings are recorded following maximal passive calcaneal inversion and eversion (Fig. 8–14A and B). Inversion and eversion amounts of motion are then determined based on the initial neutral position. Differences may be noted, depending on whether this assessment was performed in a weight-bearing or nonweight-bearing posture. Lattanza and colleagues[24] have found an average 37% increase in subtalar eversion as a component of pronation when measured in the closed chain weight-bearing posture as compared to the traditional nonweight-bearing position.

Plantar Flexion–Dorsiflexion Range of Motion

Ankle dorsiflexion range of motion must be assessed while maintaining the subtalar joint in a neutral position. If the subtalar joint is not monitored, pronator substitution may provide an inaccurate portrayal of

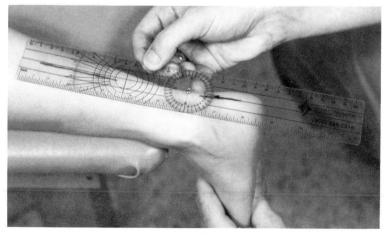

FIGURE 8–13 Measurement of subtalar neutral position.

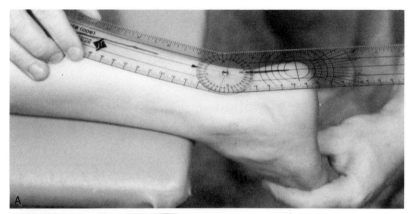

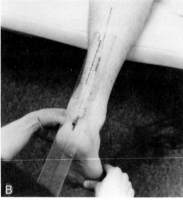

FIGURE 8–14   Measurement of subtalar calcaneal ranges of motion. *A*, Inversion. *B*, Eversion.

gastrocnemius–soleus flexibility. When the subtalar joint is pronated, midtarsal mobility is increased and dorsiflexion of the foot can occur around the oblique axis of the midtarsal joint.

A minimum of 10° dorsiflexion is needed at heel-off to allow for normal ambulation.[4] Because the knee joint is fully extended at this point in the gait cycle, the two-joint gastrocnemius muscle is fully stretched over both joints. Consequently, the knee should be placed in full extension when evaluating the range of dorsiflexion excursion available in gait. To differentiate soleus extensibility, dorsiflexion range of motion is assessed in a knee-flexed posture so that the gastrocnemius is slack. An increase of 10° dorsiflexion to a total of 20° is anticipated.

To measure ankle dorsiflexion range of motion, the athlete is placed in a prone position with the ankle extended off the end of the table. The clinician then palpates and establishes the subtalar neutral position. The distal arm of the goniometer is placed parallel with the lateral aspect of the calcaneus and the fifth metatarsal head, while the proximal arm is aligned with the bisection of the lateral aspect of the lower leg and the head of the fibula. The clinician then passively forces dorsiflexion while the athlete is actively assisting (Fig. 8–15). This active assistance provides reciprocal inhibition of the passive tension stored in the triceps surae group. Pronator substitution tendencies are manifested by calcaneal eversion. Calcaneal stabilization may have to be provided manually. This procedure should be performed with the knee

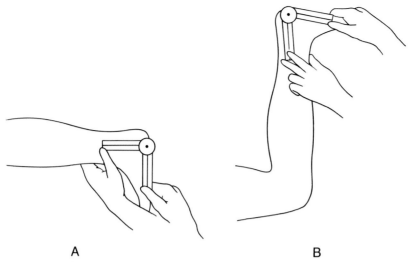

FIGURE 8–15   Goniometric assessment of ankle dorsiflexion range of motion. *A*, Knee extended. *B*, Knee flexed.

extended and flexed. If the dorsiflexion range is equal in the flexed and extended postures, ankle equinus (bony block caused by osseous lipping in the anterior ankle joint) or soleus equinus should be suspected.[4]

Plantar flexion range of motion is expected to be 50 to 60° degrees and is assessed with similar goniometric placement techniques.

Subtalar Joint Position

Subtalar joint position is determined by comparing the orientation of the calcaneus relative to the distal third of the leg when placed in its

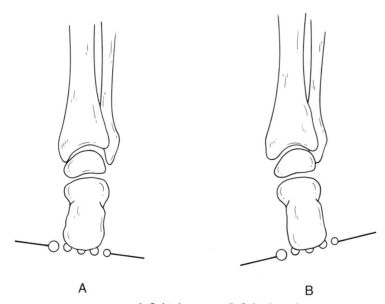

FIGURE 8–16   *A*, Subtalar varus. *B*, Subtalar valgus.

neutral position. Subtalar joint varus is defined as an inverted calcaneus when compared to the posterior bisection of the tibia in the nonweight-bearing position (Fig. 8–16A). Subtalar valgus is the opposite situation in which the calcaneus is everted relative to the tibia (Fig. 8–16B). Rearfoot varus and valgus are terms used to describe calcaneal position relative to the supporting surface. When the calcaneus is inverted relative to the floor and the subtalar joint is in neutral, the posture is defined as rearfoot varus. Rearfoot valgus then describes a weight-bearing position of calcaneal eversion relative to the supporting surface when the subtalar joint is in neutral.

In identifying an athlete's foot type it is important to evaluate the feet in their position of function. The neutral and resting calcaneal stance positions are accurate reflections of the way the lower extremity's kinetic chain interfaces with the supporting surfaces. The neutral calcaneal stance position is the angular relationship of the calcaneus and the ground with the subtalar joint in neutral. As described previously, this may be called a rearfoot varus or valgus posture. Resting calcaneal stance position is this same angular relationship in natural stance, where compensation for deviations are allowed.

Assessment is made by placing the athlete in his or her angle and base of gait and measuring this relationship by placing one arm of a goniometer parallel to the ground and the other aligned with the posterior calcaneal bisection. Measurements are made in subtalar neutral and natural relaxed stances. Ideally, these values should be the same. The diagnostic hallmark of a rearfoot varus is an inverted neutral calcaneal stance position.[31] Compensation for these deformities depends on the availability of the subtalar range of motion. Rearfoot varus is considered fully compensated if the subtalar joint allows enough calcaneal eversion to reach a perpendicular position to the floor, where

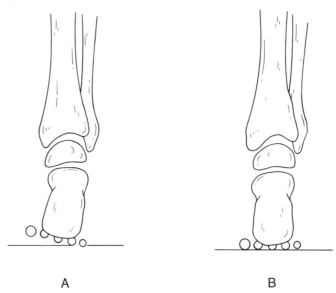

A   B

FIGURE 8–17   Rearfoot varus. *A*, Inverted calcaneus. *B*, Compensation accomplished by calcaneal eversion in natural resting stance.

forces across the heel and forefoot are equilibrated (Fig. 8–17). Uncompensated rearfoot varus is having an inverted calcaneus in the neutral calcaneal stance position and less inversion in the resting or relaxed calcaneal stance position.

Midtarsal Joint Position

Midtarsal position and foot type are determined by comparison to the subtalar joint. Forefoot varus is a structural abnormality in which the plantar plane of the forefoot is inverted relative to the plantar plane of the rearfoot, with the subtalar joint in its neutral position and the forefoot maximally pronated around both its midtarsal joint axes (Fig. 8–18A). Forefoot valgus is the opposite of forefoot varus in that the

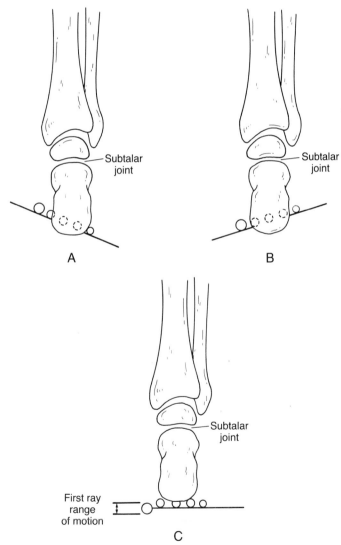

FIGURE 8–18   A, Forefoot varus, inverted forefoot. B, Forefoot valgus, everted forefoot. C, Plantar flexed first ray.

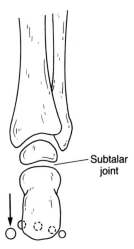

Subtalar
joint

FIGURE 8–19   Forefoot supinatus: supinated forefoot with plantar flexed first ray.

forefoot is everted relative to the rearfoot (Fig. 8–18B). An additional requirement for defining forefoot valgus is that the foot has a first ray that has normal range of motion. This differentiates forefoot valgus from a plantar flexed first ray. Often, the presence of a plantar flexed first ray gives the appearance of a forefoot valgus but can be differentiated by decreased range of motion associated with this deformity. A plantar flexed first ray shows more plantar flexion than dorsiflexion range of motion (Fig. 8–18C).

Forefoot supinatus is a relatively fixed, acquired soft tissue deformity that typically occurs in athletes whose calcaneus is maintained in an everted position. The forefoot is supinated in relation to the rearfoot because of soft tissue adaptation, and the total midtarsal range of motion is reduced. The compensatory mechanism is the plantar flexed attitude of the first ray to bring the medial forefoot in contact with the ground (Fig. 8–19).

While assessing midtarsal foot type it is important to assess the quality and quantity of midtarsal motion subjectively. Passive assessment with manual techniques can identify the relative amounts of plantar flexion–dorsiflexion and abduction–adduction around the oblique axis and inversion–eversion of the longitudinal axis. Motion should be maximal with the subtalar joint held in pronation, and should decrease as the subtalar joint is placed in a supinated position.

Postural Considerations

Tibial Varum

Tibial varum is a structural deformity in which the distal tibia is closer to the midline than the proximal tibia. Its determination quantifies the amount of frontal plane deviation of the tibia. Assessment is made with the athlete bearing weight on the measured extremity in its angle and base of gait. The goniometer is placed with one arm parallel to the ground and the other parallel with the posterior bisection of the distal tibia (Fig. 8–20). The presence of tibial varum contributes to the total varus attitude of the lower extremity.

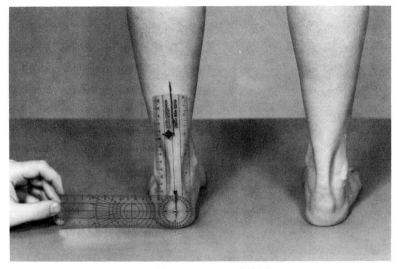

FIGURE 8–20   Measurement of tibial varum.

Tibial Torsion

To evaluate for tibial torsion, the clinician aligns the patient's legs straight so that the femoral condyles are in the transverse plane and the patella faces straight up. The clinician then assesses the amount of torsion by measuring the angle of the malleoli relative to the shaft of the tibia. The normal value is considered to be approximately 13 to 18° of external tibial torsion (Fig. 8–21).

FUNCTIONAL RELATIONSHIPS

The entire kinetic chain is intimately linked together with every movement in sport. Each segment of the body depends on the role and function of adjoining and distant structures. A prime example of this interdependence is displayed in overground ambulation. The following

FIGURE 8–21   Measurement of tibial torsion.

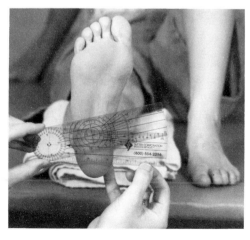

is a description of "normal" gait. Normal gait is a difficult entity to quantify, but this description can serve as a basis by which to evaluate a potentially pathologic type of movement.

Normal Gait

At heel strike, the ankle is in a neutral position and then plantar flexes to foot-flat under the eccentric control of the pretibial muscles. The subtalar and midtarsal joints are supinated at heel contact and begin the process of pronation to unlock the midtarsal joint, which allows foot adaptation to the terrain. At the knee joint, the tibia follows the directional input of the subtalar joint by internally rotating and flexing. Normal subtalar pronation during this phase of gait is a passive activity in the closed kinetic chain that directs movement and attenuates ground reaction forces.[11]

During midstance, from foot-flat to heel-off, the subtalar joint undergoes supination as the body weight shifts anterior to the weight-bearing extremity. The ankle joint is moving into its extreme of dorsiflexion. The supination movement of the subtalar joint dictates that the tibia rotate externally and allow the knee to reach full extension at the end of midstance. The posterior calf muscles eccentrically control the early pronation and concentrically shorten as the foot moves into supination. During this phase the foot reverses function from that of a mobile adaptor to a rigid lever.

Propulsion from heel-off to toe-off shows the ankle joint plantar flexing while the midtarsal joint is locking on the supinating subtalar joint. This process prepares the foot for its role as a stable platform from which to push off. The metatarsophalangeal joints extend while the knee joint flexes in preparation for the swing phase of gait.

Swing phase motion requires flexion of the knee and dorsiflexion of the ankle to provide ground clearance. The subtalar joint initially pronates in early swing to shorten the limb and assist in ground clearance. It then supinates in terminal swing to prepare for heel contact on the next step (Table 8–3, Fig. 8–22).

Dynamic Gait Assessment

Whereas assessment of lower quarter injuries with the athlete in a static posture is the benchmark for evaluation, dynamic assessment of movement patterns offers the most valid means for determining the athlete's functional ability. Assessment of gait should be incorporated into all evaluations of the lower extremity. This can be performed in any setting, but the availability of a treadmill greatly enhances the convenience of analysis.

Brandel and Williams[3] have demonstrated a statistically insignificant difference in stride length, velocity, and cadence with treadmill analysis of gait versus normal walking at 2.5 to 3.2 miles per hour. The use of a treadmill also allows easy control of gait speeds and inclination. With the recently developed vidoetape recording technology an objec-

TABLE 8-3 **NORMAL GAIT CYCLE**

	Stance Phase			Swing Phase		
	HEEL CONTACT	FOOT-FLAT	HEEL-OFF	TOE-OFF		
Joint	*Forefoot Loading*	*Midstance*	*Propulsion*	*Early Swing*	*Midswing*	*Terminal Swing*
Tibiofemoral Position	Extended → Mildly flexed →		Extended →		Maximally flexed	
Motion	Flexion, tibial internal rotation	Extension, tibial external rotation	Flexion		Extension	
Talocrural Position	Neutral → Maximally plantar flexed →		Maximally dorsiflexed →	Plantar flexed → Neutral → Dorsiflexed		
Motion	Plantar flexion	Dorsiflexion	Very rapid plantar flexion		Dorsiflexion	
Subtalar Position	Mildly supinated →	Fully pronated →	Mildly supinated →	Fully supinated		
Motion	Pronation	Supination		Pronation		Supination
Midtarsal	Everted → Unlocking to adapt	Inverted, Locking as rigid lever				
	0%	15%	30%	45%	60%	100%

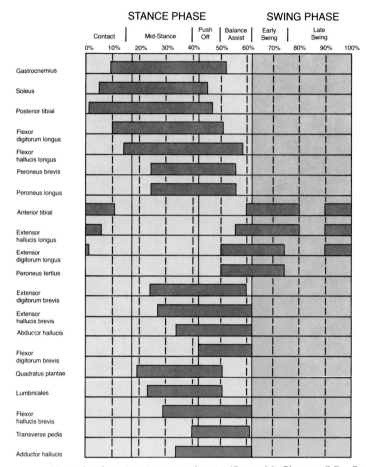

FIGURE 8-22 Muscular function in normal gait. (From McGlamry, E.D.: Fundamentals of Foot Surgery. © 1987, The Williams & Wilkins Co., Baltimore.)

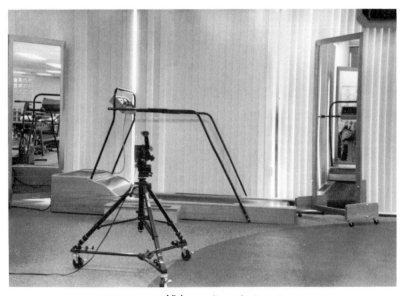

FIGURE 8-23 Video gait analysis setup.

TABLE 8–4   RECOGNITION OF SUBTALAR JOINT POSITION

View	Pronation	Supination
Posterior	Calcaneal inversion; lateral calcaneal indentation concave to midline	Calcaneal eversion; lateral calcaneal indentation convex to midline
Anterior	Internal rotation of tibia	External rotation of tibia
Lateral	Talar head adducts and plantar flexes, causing medial bulging	Medial longitudinal arch heightens

tive documentation of function is produced, and the tape can be slowed down for careful analysis. A simple clinical set-up requires only single positioning of the camera to allow anterior, posterior, and lateral views to be videotaped with the assistance of postural mirrors (Fig. 8–23).

General observations of gait should include head placement, shoulder height and position, arm swing and carry, cadence, step–stride length, weight acceptance, and single-limb stance stability. With a knowledge of normal gait mechanics, joint position and motion in the different phases of the gait cycle can be compared against expected norms. Hypotheses are then generated concerning the source of deviations and correlated with static evaluation findings. Even some of the most subtle weaknesses, inflexibilities, and postural asymmetries can be detected with this method of evaluation. Points of observation for recognizing subtalar joint position during videotape analysis of gait are presented in Table 8–4.

Pathologic Gait

Common Pronatory Disorders

By having the foot function as a rigid lever during propulsion, the weight of the body is propelled off that limb with maximum efficiency. If the subtalar joint cannot reach the neutral position, heading toward a supinated position just prior to heel-off, an unstable base of support is used for propulsion. If a condition does not allow the forefoot to lock on the rearfoot, a situation exists that is analogous to walking in sand, in which the base of support gives way under push-off forces. It takes significantly more muscle energy to push off such unstable platforms, resulting in foot and leg fatigue secondary to overuse.

It must be appreciated that pronation is a normal and necessary component of gait. Only when the amount, timing, or sequence of the pronation–supination cycle is altered is it considered abnormal.[16] An athlete with rearfoot varus demonstrates this during midstance and, as a result, can have abnormal hypermobility and shearing forces within the foot. As can be seen in Figure 8–24, the athlete with rearfoot varus does obtain some supination in propulsion but the subtalar joint is still in a pronated posture at the initiation of heel-off.

Forefoot varus is another condition that is compensated for by abnormal pronation of the subtalar joint. The subtalar joint remains pronated throughout the stance phase of gait to allow ground contact

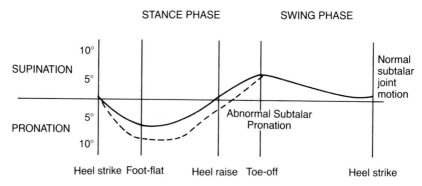

FIGURE 8–24   Graphic representation of subtalar joint motion in rearfoot varus.

on the medial forefoot and creates an apropulsive method of ambulation (Fig. 8–25).

Abnormal pronation can also be caused by factors and forces extrinsic to the foot. Flexibility deficiencies, postural deviations, and muscular weaknesses can all alter the normal pronation–supination sequence extrinsically.[37] Equinus deformities caused by a tight gastrocnemius and/or soleus tend to cause a massive subtalar joint pronation just before propulsion begins.[31] A tight Achilles complex either causes early heel-off or prolonged subtalar joint pronation to compensate for the lack of adequate talocrural dorsiflexion range of motion. In both cases the subtalar joint has not supinated to neutral prior to heel-off.

Proximal inflexibilities, such as tight medial hamstrings, which shorten stride length or affect lower extremity external rotation during swing phase, are other examples of extrinsically induced abnormal pronation.[37] These inflexibilities do not allow enough time for full resupination of the subtalar joint during the late swing phase in its preparation for heel strike.

Postural deviations such as leg length discrepancies are a final example of abnormal pronation brought on by external causes. Subtalar pronation is a method by which leg length can be shortened in the closed kinetic chain.[23] Although this chapter deals with lower leg and foot pathology, it is important to note that dysfunction may originate proximal to the structure in which it is manifested.

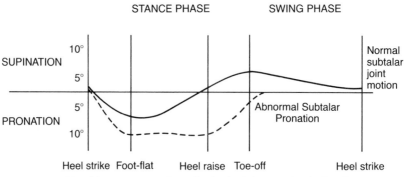

FIGURE 8–25   Graphic representation of subtalar joint motion in forefoot varus.

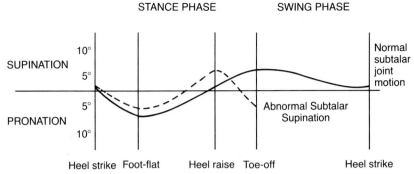

FIGURE 8–26 Graphic representation of subtalar joint motion in forefoot valgus or rigid plantar flexed first ray.

Supinatory Disorders

Abnormal supination in gait is a less common occurrence than abnormal pronation but is seen in athletes who have forefoot valgus or a rigid, plantar flexed first ray. Supinatory compensation is first found at the longitudinal axis of the midtarsal joint and then at the subtalar joint.[31] Rapid supination in midstance to bring the lateral side of the foot to the floor creates lateral instability of the ankle, making the athlete prone to inversion injuries. As can be seen in Figure 8–26, rapid supination alters the timing sequence of normal subtalar motion and the joint pronates late in propulsion.

LOWER LEG, ANKLE, AND FOOT INJURIES AND THEIR MANAGEMENT

Lower Leg Injuries

Tibiofibular Synostosis

Tibiofibular synostosis is a condition in which there is ossification of the interosseous membrane between the tibia and fibula at the inferior tibiofibular syndesmosis. The injury can occur because of a single inversion–internal rotation trauma or from recurrent, less severe episodes in which the anterior and posterior inferior tibiofibular ligaments and the interosseous membrane are damaged. Resultant spreading of the tibia and fibula allows bone formation from the periosteal insertions in the form of a flat exostosis or a synostosis which occurs proximally along the interosseous membrane.[14]

The athlete's chief complaint is that of difficulty in performing movements that require pivoting or cutting, and there is a sense of spasm and instability at the ankle joint. This injury should be suspected whenever an athlete cannot recover from an "ankle sprain" and remains symptomatic longer than usual.

Conservative management includes treatment of the initial injury with ice, compression, and rest. Rehabilitation is aimed at restoring normal joint stability. If there are continued complaints of pain and instability, a surgical synovectomy is indicated when the bone is mature to reduce risk of recurrence.

Achilles Tendon Rupture

The Achilles tendon complex is prone to injury if there is a sudden and powerful eccentric contraction of the gastrocnemius–soleus muscles (considered together as the triceps surae). This mechanism is best demonstrated in jumping and landing activities, in which the knee is extending while the ankle is dorsiflexing eccentrically. The tendon usually ruptures at a point just proximal to the calcaneus (Fig. 8–27). Vascular impairment, nonspecific degeneration leading to tissue necrosis, and the use of injectable corticosteroids may all weaken this area and predispose it to injury.

The athlete reports an audible snap and the sensation of being kicked in the leg. Immediate plantar flexion weakness and pain, swelling, and a palpable defect are usually present. The diagnosis is confirmed with a positive Thompson test, in which the athlete is in the prone position, with the knee flexed and the foot relaxed. A firm squeeze to the calf should produce calcaneal plantar flexion. A positive result is when there is no movement of the foot.

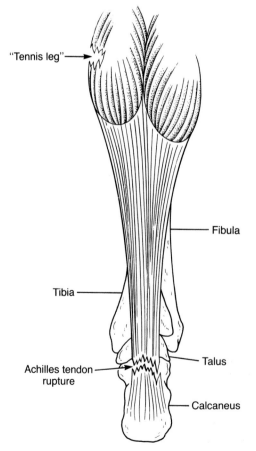

FIGURE 8–27 Tennis leg and Achilles tendon injury.

"Tennis leg"

Fibula

Tibia

Achilles tendon rupture

Talus

Calcaneus

Acute care consists of ice application, with the ankle immobilized in slight plantar flexion. A nonweight-bearing crutch gait should be used until a definitive diagnosis regarding the severity of injury has been made. Table 8–5 provides a treatment rationale for lesions of the triceps surae mechanism. Postsurgical or closed, nonsurgical care of complete ruptures usually requires 4 to 8 weeks of cast immobilization. Protected arc, active plantar flexion range-of-motion activities may be started as early as 4 weeks postinjury. This allows collagen fibers to lay down along the line of stress. A 1-inch heel lift is used when weight-bearing is allowed and is gradually decreased as the dorsiflexion range of motion improves.

Tennis Leg

Previously thought to be a tear of the plantaris muscle, "tennis leg" has now been proved through surgical exploration to be a musculotendinous lesion of the medial gastrocnemius head (Fig. 8–27).[27] The usual mechanism of injury is sudden extension of the knee with the foot in a dorsiflexed position. This places a tremendous tensile stress on the two-joint expansion of the gastrocnemius. Middle-aged athletes or those with previous degenerative changes in this area may be predisposed to this type of trauma.

The athlete feels a sudden, sharp twinge in the upper medial calf and immediately has difficulty in full weight-bearing. Typically, there is rapid swelling and ecchymosis, with point tenderness or a palpable defect at the site of the lesion.

Acute care consists of immediate first aid measures, including ice, compression, and elevation to the injured area. The ankle is placed in mild plantar flexion to alleviate stress on the area of injury. A nonweight-bearing crutch gait may be necessary, depending on the severity of the injury.

Gradual, gentle static stretching is initiated early in the subacute phase to align the healing scar tissue. Friction massage to the area also prevents random alignment of collagen fibers. As the athlete progresses to full weight-bearing, heel lifts can be used in the shoe to protect against weight-bearing stresses. As Achilles tendon flexibility improves, the height of the lifts can be gradually reduced. Table 8–5 presents further details about the rehabilitation progression of Achilles tendon-related pathology.

Tendinopathies

Tendinous lesions of the muscles of the lower leg frequently occur in athletes involved in activities of a repetitive nature. Microtraumatic damage caused by overuse, fatigue, or biomechanical abnormalities may be manifested by an inflammatory reaction of these tendons.

Achilles Tendinitis

The Achilles tendon is the common tendon of the gastrocnemius and soleus muscles. It inserts into the posterosuperior aspect of the cal-

Text continued on page 228

TABLE 8–5 GASTROCNEMIUS AND SOLEUS REHABILITATION AND TREATMENT

Parameter	Phase			
	IMMEDIATE (ACUTE)	POSTIMMOBILIZATION (SUBACUTE)	TERMINAL (CHRONIC)	RETURN TO ACTIVITY (FUNCTIONAL)
Goal	Rest; control inflammation and pain; promote healing while creating "flexible" scar tissue	Rehabilitation of gastrocnemius–soleus musculotendinous unit: Increase ROM Increase muscle contractile cabability	Increase musculotendinous tensile strength; modify, correct, or control abnormal biomechanics	Preparation and training for specific sport or activity
Modalities	Ice, compression, and elevation; oral anti-inflammatories; high voltage galvanic stimulator in "shortened" position	Heat application prior to treatment; ice application following treatment; ultrasound—continuous, pulsed	Heat prior to treatment; ice following treatment; iontophoresis or phonophoresis if prolonged or chronic inflammation; deep transverse friction massage to improve gliding function between tissue planes	Modality sequence: 1. Passive-active tissue and systemic warm-up 2. Static stretching 3. Activity or exercise 4. Stretch again 5. Cool down 6. Cryotherapy
Range of motion, flexibility	Immobilization or pain-free ROM, dependent on type and severity of damage	Pain-free AROM progressing to temperature-assisted, low-intensity, static stretching of gastrocnemius and soleus; intensity or appropriateness dictated by type of pathology: Knee straight and bent towel stretches Wall leans	Temperature-assisted, prolonged duration, low-intensity, static stretching on incline or slant board	Assess capability, tolerance, and response to mildly ballistic stretching techniques

Triceps surae exercise rationale	These exercises may have to be delayed up to 6–8 weeks in the case of surgically repaired or conservatively managed complete ruptures; isometrics progressing from submaximal to maximal intensity in protected ranges (knee flexed and/or ankle in plantar flexion)	Submaximal to maximal effort plantar flexion isokinetics in protected ranges progressing to submaximal to maximal effort plantar flexion in full arc of motion (working at highest speeds attainable and decreasing speed through velocity spectrum as comfortably tolerated)	Eccentric heel drops in gravity eliminated position progressing to eccentric isotonic heel drops in standing, foot-flat posture progressing to eccentric isotonic heel drops in standing, forefoot elevated position (speed of eccentric contraction increases as symptoms allow)	Toe walking; hopping on toes; sports-specific training—heel raises in position of forward trunk lean; plyometric drills: multiple jumps and hops, in-depth jumps and box drills
Closed chain, proprioceptive exercise	BAPS in nonweight-bearing positions, if not immobilized	BAPS in partial to full weight-bearing with increasing levels of ROM difficulty	BAPS board in full weight-bearing with overload posteriorly	Balance boards
Complementary exercise	Hip–knee–trunk strengthening and conditioning activities	Dorsiflexion, inversion, and eversion strengthening in pain-free ranges; intrinsic exercise	Lower extremity stretching and continuance of previous phases' activities	Ensure normal plantar flexion to dorsiflexion strength ratios—3–4:1 at slow speeds of contraction
Alternative conditioning	Upper body ergometer	Pool running with flotation device	Pool running in chest to waist-deep water; cycling; stationary cross-country skiing with heel wedge	Stationary cross-country skiing at increasing levels of inclination
Activity modifications and education	Controlled immobilization and rest, as necessary	Progression of ambulation from non- to partial to full weight-bearing; trial of low-amplitude rebounder running	Flat training surfaces only, avoiding hilly and cambered terrains or muddy surfaces	Careful increases in training regimen; not increasing by more than 5% per week in intensity, frequency, or duration
Assistive devices, orthotics	Crutches as necessary; weight-bearing status dictated by severity of pathology	Sorbathane–PPT heel lift insert reduces stress on Achilles tendon and decrease ground reaction forces	Orthotic insert to control any excessive, abnormal compensatory pronation	Orthotic and/or Achilles tendon taping techniques

TABLE 8–6 LOWER LEG TENDINOPATHY TREATMENT

Parameter	Phase			
	IMMEDIATE (ACUTE)	INTERMEDIATE (SUBACUTE)	TERMINAL (CHRONIC)	RETURN TO ACTIVITY (FUNCTIONAL)
Goal	Rest; control inflammation and pain; promote healing while creating "flexible" scar tissue	Rehabilitation of musculotendinous unit: Increase ROM Increase muscle contractile capability	Increase musculotendinous tensile strength; modify, correct, or control abnormal biomechanics	Preparation and training for specific sport or activity
Modalities	Ice massage; oral anti-inflammatories; gentle transverse friction massage to prevent adhesion formation	Heat prior to treatment; ice following treatment; ultrasound—pulsed, continuous; myofascial techniques to muscle belly: J stroking, kneading, cross-hand lateral shear	Heat prior to treatment; ice following treatment; iontophoresis, phonophoresis; deep transverse friction massage to improve gliding function between tissue planes	Modality sequence: 1. Passive-active tissue and systemic warm-up 2. Static stretching 3. Activity or exercise 4. Stretch again—mildly ballistic 5. Cool down 6. Cryotherapy
Range of motion, flexibility	Pain-free active range of motion	Temperature-assisted, prolonged duration, low-intensity, static stretching of antagonist	Low-intensity, static stretching of involved musculotendinous unit	Assess capability, tolerance, and response to ballistic motion of involved tissue
Exercise rationale	Isometrics	Submaximal to maximal effort isokinetics in progressively larger arcs	Eccentric exercise at increasing speeds of contraction, as tolerated	Functional rehabilitation: toe and heel walking; inversion board

Closed chain, proprioceptive rehabilitation	BAPS board in nonweight-bearing positions	of motion; concentric isokinetic contractions at highest attainable speeds in a velocity spectrum to minimize tensile stress early in this phase	by tissue symptomatic response	ambulation; hopping and bounding; sports-specific training
		BAPS board in partial to full weight-bearing with increasing levels of range-of-motion difficulty	BAPS board in full-weight bearing with resistance overload to appropriate muscle groups	Balance boards
Complementary exercise	Hip–knee–trunk strengthening and conditioning activities	Exercise of foot intrinsic musculature	Lower extremity stretching and continuance of previous phases' activities	Ensure normal agonist–antagonist strength ratios and muscle balance
Alternative conditioning	UBE	Pool running with assistance of flotation device	Pool running in chest to waist-deep water; stationary recumbent cycling	Stationary cross-country skiing
Activity modification, education	Controlled immobilization and rest, as necessary; examine athletic shoes, training surfaces, and training regimens	Trial of low-amplitude, rebound running	Flat training surfaces only, avoiding hilly and cambered terrains or muddy surfaces	Careful increases in training regimens; not increasing program by more than 5% per week in intensity, duration, or frequency
Assistive devices, orthotics	Heel lift, if appropriate	Viscoelastic inserts to decrease ground reaction forces (especially in rigid cavus feet)	Orthotic insert to control any excessive or abnormal compensatory subtalar joint motion	Orthotic and/or taping techniques

caneus and is a frequent site of pathology in competitive and recreational athletes.[6, 18] It is surrounded by the paratenon, which functions as an elastic sleeve that envelops the tendon and allows free movement against surrounding tissues. In areas in which the tendon passes over zones of potential pressure and friction, the paratenon is replaced by a synovial sheath or bursa.[7]

The major blood supply to the Achilles tendon is provided through the paratenon. An area of reduced vascularity is found 2 to 6 cm proximal to the insertion.[32] This region of relative avascularity may play an etiologic role in the frequent onset of symptoms at this level.[32]

Although an Achilles tendon overuse injury is a common problem, the nomenclature used to identify these injuries is often confusing. Classification is based on whether the Achilles tendon itself or the peritendinous tissue that surrounds it is involved. Achilles tendinitis is defined as disruptive lesions within the substance of the tendon itself, whereas peritendinitis involves inflammation in the paratenon.[7] These conditions could occur simultaneously or in isolation.

The onset of Achilles tendinitis and/or peritendinitis is usually gradual and insidious, although some precipitating factor may be identified. The athlete complains of a dull, aching pain during or after activity. On physical examination, slight edema or tendon thickening may be present. Point tenderness is usually elicited 2 to 3 cm proximal to the calcaneal attachment. Because this is a contractile lesion, pain usually increases with passive dorsiflexion and resisted plantar flexion.[9] Crepitation may be noted in plantar flexion movements in the subacute and chronic stages.[21]

Table 8–6 presents a suggested rationale for the conservative management and treatment of tendinitis and peritendinitis. The four stages of injury define potential entry points into the treatment system. An athlete could initially be seen at any one of these stages. Progression from one stage to the next is variable and is dictated by time, symptoms, and the individual athlete's response.

As is usually true, the best treatment for microtraumatic injuries such as Achilles tendinitis is prevention of onset. The frequency and/or severity of inflammatory Achilles injuries may be reduced if some suggested guidelines are followed:

1. Select appropriate footwear. The athletic shoe should have a firm, notched heel counter to decrease tendon irritation and control rearfoot motion. The midsole should have a moderate heel flare, provide adequate wedging, and allow flexibility in the forefoot. It is also important to maintain a relatively consistent heel height in all shoes worn during the day.
2. Avoid training errors. Achilles tendon microtrauma can be induced extrinsically because of training errors. Steady, gradual increases of no more than 5 to 10%/week in training mileage and speed on appropriate terrains should be emphasized. Use of cross-training principles may also reduce cumulative stresses on the Achilles tendon.
3. Ensure gastrocnemius–soleus flexibility. The talocrural joint should have 10° of dorsiflexion with the knee joint extended

and 20° with the knee flexed. Normal gait requires 10° of dorsiflexion just prior to heel-off, when the subtalar joint is in neutral and the knee is extending in stance phase.[4]

4. Control pronation forces. Abnormal compensatory pronation forces can cause a whipping or bowstring effect on the medial edge of the Achilles tendon. Orthotic correction may be indicated if this abnormal pronation is of intrinsic origin.[7]

5. Ensure adequate strength. The triceps surae musculotendinous unit must have adequate concentric and eccentric contractile capabilities. This includes dynamic symmetry in bilateral comparisons and appropriate balance with its ipsilateral antagonist. A plantar flexion to dorsiflexion ratio of 3:1 or 4:1 has been suggested for slow isokinetic speeds of contraction.[12]

6. Carry out postural screening for biomechanical malalignments. This may detect any abnormalities that could adversely affect the kinetic chain and increase stress on the Achilles tendon. Such conditions include leg length discrepancies, cavus foot resulting from metatarsal forefoot equinus, ankle equinus, tibial varum, and rotational influences of the femur or tibia.[4]

Anterior Tibialis Tendinitis

An inflammatory response of the anterior tibialis tendon occurs when it cannot absorb deceleration forces in the heel strike to foot-flat phase of gait. Uncontrolled or excessive pronation following heel strike stretches the anterior tibialis as it attempts to control the speed of forefoot loading.

Conditions that predispose the anterior tibialis to overuse usually include training errors and physical abnormalities. Frequently, the combination of excessive extrinsic forces placed on intrinsic abnormalities produces stresses that cannot be dissipated or tolerated by the athlete. Extrinsic factors include dramatic increases in mileage, overstriding, and excessive hill running, which can all cause fatigue and injury. The athlete with a tight Achilles complex requires increased muscular output of the anterior tibialis to overcome the inherent posterior tautness. This condition is then magnified with uphill running, which necessitates full dorsiflexion range of motion. In downhill running, increased eccentric forces are necessary to control forefoot loading over an increased range of motion. If the anterior tibialis has undergone adaptive shortening in response to chronic hyperpronation, the musculotendinous unit cannot provide the necessary range of motion and absorption of tensile forces needed during the early stance phase.

This injury is characterized by pain and swelling over the dorsum of the foot. Crepitation along the tendon or where it inserts onto the navicular may be present. Examination reveals pain with stretching into the extremes of plantar flexion and pronation, and pain-inhibited weakness with manual muscle testing of anterior tibialis function.

Table 8–6 summarizes the treatment rationale for lower leg tendinopathies. Prime consideration should be given to correcting soft tissue imbalances, improving eccentric muscular capabilities, and selecting appropriate footwear. Shoe selection should focus on midsole materials that attenuate shock and accommodate orthotic additions. A heel lift may be used for the athlete with structural equinus, or varus posting may be indicated if a forefoot varus or supinatus is prolonging the pronation process.

Peroneal Tendinitis

Inflammatory lesions of the peroneal tendons or of its protective sheath are common in athletes who, for compensatory reasons, overuse this musculature. The pathology is seen secondary to chronic lateral ankle sprains or in athletes with mobile, plantar flexed first rays. In both these situations, the peroneal tendons are worked excessively in an attempt to provide stability. Any mechanical stress caused by abnormal forefoot structures, which forces the foot into a valgus position, can also amplify this inflammatory response.

Pain and swelling typically occur in the area just posterior to the lateral malleolus. Occasionally, symptoms are manifested at the musculotendinous junction.[9] Tendon crepitus may be present in more chronic conditions. Pain and weakness are evident with passive overstretching of these contractile structures and when resistance is provided to plantar flexion and eversion of the first ray. Peroneal brevis tendinitis is more affected by resistance to calcaneal eversion and ankle plantar flexion. The differential diagnosis must be made among subluxing peroneals, inversion ankle sprains, sural nerve entrapment, and subacute lateral compartment syndrome, because subsequent management differs for each of these conditions.

Rehabilitation is aimed at providing symptomatic relief and identifying the causative factors. Muscular imbalances between the anterior or posterior tibialis and peroneals should be explored. Orthotic relief of structural abnormalities can be provided by a metatarsal pad with a first ray cut out. Transverse friction massage can be used as a means of symptom reduction and promotion of healing.[9] Table 8–6 presents further treatment considerations.

Posterior Tibialis Tendinitis

Posteromedial shin pain secondary to athletic overuse can indicate inflammatory microtrauma to the tendon of the posterior tibialis. Periosteal irritation and tibial stress reactions may also be suspected.

Medial tibial stress, whether tendinitis or periostitis, is generally the result of abnormal hyperpronation biomechanics (Fig. 8–28). The muscles in the superficial posterior compartment contract in a stretched position and are overworked in an attempt to stabilize the foot during propulsion. Common predisposing factors include improper training on crowned or banked surfaces, inappropriate footwear, and any structural condition that increases the varus attitude of the lower extremity.

Pain and swelling are present over the posteromedial crest of the tibia along the origin of the posterior tibialis. Tenderness and crepitation may be found anywhere along the course of the tendon as it passes behind the medial malleolus and inserts distally on the navicular and first cuneiform. Manual resistance to plantar flexion and inversion localizes

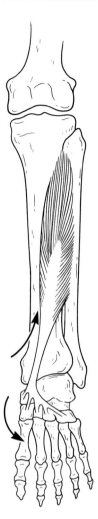

FIGURE 8–28 Etiology of posterior tibialis tendinitis: excessive traction stress placed on the posterior tibialis tendon with hyperpronation.

the complaint. In subacute phases, repeated unilateral heel raises, which require plantar flexion and supination of the calcaneus, can be a source of symptom aggravation.

Differential diagnosis is important to rule out a tibial stress reaction, in which there is pain at the junction of the lower and middle thirds of the posteromedial tibia. Tibial stress fractures can occur in this area if the bony osteoblastic activity cannot keep pace with the osteoclastic stress placed on it. At approximately 2 weeks postsymptom awareness, a fracture through the tibial cortex may become evident on x-ray. Previous to this finding, a bone scan reveals increased calcium uptake in the area of injury. Clinical differentiation is accomplished by detection of tenderness in areas devoid of muscle on the tibial shaft or by the use of percussion and tuning fork vibration techniques.

Treatment is aimed at alleviating abnormal pronation using a semi-rigid orthotic with a medial heel wedge. Attention should also be given to the training regimen and to finding shoes with a stable, firm, and snug heel counter.

Flexor Hallucis Longus Tendinitis

The athlete who must perform repetitive push-off maneuvers is especially prone to developing tendinitis in the long flexor of the great toe. Hyperpronation during propulsion also places excessive stress on the tendon as it contracts from a lengthened position. This condition is similar to posterior tibial tendinitis and can be differentiated through selected manual muscle testing. Pain with passive extension of the first metatarsophalangeal (MTP) joint while the ankle is dorsiflexed confirms the diagnosis. The condition is managed with appropriate varus posting and tape restriction for excessive dorsiflexion of the first MTP joint.

Flexor Digitorum Longus Tendinitis

The flexor digitorum longus is another musculotendinous unit in the superficial posterior compartment that is susceptible to overuse microtrauma. Pain is usually found in the posteromedial third of the leg as a result of overuse from forced, resistive dorsiflexion of the toes during propulsion.[15] The resultant cramping sensation present in the forefoot and toes can be relieved with the use of a viscoelastic metatarsal pad, which dorsally displaces the metatarsal heads and reduces the extension angle of the lesser four MTP joints. A more rigid sole in the athletic shoe may also help prevent excessive forced hyperextension of the digits in propulsion. Exercise rehabilitation focuses on correcting any intrinsic muscular imbalances that allow toe clawing deformities and that require the flexor digitorum longus to work harder.[15] The intrinsic muscles of the foot can be isolated for emphasis during toe curling exercises. This is accomplished by contracting the extensor hallucis longus to inhibit the long toe flexor's ability to contract. (Fig. 8–29).

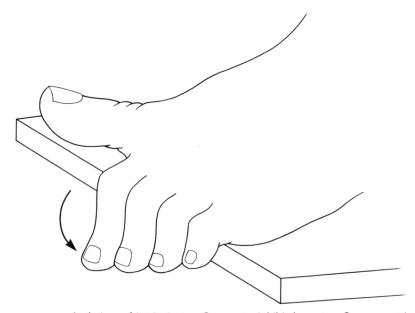

FIGURE 8–29   Isolation of intrinsic toe flexors to inhibit long toe flexor contribution.

Compartmental Compression Syndromes

There are four osseofascial compartments in the lower leg—the anterior, lateral, superficial posterior, and deep posterior compartments. The anterior compartment is the most common site for compression ischemia. It is bordered by the interosseous membrane posteriorly, the tibia and fibula medially and laterally, and a tough, nonexpansive fascial covering anteriorly. If pressure increases within the compartment there is no space for expansion or accommodation. With increasing pressure, circulation and tissue function can be quickly compromised. There are two types of anterior compartment compression syndrome, acute and recurrent.

Acute Anterior Compartment
Compression Syndrome

This condition is usually traumatic in its onset. Contusions, crush injuries, fractures, or severe overexertion can cause a rapid increase in compartmental volume from bleeding or muscular swelling. Increased intercompartmental pressure leads to venous collapse and increased resistance to arterial circulation. These physiologic changes produce an ischemic pain complaint and, ultimately, tissue necrosis if the process is left uninterrupted.

The athlete's chief complaint is intense pain disproportionate to the injury, which is not relieved by rest. Palpation reveals a "woody tension" over the muscles of the anterior compartment and passive plantar flexion evokes pain. In the advanced stages, neurologic changes may be evident, and the dorsalis pedis and anterior tibial pulses may be diminished. Table 8–7 presents the neurologic changes manifested in the later stages of lower leg compartment syndrome.

This condition is considered a medical emergency, because early muscle damage occurs in the first 4 to 6 hours and irreversible tissue damage occurs within 18 hours after injury. Acute care consists of ice application without compression and monitoring of the neurovascular status. If pain and swelling do not respond to conservative treatment, an emergency surgical fasciotomy must be performed.

Recurrent Compartment Syndrome

Chronic, exertional compartment syndrome has the same pathophysiology as acute compartment syndrome, but its presentation and care are different (Table 8–8). The athlete complains of lower leg pain and tightness that occurs at a constant interval following the initiation of

TABLE 8–7 **LATE NEUROLOGIC CHANGES IN COMPRESSION SYNDROMES**

Compartment	Area of Paresthia	Areas of Weakness
Anterior	First dorsal web space	Dorsiflexors (drop foot)
Lateral	Anterior lateral of leg	Eversion (peroneals)
Deep posterior	Medial arch	Inversion
Superficial posterior	Sural nerve distribution	Plantar flexion

TABLE 8–8 **SYMPTOM PRESENTATION OF ACUTE VERSUS RECURRENT COMPARTMENT SYNDROMES**

Type	Recurrent	Acute
Pathology	Reversible changes	Irreversible tissue damage possible
Effect of rest	Symptoms decrease	No change in symptoms
Nature of complaint	Cramping, aching	Intense pain
Involvement	Often bilateral	Usually unilateral

physical activity. The symptoms subside with rest but return on resumption of the activity. Most patients have bilateral involvement with mild edema, tenderness, and occasional paresthesia. The diagnosis is confirmed with wick catheter measurement of intercompartmental pressure at rest and during activity.

Conservative management includes ice application before and after exercise, lower leg stretching, and balancing plantar flexion–dorsiflexion strength. Any alterations in the training program that decrease muscular workloads may also be helpful. Bevel-heeled shoes, softer training surfaces, and energy-absorbing orthotics may accomplish this goal. If conservative measures fail, a surgical fasciotomy is indicated.

Ankle Injuries

Pathologic trauma to the ligamentous structures of the ankle is a common athletic injury. The vast majority of these injuries occur to the lateral side of the joint with an inversion component of motion. In the neutral position of 0° dorsiflexion, the calcaneofibular ligament is taut but, as the foot plantar flexes, the anterior talofibular ligament tightens as its fibers become parallel to the axis. Eighty to 90% of ankle sprains occur as the result of this plantar flexion–inversion mechanism. The direction of force initially damages the anterior talofibular ligament and further stress affects the calcaneofibular and posterior talofibular ligaments, in that order. The posterior talofibular ligament is not involved or injured until the other two ligaments have ruptured and some degree of lower extremity rotation has occurred. Injuries to the medial side of the joint and the deltoid ligament are less frequent and typically involve a hyperpronation force, such as when an athlete plants the foot and then cuts in the opposite direction. Table 8–9 outlines the common mechanisms of injury for bony and ligamentous structures of the ankle.

Inversion Sprains

The signs and symptoms of ankle ligamentous injuries vary according to the severity of injury, the tissues involved, and the extent of their involvement. Varying degrees of pain, swelling, point tenderness, and functional disability are usually evident. Following inversion trauma, radiographic studies of the joint and bone structure are of paramount importance. Bony lesions must be ruled out before decisions about appropriate management of the injury can be determined. Unstable bimalleolar fractures, proximal fibular fractures, and avulsion-type frac-

TABLE 8–9   MECHANISM OF ANKLE INJURIES

Mechanism of Injury	Comments	Ligamentous Injury (Progression of Increasing Severity of Pathology)*	Potential Bony Lesions
Plantar flexion–inversion	Typical ankle sprain	ATF→ATF & CF→ATF & CF & PTF	Transverse fracture of lateral malleolus Avulsion fracture of base of fifth metatarsal
Supinated position—adduction force			Medial malleolus fracture
Plantar flexion—inversion and rotation Supinated position—eversion force	Crossover cut on a plantar flexed and inverted foot	ATF & tibfib→ATF & tibfib & CF	Spiral fracture of lateral malleolus or fracture of neck of fibula
Pure inversion	Rare; landing on another's foot	CF→CF & ATF→CF & ATF & PTF	
Pronation: abduction—eversion—dorsiflexion Pronated position—eversion force	Open cut	Deltoid→deltoid & tibfib & interosseus membrane	Avulsion fracture of medial malleolus Fibular fracture above the mortice line

* ATF, anterior talofibular ligament; CF, calcaneofibular ligament; PTF, posterior talofibular ligament; tibfib, anterior and posterior tibiofibular ligaments.

TABLE 8–10 SIGNS AND SYMPTOMS OF LATERAL ANKLE SPRAINS

Grade	Severity	Involvement*	Functional Status	Swelling	Pain, Tenderness	Ligament Laxity
I	Mild	Usually only ATF	Maintenance of joint integrity produces minimal functional disability	Variable, but usually slight	Mild, localized pain over ATF	Negative anterior drawer and talar tilt
II	Moderate	ATF & CF	Moderate disability, with difficulty in heel and toe walking	Variable, but more than in grade I, and resultant ecchymosis	Moderate pain and tenderness over involved ligaments	Laxity evident, but distinct end points to stress
III	Severe	ATF & CF; possibly PTF	Functional disability, with loss of ROM and complete inability to bear weight	Anterolateral and spreading diffusely around the joint	Marked tenderness to palpation	Positive anterior drawer and/or talar tilt

* ATF, anterior talofibular ligament; CF, calcaneofibular ligament; PTF, posterior talofibular ligament.

tures are all possible and may require surgical fixation or longer periods of immobilization.

Table 8–10 outlines some criteria for assessing the severity of injury in lateral ankle sprains. This grading process provides a basis for making logical estimates about the rate and intensity that can be used in progressing the athlete through the phases of treatment and rehabilitation, as well as an initial estimate of length of time that is necessary before the athlete can return to full participation.

Treatment and Rehabilitation

The etiology of functional or chronic disability associated with ankle sprains can be the result of various pathologic abnormalities. These include anterior, posterior, or varus instability of the talus in the ankle mortice, instability, or adhesion formation of the subtalar joint, inferior tibiofibular diastasis, peroneal muscle weakness, and motor incoordination secondary to articular deafferentation.[5, 12, 13, 16, 22, 28]

Each potential problem must be addressed in the treatment and rehabilitation program. The damaged ligaments must be allowed to heal as a "flexible" restraint, the contractile elements must regain dynamic stabilization capabilities, and the proprioceptive system must be completely restored. Table 8–11 suggests a treatment plan for the conservative management of inversion ankle sprains. Each athlete's injury is unique and progression through the various stages of rehabilitation may have to be altered, depending on the severity of tissue trauma, previous history, and goals of rehabilitation. Figures 8–30 to 8–39 illustrate some of the rehabilitation procedures used in the restoration of normal ankle joint function following ligamentous injury.

The goal of management is to provide dynamic stability to a potentially unstable joint. During the acute immobilization phase, emphasis is placed on controlling symptoms and on maintaining general conditioning and neuromuscular continuity. Various modalities are used to minimize effusion and decrease pain. Ice, compression (intermittent or constant), electrotherapy, and gentle effleurage with the ankle elevated all facilitate anesthesia and absorption of edema. Support to the injured ligaments is provided by the use of a neutral orthotic, Gibney's strapping (open basketweave taping with a horseshoe pad to compress extracellular fluids back into circulation), and a posterior splint to maintain Achilles tendon flexibility. Because strict immobilization is no longer recommended, cautious and gentle motion in protected arcs can be initiated through Biomechanical Ankle Platform System* (BAPS) board activity (Fig. 8–30). Isometric exercises are also started during this phase to minimize or retard atrophy.

The weight-bearing status of the athlete is progressed as symptoms and healing allow. Insistence should be made on a normal heel-to-toe gait and on keeping weight-bearing forces below the pain symptom level. Early, pain-free weight-bearing will maintain proprioceptive input, prevent stiffness, and provide a means for an active muscle pump to mobilize effusion.

---

* Available from Camp International, Jackson, Michigan.

TABLE 8-11 **CONSERVATIVE MANAGEMENT OF ANKLE SPRAINS**

Parameter	Phase			
	IMMEDIATE (ACUTE) IMMOBILIZATION	INTERMEDIATE (SUBACUTE) POSTIMMOBILIZATION	TERMINAL (CHRONIC)	RETURN TO ACTIVITY (FUNCTIONAL)
Goals	Protect joint integrity; control inflammatory response; control pain, edema, and spasm	Prevent or minimize contracture and adhesion formation; maintain soft tissue and adjacent joints' mobility	Functional progression of closed chain activities; proprioceptive retraining; correct or control abnormal biomechanics	Preparation for return to sport
Weight-bearing status	Non- to touch-down weight-bearing	Crutch partial weight-bearing progressing toward full weight-bearing	Full weight-bearing	Full weight-bearing
Modalities	Ice; compression (intermittent and/or constant); elevation; TENS and high voltage galvanic stimulator; gentle effleurage in elevated positions	Cryotherapy (Ice-ROM-Ice-ROM, etc.); contrast baths; friction massage at site of lesions	Cryokinetics (Ice-closed chain motion-Ice, etc.); manipulative ruptures of adhesions, if necessary	Ice postparticipation
External support	Neutral orthotic; Gibney open basketweave taping technique; posterior splint	Stirrup splint with heel lock support	Stirrup splint with heel lock protection	Taping; air splint or lace-up ankle support; orthotics
Range of motion, flexibility	Early pain-free mobilization in sagittal plane if not in strict immobilization	Grades I-II joint mobilizations; Achilles tendon stretching in sitting and standing	Achilles tendon stretching in supinated postures	

Open kinetic chain exercise	Isometrics	Alphabet ROM; toe curls and marble pick-ups; surgical tubing exercise in all planes; submaximal isokinetics in protected arcs	Full arc isokinetics	Ensure normal inversion–eversion strength ratios—3:2 at slow speeds of concentric isokinetic contraction
Closed kinetic chain exercise		Heel raises in nonweight-bearing positions; soleus pumps; body weight transfers in bilateral stance from medial to lateral	Heel raise progression; body weight transfers with elastic tubing resistance	Body weight transfers in position of inversion or eversion with tubing overload resistance; marching, running, backpedaling against elastic tubing resistance
Proprioception, agility, balance drills	BAPS board in nonweight-bearing positions	BAPS board in partial weight-bearing; stork stands	BAPS board in full weight-bearing; jumping rope; ProFitter; tilt or balance boards	BAPS board with weighted overload; four-square hopping; functional running program—backpedaling, sidesteps, cariocas
Complementary and alternative exercises	Gluteus medius strengthening	Pool therapy; stationary cycling	Rebounder minitramp; single-leg recumbent or stationary cycling; stationary cross-country skiing	Versa-Climber, StairMaster, or lateral step-ups

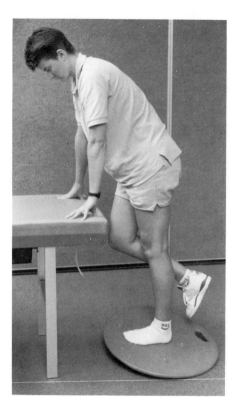

FIGURE 8–30 Biomechanical ankle platform system—BAPS board.

In the intermediate or postimmobilization phase, attention is focused on the healing ligaments. Subpathologic stress through joint mobilization is placed on the injured ligaments to stimulate organized collagen formation along the lines of normal fiber direction. Care must

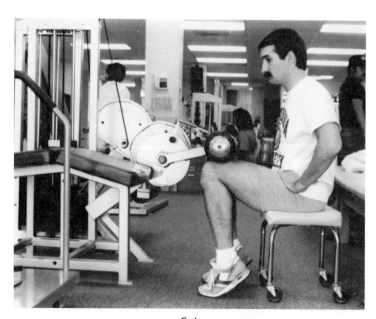

FIGURE 8–31   Soleus pumps.

be taken not to place traction forces on the joint with ankle weight resistance on the foot. Closed chain rehabilitation in a weight-bearing position is preferred because it can provide compressive forces that augment stability.

Weight-bearing is progressed in this stage to full weight-bearing without ambulation assistance. The use of stirrup-type splints with heel lock protection to limit excessive calcaneal inversion is indicated. Exercise rehabilitation may include Achilles tendon stretching; open chain, cryotherapy-assisted active range of motion progressing toward submaximal effort isokinetics in limited arcs; and closed chain functional activities such as soleus pumps, stork stands, and body weight transfers over the injured extremity (Figs. 8–31 to 8–33).

In the terminal phase of rehabilitation, progressive closed chain activities with emphasis on restoring kinesthetic awareness is given priority. Other modalities at this point are only used as needed, but ice

FIGURE 8–32   Stork stands.

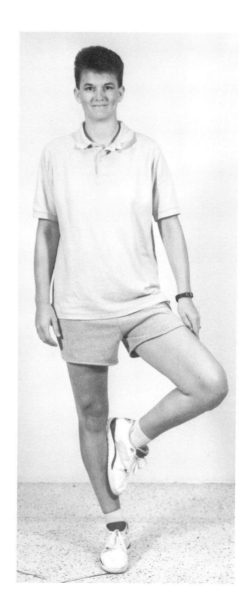

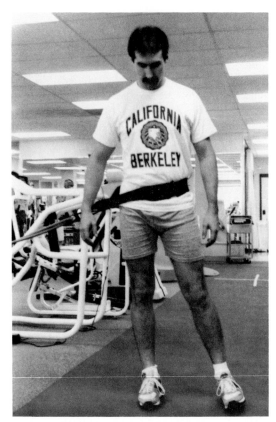

FIGURE 8–33   Body weight transfers with surgical tubing.

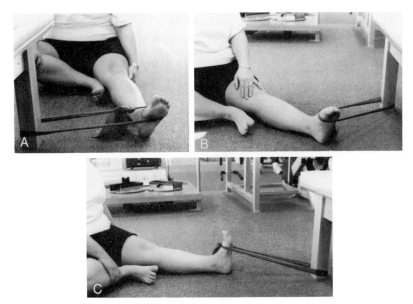

FIGURE 8–34 Surgical tubing resisted exercises. *A*, Eversion. *B*, Inversion. *C*, Dorsiflexion.

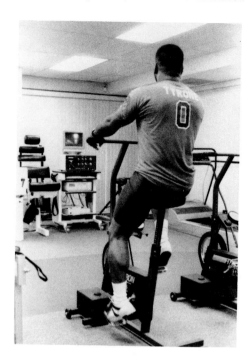

FIGURE 8–35 Ankle rehabilitation on stationary bike.

following rehabilitation is usually necessary. Exercise rehabilitation becomes aggressive and includes slant board Achilles tendon stretching without allowing subtalar joint substitution, full arc isokinetics, and heel raise progression. Balance and motor coordination are enhanced by the use of a ProFitter,* balance board, and rebounder minitrampoline (Figs. 8–34 to 8–39).

---

* Available from ProFitter, Calgary, Canada.

FIGURE 8–36 Ankle rehabilitation on cross-country skier.

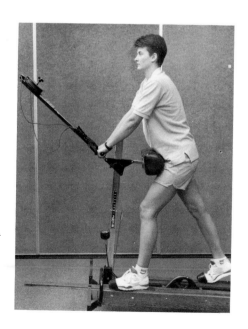

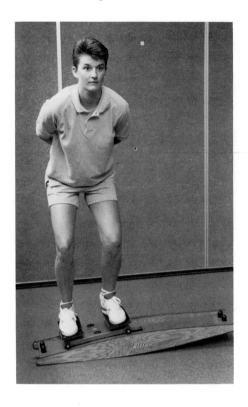

FIGURE 8–37   Ankle rehabilitation on ProFitter.

FIGURE 8–38   Ankle rehabilitation with surgical tubing.

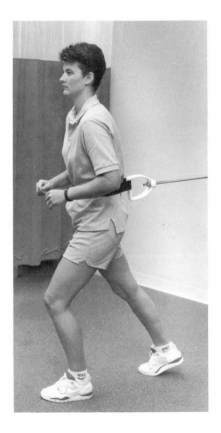

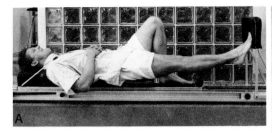

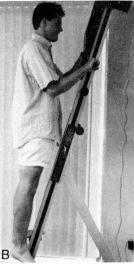

FIGURE 8–39   Closed chain plantar flexion strengthening. *A,* Supine with gravity eliminated on Shuttle 2000. *B,* Standing on Versa-Climber.

As the athlete prepares to return to athletic participation, a functional progression should be used to simulate those stresses, forces, and motions inherent to the sport that caused the original injury. Elastic tubing resistance to weight-bearing activities improves ankle strength and coordination, and stimulates proprioception for the entire lower extremity. Progression from resistance in marching to running to running on inclines can be employed. Tubing resistance can come from all directions, and progression is based on pain-free exercise without effusion or tendency for the ankle to roll over.[28] Tape or external support should not be used during these controlled activities to allow full rehabilitative benefit. Clinical plyometrics such as four-square hopping also represents an excellent means of recreating athletic activity (Fig. 8–40). Finally, a functional movement progression that includes backpedaling, sidestepping, cariocas, pivoting, and cutting should be used in assessing the athlete's readiness for return to play.

Orthotic and external support should be used to prevent recurrence of trauma. The athlete with an uncorrected rearfoot varus and forefoot valgus with a plantar flexed first ray compensates with prolonged or excessive supination in midstance and is extremely susceptible to reinjury. Because it takes at least 20 weeks for a ligament to regain its normal histologic characteristics, ankle taping and/or ankle support should be provided for at least 5 to 6 months postinjury during athletic participation.

Postsurgical Management of Lateral Ankle Reconstructions

Sometimes surgical reconstruction of the lateral ligaments using the peroneals is performed to provide joint stability. The postoperative therapeutic management of these procedures involves principles similar to those used in the conservative care of grade III ankle injuries. Typically, a short leg cast or brace is applied for 6 weeks with the ankle

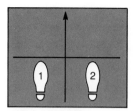

Side to side: Hop laterally between two quadrants.

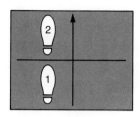

Front to back: Hop forward and backward between two quadrants.

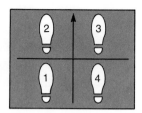

Four square: Hop from square to square in a circular pattern. Sets are performed clockwise and counterclockwise.

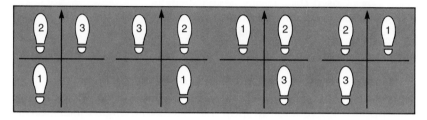

Triangles: Hop within three different quadrants. There are four triangles, each requiring a different diagonal hop.

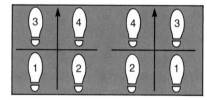

Crisscross: Hop in an X pattern.

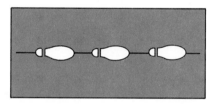

Straight-line hop: Hop forward and then backward along a 15 to 20 ft. line.

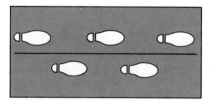

Line zigzag: Hop from side to side across a 15- to 20-ft. line while moving forward and then backward.

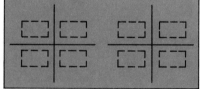

Disconnected squares: While performing the first five patterns, hop into squares marked in the quadrants.

FIGURE 8–40   Four-square hopping ankle rehabilitation. The eight basic hopping patterns in the four-square ankle rehabilitation program are arranged in order of increasing difficulty. The arrow denotes the direction the athlete is facing. The number 1 is the starting point. (From Toomey, S.J. (1986): Four-square ankle rehabilitation exercises. Physician Sportsmed., 14:281.)

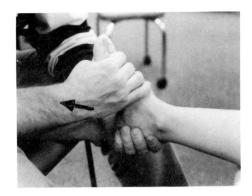

FIGURE 8-41 Talocrural joint traction to increase general mobility of ankle.

in 0° dorsiflexion and mildly everted. During the first 2 weeks the athlete uses a nonweight-bearing crutch gait. The final 4 weeks of immobilization allows partial weight-bearing on the crutches. Strict immobilization is discontinued at 6 weeks and active assistive range-of-motion exercises in the sagittal plane are begun. At 8 weeks, active range-of-motion exercises for calcaneal inversion and eversion are begun, along with resistive exercises for the plantar flexors and dorsiflexors. When the athlete can walk without a detectable limp, functional rehabilitation progression may commence. Return to activity is expected after 4 to 6 months.

Rehabilitation of Postimmobilization Fractures

Rehabilitation following cast removal of ankle fractures is focused on restoring joint mobility. The immobilization time necessary for ensuring fracture union causes capsular restrictions, muscular atrophy, and proprioceptive deficits. Emphasis is then placed on joint mobilization and appropriate exercises to strengthen and mobilize the soft tissues. The mechanics of the fracture and its surgical fixation must be understood and appreciated to avoid excessive force or stress on the initial injury. Figures 8–41 to 8–50 demonstrate joint mobilization techniques that may be used carefully and rationally to restore accessory joint motion and normal joint arthokinematics.

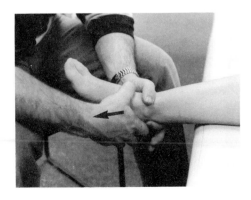

FIGURE 8-42 Subtalar joint traction to increase general mobility of subtalar joint.

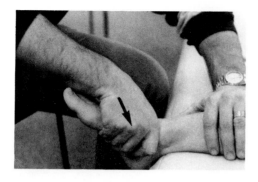

FIGURE 8–43 Talocrural joint: posterior glide of the talus to increase plantar flexion range of motion.

FIGURE 8–44 Talocrural joint: anterior glide of talus to increase plantar flexion range of motion.

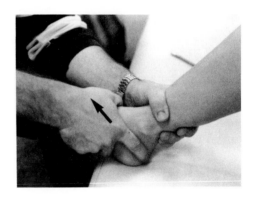

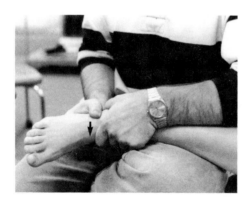

FIGURE 8–45 Medial glide of calcaneus to increase calcaneal eversion (pronation).

FIGURE 8–46 Lateral glide of calcaneus to increase calcaneal inversion (supination).

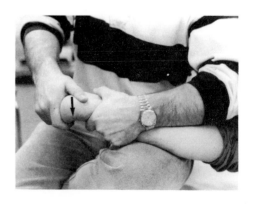

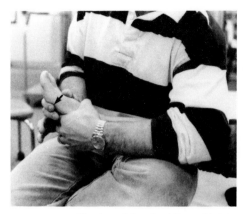

FIGURE 8–47   Plantar glide of midtarsal joint.

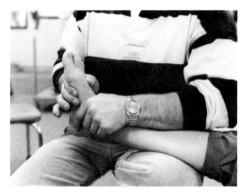

FIGURE 8–48   Dorsal glide of midtarsal joint.

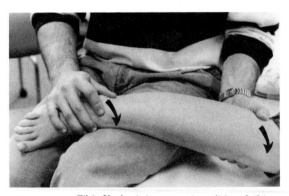

FIGURE 8–49   Tibiofibular joint: anterior glide of tibia.

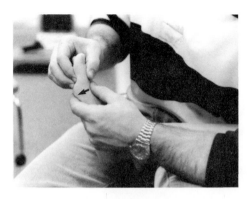

FIGURE 8–50 Dorsal glide of first MTP joint.

Peroneal Tendon Subluxation

The peroneal tendons lie in a deep groove posterior to the lateral malleolus. They are subject to subluxation out of this groove if the peroneal retinaculum is ruptured by sudden and violent dorsiflexion and eversion forces. This is commonly seen when a novice skier falls forward while loading the inner edge of the skis.

This injury is commonly confused with inversion ankle sprains because of the similarity in symptoms. The athlete relates a feeling of tenderness, instability, and swelling in an area around the lateral malleolus. Differential diagnosis can be determined if there is complaint of intense retromalleolar pain with resistive dorsiflexion and eversion or, in those with a chronic condition, marked instability and audible snapping of the tendon in and out of its groove.

Conservative management involves reducing the inflammatory response with ice, compression, and elevation. Peroneal stabilization can be attempted with taping techniques that limit excessive motion and incorporate a J-shaped pad that compresses the tendons as they pass around the lateral malleolus (Fig. 8–51). If conservative management fails to control the symptoms, surgical intervention may be elected. Surgical procedures generally attempt to reconstruct or reinforce the damaged peroneal retinaculum or use bony procedures to deepen the groove behind the lateral malleolus.

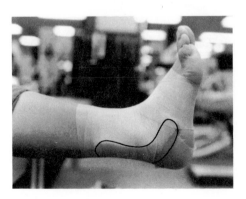

FIGURE 8–51 J-pad stabilization of peroneal tendons.

Calcaneal Injuries

Heel Bruises

Contusion injuries to the heel and calcaneal fat pad are among the most disabling in sports. Athletic activities that require frequent jumping or changes of direction seem to be especially prone to producing this type of injury. Runners with leg length discrepancy who overstride on the short leg side and have resultant increased impact forces at the heel strike area are also especially vulnerable to this type of trauma. Contusion injuries that cause subperiosteal bleeding and tender scar formation are sensitive to tissue compression monitored by pressure nerve endings in the area.

The athlete will complain of severe pain in the plantar aspect of the calcaneus, which is greatly aggravated by weight-bearing. Treatment must include some element of rest to minimize continued, repetitive trauma. As the athlete returns to play, the heel should be taped and placed in a heel cup. It is also helpful if a shoe with a firm, well-fitting heel counter is selected for participation. The tape and heel cup strengthen and support the columnar septae and lobules, which provide the calcaneal fat pad with its impact-absorbing qualities.

Os Trigonum Injury

Injury to the os trigonum is common in athletes who function on their toes (e.g., ballet dancers) or who encounter resistance to dorsiflexion while in the extreme of plantar flexion (e.g., soccer player having a kick blocked). Accessory bone fracture or soft tissue pinching produces severe local pain in the posterior portion of the ankle. Conservative treatment involves taping techniques to limit end-range plantar flexion. If this motion is necessary for performance, surgical excision may be necessary.

Calcaneal Epiphysitis

Traction epiphyseal injuries in active adolescents are common when they wear cleated shoes or rapidly alter the heel height of their athletic shoe. The tight Achilles tendon pulls on the calcaneal epiphyseal attachment, producing a disruption of circulation and possible fragmentation (also known as Sever's disease). The young athlete complains of pain on the posterior heel at the insert of the Achilles tendon, which is aggravated by activity and relieved by rest. This condition ends at skeletal maturity, when the epiphysis closes. Until then, judicious rest and the insertion of bilateral heel lifts can help alleviate injurious stresses.

Retrocalcaneal Bursitis

Long distance running and repetitive jumping can create a bursal inflammation between the Achilles tendon and calcaneus. This condition is aggravated by excessive compensatory pronation, which results in cumulative trauma and pressure to the posterolateral aspect of the

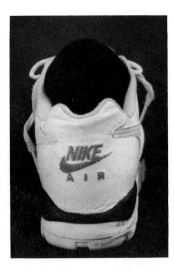

FIGURE 8–52   Notched heel collar on running shoe.

heel. A structural predisposition to bursal inflammation may exist in the cavus foot if there is spurring on the posterior superior aspect of the calcaneus.

This condition is characterized by pain, swelling, and discoloration on the posterolateral and superior aspects of the heel. Tenderness is elicited anterior to the Achilles tendon but posterior to the talus.

Ice, anti-inflammatories, and orthotic control of the hypermobile calcaneus are used. If the subcutaneous bursa is involved, heel counter collar modification should also be employed (Fig. 8–52). Shoe selection should place a high priority on a stable heel counter. Structural predisposition may be alleviated by a heel lift, or surgical excision of bony spurs in chronic conditions that do not respond to conservative management may be necessary.

Plantar Fasciitis

The plantar fascia is a dense band of fibrous connective tissue that originates from the calcaneal tuberosity and runs forward to insert on the metatarsal heads. As a tension band, it supports the medial longitudinal arch and assists in the push-off power of running and jumping.[34] Biomechanical abuse of this tissue results in microtrauma and inflammation. Chronic overuse and irritation can lead to bone formation in response to the traction forces of the plantar fascia and the muscles attaching to the calcaneal tuberosity.

This condition is most often seen in the running athlete who hyperpronates or has a rigid cavus foot and tight Achilles tendon. In both instances, excessive traction is placed on the fascia, which can be magnified with uphill or hard surface training terrains. Creighton and Olson[8] have noted that decreased active and passive ranges of motion at the first MTP joint correlate with the onset of plantar fasciitis. Inadequate or inappropriate MTP motion can alter the windlass effect of the plantar fascia and decrease the inherent stability of the foot as the heel comes off the ground.

A gradual, insidious onset of pain is present along the plantar aspect of the foot, which can radiate along the path of the fascia. Tenderness to palpation can be found at the medial aspect of the calcaneal tuberosity, in the medial arch, and occasionally at the distal insertion of the fascia on the metatarsal heads. The most consistent finding is that of exquisite pain with weight-bearing forces of the first few steps in the morning. The phenomenon of "physiologic creep," in which the tissues contract while nonweight-bearing during the night and then are forcefully stretched with initial morning weight-bearing, may explain this common complaint. Because it is a noncontractile structure, active or passive dorsiflexion of the great toe usually elicits the symptoms. These signs and symptoms can mimic those of other pathologies but should be differentiated from medial plantar nerve irritation, tarsal tunnel syndrome, and infracalcaneal bursitis.

Initially, treatment should be directed at controlling the inflammatory response and then at alleviating or reducing the excessive tension being placed on the plantar fascia and its associated structures, which have their origin at the calcaneal tuberosity. During the acute state, ice massage, anti-inflammatory medications, and rest from aggravating activities are prescribed. Sponge rubber heel lifts with a doughnut-shaped cutout may provide weight-bearing relief on the injured structures. In the subacute stage, pulsed phonophoresis, cross-fiber friction massage, and heel cord stretching are used to manage symptoms. Correction of abnormal stresses can be provided through low-dye taping for the hyperpronator (Fig. 8–53), shock-absorbing inserts for the rigid cavus foot, and joint mobilization for the hypomobile first MTP joint (Fig. 8–54).

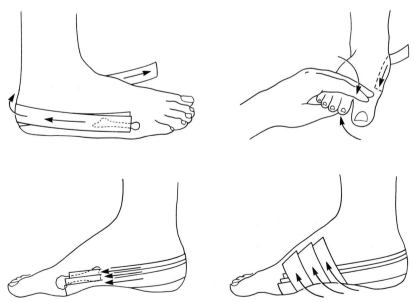

FIGURE 8–53 Modified LowDye taping technique to decrease traction stress on plantar fascia. (Steven Roy/Richard Irvin, SPORTS MEDICINE: Prevention, Evaluation, Management, and Rehabilitation, © 1983, p. 58. Reprinted by permission of Prentice-Hall, Inc., Englewood Cliffs, New Jersey.)

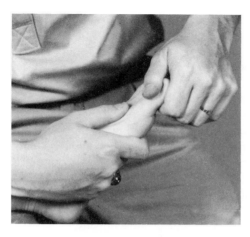

FIGURE 8–54 Traction mobilization on first MTP joint to increase mobility.

Foot Injuries

Tarsal Tunnel Syndrome

Tarsal tunnel syndrome is an entrapment neuropathy of the posterior tibial nerve as it passes through the osseofibrous tunnel between the flexor retinaculum and medial malleolus (Fig. 8–55). The typical mechanism of injury in athletes is excessive pronation, which causes a tightening of the flexor retinaculum. Hyperpronation of the forefoot can also cause the calcaneonavicular ligament to compress the medial plantar branch of the posterior tibial nerve. Direct trauma or chronic inflammation in this area produces a space-occupying lesion that can alter neurologic function.

The athlete reports intermittent burning, pain, tingling, and numbness in the medial foot, which are aggravated by weight-bearing. A positive Tinel's sign may be elicited with tapping or compression over the affected nerves to reproduce the symptoms. In advanced stages, weakness in toe flexion and abductor hallucis atrophy may be evident.

The athlete should be placed in a neutral-position orthotic to control pronation and instructed in activity modifications. Therapeutic mo-

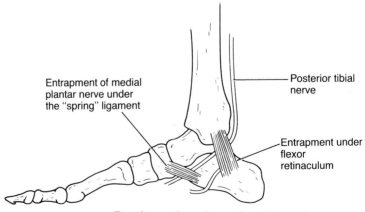

Entrapment of medial plantar nerve under the "spring" ligament

Posterior tibial nerve

Entrapment under flexor retinaculum

FIGURE 8–55 Tarsal tunnel syndrome (medial view).

dalities such as ultrasound and phonophoresis may be tried to reduce edema and fibrosis in the area of entrapment. Resistant cases may require surgical release of the tissue that is causing compression.

Cuboid Syndrome

Cuboid syndrome describes a partial displacement of the cuboid bone by the pull of the peroneus longus. The onset can be gradual or traumatic. Acute pain and hypomobility can be induced with trauma or with a powerful contraction, with the foot in a plantar flexed and inverted position. Gradual onset is more typical in the hyperpronated foot. Under these circumstances the peroneus longus is at a mechanical disadvantage, and it pulls the lateral portion of the cuboid dorsally and the medial portion in a plantar direction.[38]

The signs and symptoms of this injury include tenderness along the cuboid, peroneus longus, and lateral metatarsal heads. Treatment is directed at restoring normal osteokinematics and protecting against further trauma or aggravation. Following ice massage or a cold whirlpool bath, the athlete is prepared for bony manipulation. With the athlete in a prone position, with the knee mildly flexed to protect against excessive traction of the superficial peroneal nerve, a downward thrust of the thumbs is used to relocate the cuboid into its appropriate position (Fig. 8–56). Following restoration of bony anatomy, a segmental balance pad may be used to unload stress on the fourth metatarsal and its cuboid articulation.[38] In athletes with chronic hyperpronation, low-dye taping or medial heel wedges can be used to counteract the damaging pull of the peroneus longus.

Metatarsal Stress Fractures

Metatarsal stress fractures occur when osteoclastic activity is greater than osteoblastic activity. Stress overload caused by prolonged pronation and excessive hypermobility of the first ray can begin a cycle of injury (Fig. 8–57). Hughes[17] has noted that predisposition to stress fractures is greatest in the presence of forefoot varus and decreased ankle dorsiflexion range of motion. Both these conditions result in

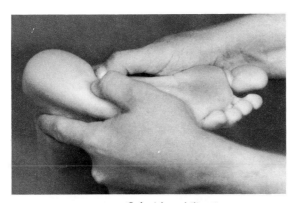

FIGURE 8–56   Cuboid mobilization.

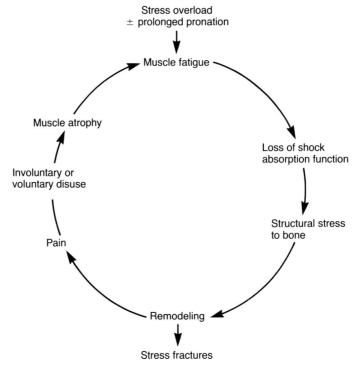

FIGURE 8–57   Stress Fracture injury cycle. (From Taunton, J.E., Clement, D.B., and Webber, D. (1981): Lower extremity stress fractures in athletes. Physician Sportsmed., 9:85.)

pronation during the propulsive phase of gait, placing considerable stress on the central three metatarsals, especially the second. Metatarsal stress fractures are most likely to occur at the beginning of the season in the deconditioned athlete or with sudden changes in training surfaces or athletic footwear.

There is localized pain and swelling over the metatarsal, which increase with activity and decrease with rest. Percussion and active flexion–extension of the toes also exacerbate the complaint.

Treatment is straightforward. The athlete must rest from weight-bearing or aggravating activities and find alternative methods of maintaining conditioning. In those in whom pain is present with ambulation, or if there is suspicion of noncompliance with reducing activity levels, a short-leg walking cast may be appropriate. On return to activity, orthotics, tape, or a felt cutout to float the affected metatarsal should be used to relieve osteoclastic stresses.

During the subacute phase it is important for the athlete to correct the muscular, flexibility, and conditioning deficits that may have lead to the initial injury.

Proximal Diaphysis Fracture of the Fifth Metatarsal

Weight-bearing forces are great on the fifth metatarsal because of its many soft tissue attachments. Tension on the bone from the peroneus

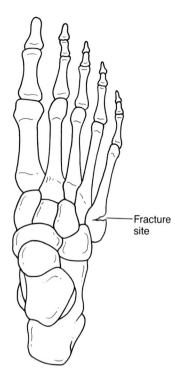

Fracture
site

FIGURE 8–58 Proximal diaphysis fracture of fifth metatarsal (dorsal view).

brevis, cubometatarsal ligament, lateral band of the plantar fascia, and peroneus tertius can lead to stress reactions, which can become a complete fracture with inversion trauma or a nonunion stress fracture with repetitive forces.[10] These lesions normally occur just distal to the base of the fifth metatarsal and are notoriously unpredictable in their healing (Fig. 8–58). Nonunion and reinjury are frequent. Management is therefore controversial and must be individualized to the athlete. Some recommend early, aggressive surgical intervention with the use of a malleolar leg screw across the fracture site, whereas others simply use nonweight-bearing immobilization.[19] Conservative management allows 4 to 6 weeks of healing; the cast is then removed to determine whether the athlete can function with a nonfibrous union. Full athletic participation is contraindicated until there is full consolidation of the fracture site. When healing is complete, orthotic therapy should be considered to redistribute injurious forces.

Interdigital Neuroma

Compression and shearing forces at the bifurcation of the neurovascular bundle between the metatarsal heads can result in the formation of a benign tumor of fibrous tissue, called a Morton's neuroma (Fig. 8–59). Pinching and squeezing of the neurovascular bundle between the metatarsal heads and transverse metatarsal ligament occur in the hypermobile foot during midstance and propulsion.

The chief complaint is that of a burning or electric-shock sensation in the forefoot that radiates into the toes. The lesion is usually located between the third and fourth metatarsals and is often mistaken for a

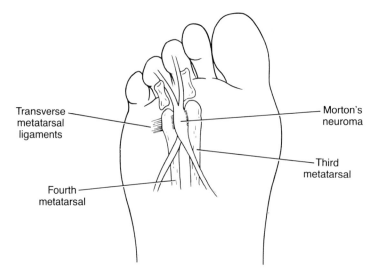

Transverse metatarsal ligaments

Morton's neuroma

Third metatarsal

Fourth metatarsal

FIGURE 8–59   Plantar view of interdigital neuroma.

stone in the shoe by the athlete. Pain can be relieved by removal of shoes and aggravated by manual metatarsal head compression. A clicking or reproduction of symptoms can be elicited with simultaneous compression of the metatarsal heads in the transverse plane and plantar flexion of the affected MTP joints (Fig. 8–60).

Some success has been achieved with the use of a metatarsal pad placed just proximal to the metatarsal heads, which increases their spatial spread and increases toe flexion. Shoe selection should ensure a wide toe box, and orthotic inserts may be used to control hypermobility. Corticosteroid and anesthetic injections or oral anti-inflammatory medications can also be tried. Surgical excision of the neuroma is indicated when conservative measures fail.

Turf Toe

Acute hyperdorsiflexion injuries to the first MTP joint occur as the toes are pressed down into an unyielding surface just prior to toe-off. This

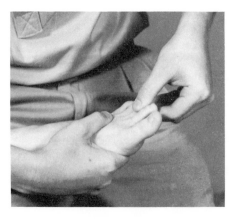

FIGURE 8–60 Metatarsal head compression in combination with plantar-dorsal glide to elicit pain from an interdigital neuroma.

force causes hyperextension of the MTP joint as the phalanx is jammed into the metatarsal.[35] Repetitive trauma of this nature results in plantar capsule tears, articular cartilage damage, and possible fracture of the medial sesamoid bone. Chronic trauma can lead to metatarsalgia, with ligamentous calcification and hallux rigidus.[30]

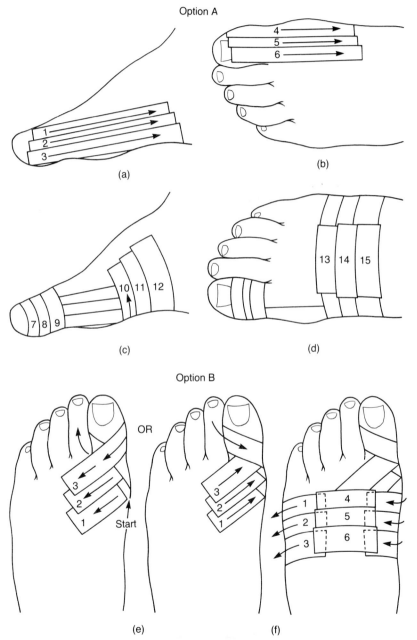

FIGURE 8–61 Turf toe taping technique to prevent excessive hyperextension of the first MTP joint. (Steven Roy/Richard Irvin, SPORTS MEDICINE: Prevention, Evaluation, Management, and Rehabilitation. © 1983, p. 57. Reprinted by permission of Prentice-Hall, Inc., Englewood Cliffs, New Jersey.)

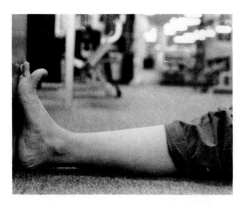

FIGURE 8–62 Active range of motion of first MTP joint, with first metatarsal head stabilized.

Sudden acceleration under high loads against unyielding Astroturf is the usual mechanism of injury. Athletes who wear shoes that are extremely flexible and offer minimal support are especially prone to this injury. Also, athletes who wear a longer shoe to achieve greater width effectively lengthen the lever arm forces acting on the joint, and the feet are subject to repetitive trauma.

The athlete presents with a tender, red, and swollen first MTP joint that has increased pain with passive toe extension. Initial management calls for rest, ice, compression, elevation, and support to the injured joint. Tape immobilization can be used to check excessive extension and valgus stresses that irritate the joint (Fig. 8–61). Rehabilitation procedures may include whirlpool range-of-motion exercises, ultrasound to mobilize scar tissue formation, and active range-of-motion exercises with the first ray stabilized. Figure 8–62 demonstrates an exercise used to increase active range of motion for the hypomobile first MTP joint.

In the subacute stage, gentle plantar-dorsal glides of the first phalanx may be indicated to improve arthrokinematic mobility. On return to activity, the athlete should possess at least 90° of painless passive toe extension and have been screened for appropriate shoe selection.[30] A steel spring plate in the toe box or rigid taping into plantar flexion should be used initially when resuming full participation.

Sesamoiditis

The two small sesamoid bones of the foot are found on the plantar surface of the first metatarsal head, embedded within the tendon of the flexor hallucis brevis. The sesamoid bones enhance the windlass mechanism and help distribute and disperse weight-bearing forces during propulsion. The medial or tibial sesamoid is often bipartate, and its appearance can be confused with a fracture.[36] Sesamoiditis describes an inflammatory condition of the tissues surrounding the sesamoids.

The athlete most prone to medial sesamoid pathology is the one with a rigid cavus foot, tight Achilles tendon, and plantar flexed first ray.[2] Sesamoid pain also occurs in athletes with normal foot structure but whose activities require maximal dorsiflexion of the first MTP joint, which allows excessive impact loading stresses on the sesamoids.

The athlete usually presents with tenderness and swelling of the first metatarsal head and pain with passive dorsiflexion. Pressure from improper cleat placement on the athletic shoe may also be a source of further aggravation.

Initial treatment in the acute stage involves ice massage, anti-inflammatory medications or cortisone injections, and rest. Pulsed phonophoresis and iontophoresis are alternative methods of combatting the inflammatory response, which may be of symptomatic value. Definitive treatment must include relief of weight-bearing stresses on the affected area. A semirigid orthotic with the first ray cut out and a Morton's extension can provide this relief.

ORTHOTIC THERAPY

The intent of orthotic therapy is to allow the subtalar joint to function near and around its neutral position. This is accomplished by balancing the forefoot to the rearfoot and by balancing the rearfoot with its supporting surface. There are a number of indications for the use of biomechanical orthotics:

1. Support and correction of intrinsic rearfoot and forefoot deformities
2. Support or restriction of range of motion
3. Treatment of postural problems
4. Dissipation of excessive ground reaction forces
5. Decrease of shear forces or tender spots on the plantar surface of the foot by redistribution of weight-bearing to more tolerant areas
6. Control of abnormal transverse rotation of the lower extremity

Contraindications to the use of orthotic therapy in the management of lower extremity injuries include the following:

1. Lack of intrinsic foot abnormality
2. Correction of soft tissue induced equinas
3. Incomplete lower quarter biomechanical examination

The anatomy of the orthotic consists of the module (shell) and the post (Fig. 8–63). The module is the body of the orthotic, which con-

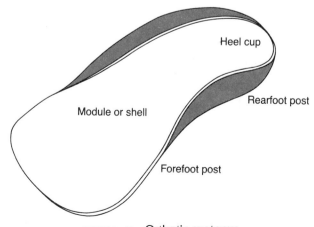

FIGURE 8–63   Orthotic anatomy.

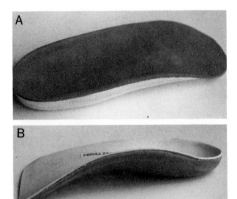

FIGURE 8–64   Orthotics. *A,* Semi-rigid. *B,* Rigid.

forms to the foot's plantar contours. The post is the "shim"; this is placed on the front or rear of the module, which brings the ground up to the foot and places the subtalar joint in its neutral position.

Two main types of orthotics are used. The biomechanical orthotic is constructed of rigid materials such as high-density plastics or semirigid materials called thermoplastics (Fig. 8–64*A* and *B*). Biomechanical orthotics control and resist abnormal foot forces. Accommodative orthotics are constructed of soft materials, such as Plastazote. These orthotics allow the foot to compensate, and the materials used in construction yield to abnormal foot forces. Posting on accommodative orthotics is referred to as bias.

The post is the corrective portion of the orthotic and is analogous to the corrective lens of eyeglasses. Posts can be located in the rearfoot or forefoot and can be constructed intrinsically or extrinsically to provide a varus (medial) or valgus (lateral) angulation. In order for the biomechanical orthotic to be effective and the athlete to comply in its use, it must meet the following requirements:

1. Must conform precisely to all contours of the foot, especially the heel seat and calcaneal and forefoot inclinations
2. Must be rigid enough to maintain the shape, contour, and imposed angular relationships of the foot
3. Must control abnormal motion, allow normal motion, and provide proper sequencing and timing of motion
4. Must be able to withstand stress and wear
5. Must be comfortable and ensure wear compliance
6. Must be adjustable
7. Must end proximal to the weight-bearing surfaces of the metatarsal heads
8. Must be narrow enough to fit on the shoe last and allow the first and fifth rays to function independently

If an athlete is using orthotics, shoe selection should be appropriate. Criteria for shoe selection include a straight-last shoe with a snug, deep, and stable heel counter. The shoe should have minimal heel height and adequate shoe depth. For the narrow-shank shoe, the insoles and arch cookies may have to be removed and replaced with a "cobra pad" orthotic,[26] in which the entire insert consists of posting

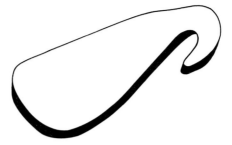

FIGURE 8–65   Cobra pad orthotic.

(Fig. 8–65). Feet that are high-arched or have an equinus attitude are difficult to fit with orthotic inserts.

Once the orthotic has been fabricated, it should be placed in the athlete's shoe for a 5- to 10-minute running trial. Areas of irritation may have to be ground down and assessment of correction of gait deviations determined. The athlete should be instructed about gradually breaking in the orthotic, with the wear time not to exceed 1 additional hour of wear for each day the orthotic has been worn.

RETURN TO COMPETITION

The final component of lower leg rehabilitation is the functional progression and testing program, which must precede return to athletic competition. The concept of functional progression mandates a logical and ordered sequence of rehabilitative activities leading back to previous performance. Athletes must be educated to appreciate that they cannot simply resume the activities that led to the initial injury when pain and swelling have subsided. Even the return of normal strength, flexibility, and endurance does not automatically ensure safe resumption of activity. Exercise programs cannot duplicate the speeds, forces, and stresses that normal high-speed athletic activities demand.

For these reasons, the athlete must be guided gradually back to activity by breaking down the component movements of the sport and addressing them in inverse order of difficulty. An example of this progression for an athlete with a lower extremity injury might be the following:

Nonweight-bearing exercise
Partial weight-bearing exercise
Full weight-bearing exercise
Walking
BAPS or balance board activities
Rebounder running
Jogging
Running
Jumping and hopping
Backpedaling
Figure-eight running
Cutting and twisting
Zigzag running
Plyometrics

NAME _____ INVOLVED EXTREMITY _____
DATE _____

	( )UNINVOLVED SIDE	( )INVOLVED SIDE	% DEFICIT
Unilateral Standing Long Jump (inches)	Trial 1 ____ Trial 2 ____ Trial 3 ____ Mean=___ inches	Trial 1 ____ Trial 2 ____ Trial 3 ____ Mean=___ inches	___%
Unilateral Vertical Jump (inches)	Trial 1 ____ Trial 2 ____ Trial 3 ____ Mean=___ inches	Trial 1 ____ Trial 2 ____ Trial 3 ____ Mean=___ inches	___%
20 inch hop for time (seconds)	Trial 1 ____ Trial 2 ____ Trial 3 ____ Mean=___ seconds	Trial 1 ____ Trial 2 ____ Trial 3 ____ Mean=___ seconds	___%
Stork Stand (seconds)	Trial 1 ____ Trial 2 ____ Trial 3 ____ Mean=___ seconds	Trial 1 ____ Trial 2 ____ Trial 3 ____ Mean=___ seconds	___%
4-square hop (# of repeats in 30 seconds)	_____	_____	___%
Unilateral Heel Raises (single lift capacity in pounds)	_____	_____	___%
Deep Squat (point of heel off)	Symmetry present: Yes No		
BAPS Board Evaluation: Level ____ Overload ____	_____	_____	____

(# of reps in 30 seconds)

SUBJECTIVE ASSESSMENT:

Sprinting _____

Backpedaling _____

Carioca _____

Box Run Right and Left _____

Video Gait Analysis _____

_____

_____

RECOMMENDATIONS: No participation   Participation with   Full Participation
                                                   restrictions

EVALUATOR _____

FIGURE 8–66   Sample form for evaluation of lower leg injuries.

The program is structured according to the specific demands of the athlete's sport. Modifications are appropriate depending on the goals and aspirations of the athlete. Specific criteria that dictate graduation from one functional level to the next must be defined precisely. It is the responsibility of the rehabilitation professional to provide the framework and specifics by which the athlete will function and progress.

Once the athlete has completed the functional progression program and is psychologically prepared to return to competition, an objective evaluation of physical readiness should be performed. Criteria for return to activity should include absence or control of pain, swelling, and spasm; isokinetic symmetry in peak torque, total work, and average power; and functional normality. Figure 8–66 is a sample functional evaluation form for lower leg injuries. It contains testing maneuvers and activities that can be used to judge an athlete's readiness to perform with symmetric functional normality.

References

1. American Academy of Orthopaedic Surgeons (1965): Joint Motion: Methods of Measuring and Recording. Chicago, American Academy of Orthopaedic Surgeons.
2. Axe, M., and Ray, R. (1988): Orthotic treatment of sesamoid pain. Am. J. Sports Med., 16:411–416.
3. Brandel, B.K., and Williams, K. (1974): An analysis of cinematographic and electromyographic recordings of human gait. In: Nelson, R., and Morehouse, C. (eds.): Biomechanics, Vol. IV. Baltimore, University Park Press.
4. Bouche, R.T., and Kuwanda, K.T. (1984): Equinus deformity in the athlete. Physician Sportsmed., 12:81–91.
5. Bosien, W.R. (1955): Residual disability following acute ankle sprains. J. Bone Joint Surg. [Am.], 37:1237–1243.
6. Clancy, W.G., Neidhart, D., and Brand, D.L. (1976): Achilles tendinitis in runners. A report of five cases. Am. J. Sports Med., 4:46–57.
7. Clement, D.B., Taunton, J.E., and Smart, G.E. (1984): Achilles tendinitis and peritendinitis: Etiology and treatment. Am. J. Sports Med., 12:179–184.
8. Creighton, D., and Olson, V. (1987): Evaluation of range of motion of first metatarsophalangeal joint in runners with plantar fasciitis. J. Orthop. Sports Phys. Ther., 8:357–361.
9. Cyriax, J. (1978): Textbook of Orthopedic Medicine, 7th ed. London, Bailliere Tindall.
10. Dameron, T.B. (1975): Fractures and anatomical variations of the proximal portion of the fifth metatarsal. J. Bone Joint Surg. [Am.], 57:788–792.
11. Donatelli, R. (1985): Normal biomechanics of the foot and ankle. J. Orthop. Sports Phys. Ther., 7:91–95.
12. Davies, G. (1984): A Compendium of Isokinetics in Clinical Usage. Lacrosse, WI, S & S.
13. Freeman, M.A.R., Dean, M.R.E., and Hanham, I.W.F. (1965): The etiology and prevention of functional instability of the foot. J. Bone Joint Surg. [Br.], 47:678–685.
14. Friedman, M. (1986): Injuries to the leg in athletes. In: Nicholas, J., and Hershman, E. (eds.): The Lower Extremity and Spine in Sports Medicine. St. Louis, C.V. Mosby.
15. Garth, W., and Miller, S. (1989): Evaluation of toe claw deformity, weakness of foot intrinsics, and posteromedial shin pain. Am. J. Sports Med., 17:821–827.
16. Gray, G. (1984): When the Foot Hits the Ground Everything Changes. Toledo, OH, American Physical Rehabilitation Network.
17. Hughes, L.Y. (1985): Biomechanical analysis of the foot and ankle to developing stress fractures. J. Orthop. Sports Ther., 7:96–101.
18. James, S.L., and Brubaker, C.E. (1973): Biomechanics of running. Orthop. Clin. North Am., 4:605–615.

19. Johnson, B. (1982): Case report: The Jones fracture—Review of proximal diaphyseal fractures of the fifth metatarsal in five athletes. Athletic Training, 17:268–270.
20. Kapandji, I.A. (1970): The Physiology of Joints, Vol. II. Edinburgh, Churchill-Livingston.
21. Keene, S. (1985): Ligament and muscle-tendon unit injuries. *In:* Gould, J., and Davies, G. (eds.): Orthopedic and Sports Physical Therapy. St. Louis, C.V. Mosby.
22. Kisner, C., and Colby, L.A. (1985): Ankle and foot. *In:* Therapeutic Exercise: Foundation and Techniques. Philadelphia, F.A. Davis.
23. Klein, K. (1990): Biomechanics of running. Presented at Metroplex Trainer's Meeting, Fort Worth, TX, January, 1990.
24. Lattanza, L., Gray, G., and Katner, R. (1988): Closed vs. open kinematic chain measurements of subtalar joint eversion: Implications for clinical practice. J. Orthop. Sports Phys. Ther., 9:310–314.
25. Magee, D.J. (1987): Orthopedic Physical Assessment. Philadelphia, W.B. Saunders.
26. McPoil, T., and Brocato, R. (1985): The foot and ankle: Biomechanical evaluation and treatment. *In:* Gould, J., and Davis, G. (eds.): Orthopedic and Sports Physical Therapy. St. Louis, C.V. Mosby.
27. Miller, W.A. (1977): Rupture of musculotendinous junction of medial head of gastrocnemius. Am. J. Sports Med., 5:191–193.
28. Rebman, L. (1986): Suggestions from the clinic: Ankle injuries: Clinical observations. J. Orthop. Sports Phys. Ther., 8:153–156.
29. Root, W.L., Orient, W.P., and Weed, J.N. (1977): Clinical Biomechanics, Vol. II: Normal and Abnormal Function of the Foot. Los Angeles, Clinical Biomechanics.
30. Sammarco, G.J. (1988): How I manage turf toe. Physician Sportsmed., 16:113–199.
31. Seibel, M.O. (1988): Foot Function. Baltimore, Williams & Wilkins.
32. Smart, G.W., Tauton, J.E., and Clement, D.B. (1980): Achilles tendinitis and peritendinitis. Med. Sci. Sports Exerc., 17:731–743.
33. Subotnick, S. (1989): Sports Medicine of the Lower Extremity. New York, Churchill-Livingstone.
34. Tanner, S., and Harvey, J. (1988): How we manage plantar fasciitis. Physician Sportsmed., 16:39–48.
35. Visnick, A. (1987): A playing orthosis for turf toe. Athletic Training, 22:215.
36. Vogelbach, D. (1989): The foot and ankle. Presented at HEALTHSOUTH Continuing Education Program. Birmingham, AL.
37. Wallace, L. (1986): Lower quarter pain: Mechanical evaluation and treatment. Presented at Seventh Annual Conference of the Sports Physical Therapy Section, Williamsburg, VA.
38. Woods, A., and Smith, W. (1983): Case report: Cuboid syndrome and the techniques for treatment. Athletic Training, 18:64–65.

CHAPTER 9

♦

Knee Rehabilitation

Gary L. Harrelson, M.S., A.T.,C.

The knee joint is one of the most frequently injured joints in the body, especially in those engaging in athletic activity. The incidence of permanent and progressively residual instability is higher from knee injury than from any other traumatic joint injury sustained in sports.[133] Even though it appears to be a relatively simple joint, the biomechanics of the knee and its surgical treatment have long been subjects of discussion in the literature and professional circles. The advent of arthroscopy has led to a greater understanding of these topics, and more is known about knee evaluation, treatment, and surgical intervention. Concurrently, the field of rehabilitation has also grown, and many traditional ideas and methods have been abandoned. Indications and contraindications for specific exercises are now research-based. This chapter emphasizes knee rehabilitation of the entire kinematic chain, early controlled motion, and return to participation along a functional progression, and restoration of lower extremity muscular strength, power, endurance, and neuromuscular control.

ARTHROLOGY AND ARTHROKINEMATICS

The knee joint is not only involved in carrying out activities of normal daily living, but is also subjected to greater forces during athletic participation than other joints. The knee is actually composed of two joints, the tibiofemoral and patellofemoral, and each affects the other. The knee joint possesses a large range of motion in only one plane, so its bony and soft tissue structures must be able to withstand considerable loads and/or externally applied forces.[140] The knee is inherently unstable because of its location between the two longest bones in the body, so it is subject to large torque forces. Knee stability is maintained through static restraints (e.g., ligaments) with dynamic restraints (e.g., muscles) attempting to compensate when there is static instability, as in the anterior cruciate ligament—deficient knee. Unfortunately, the ability

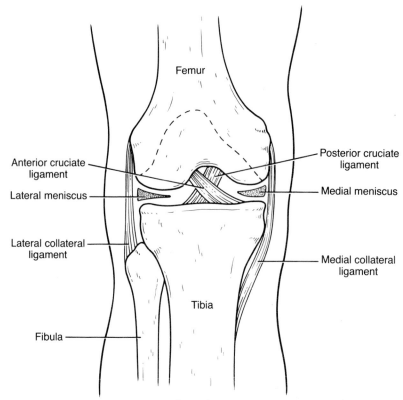

FIGURE 9–1   Static knee restraints.

of dynamic restraints to maintain knee stability is evident by the small number of athletes with anterior cruciate ligament–deficient knees who can return to full and unlimited sports participation without modifying their activity or later undergoing a surgical reconstruction of this ligament.[35]

The four main ligaments that provide the knee's static stability are the medial collateral ligament (MCL), lateral collateral ligament (LCL), anterior cruciate ligament (ACL), and posterior cruciate ligament (PCL) (Fig. 9–1). The MCL and LCL are responsible for resisting valgus and varus forces, respectively. The ACL deters anterior translation of the tibia on the femur, whereas the PCL checks posterior excursion of the tibia on the femur. The ACL suffers the highest incidence of injury of these four ligaments.

Additional static stability is provided by the joint capsule, specifically the posterior aspect. Of this, the posterolateral portion is most frequently damaged in traumatic injuries.[140] The posterolateral corner of the knee is reinforced by the arcuate, fabellafibular, and lateral collateral ligaments.[135] The posterior capsule is less prone to injury when the knee is in the flexed position because the structure is relatively slack.[59]

Also located within the knee joint are two menisci that help maintain some knee stability and act as shock absorbers for forces transmitted through the joint. These menisci also aid in distributing weight-bearing forces and increasing joint congruency, and possibly in improving articular cartilage nourishment capability.[65] The medial meniscus is the most often injured and is attached to the semimembranous and MCL, which may contribute to its greater incidence of injury. Conversely, the lateral meniscus has more freedom, conceivably contributing to its lower incidence of injury (although it is attached to the popliteus muscle).

Biomechanically, the menisci move in an anteroposterior direction and follow the tibia with flexion and extension but, during rotation, the menisci follow the femur.[75] Meniscal movement during knee flexion and extension is a result of the dynamic effects of the semimembranous and popliteus insertions during flexion and of the extensor mechanism with extension.[98]

Because the meniscus is basically avascular, except peripherally, healing does not occur once it is damaged and surgery is required to remove the torn piece of meniscus. This can usually be accomplished by arthroscopy. Peripheral tears can sometimes be repaired by arthroscopy or through a small incision. Research[98, 137] has documented the role of the knee meniscus in deterring degenerative joint changes and contributing to knee stability. Once all or part of a meniscus is removed, there is an increased area for articular cartilage degradation and tibiofemoral joint motion.

Although the greatest magnitude of movement is in the sagittal plane (e.g., flexion-extension), rotational movements are crucial to normal function.[140] During extension of the nonweight-bearing knee, 5° to 7° of tibial external rotation occurs during the last 30° of extension. Because the distal segment is fixed (closed chain), in the weight-bearing position the 5° to 7° of rotation that occurs probably results from combined tibial external rotation and femoral internal rotation. The overall effect of this motion is a closed-pack position, referred to as the "screw-home" mechanism. This is the position of maximum stability and negates rotation and valgus or varus motions.

Ligaments

The effect of knee motion on ligaments has been studied extensively, as has the role of secondary restraints in compensating for increased knee motion when a ligament is torn and in deterring abnormal forces. The contribution of the primary restraints increases as the secondary structures become slack with flexion.[18] The effect of knee motion on liga-

TABLE 9–1   SUMMARY OF KNEE LIGAMENT FUNCTION

Medial Collateral	Lateral Collateral	Anterior Cruciate	Posterior Cruciate
Tight in extension and external rotation; perhaps some participation in anteroposterior motion	Tight in extension and probably external rotation	Tight in extension; controls anterior glide of tibia on femur	Tight in flexion; limits posterior glide of tibia

* From Soderberg, G.L.: Kinesiology: Application to Pathological Motion. © 1986, the Williams & Wilkins Co., Baltimore.

ments has implications for the indications and contraindications of treatment, and many investigators[17, 21, 52, 58, 76, 79, 101, 144, 156] have examined the effects of knee motion on ligaments (Table 9–1). The cruciate and collateral ligaments provide the primary ligamentous restraining force in a single plane, but can act as secondary restraints in other planes.[21, 59, 114, 118]

The MCL is the primary restraint to medial opening of the knee at both 5° and 25° of flexion.[53] The MCL is tight in extension and external rotation.[140] The other cruciate ligaments and posteromedial capsule provide secondary restraints. [53, 138] The LCL is the predominant restraint to lateral opening, with the other cruciate ligaments, lateral capsule, and tendons of the iliotibial tract and popliteus acting as secondary restraints.[18] The LCL is tight in extension and probably also in external rotation.

The ACL resists anterior displacement of the tibia on the femur and has a vital role in resisting internal rotation.[22] This is verified by sectioning of the ACL, which results in increased tibial rotation.[88, 128] Grood and colleagues[59] have reported that the ACL provides 85% of the ligamentous restraining force to anterior drawer at 30° and 90° of flexion. The medial and lateral capsules, collateral ligaments, and iliotibial tract and band also contribute to anterior stability.[60, 129] The ACL becomes tight in extension.[140] Conversely, the primary function of the PCL is resisting posterior displacement of the tibia on the femur. The posterior medial and lateral capsules, collateral ligaments, and popliteus complex help deter posterior tibial excursion.[60, 138, 140] The PCL becomes tight in flexion, but less is known about its rotation function. Fukubayashi and associates,[54] however, have reported a marked loss of rotation with insufficiency of the cruciate ligaments, and concluded that intact cruciate ligaments produce concurrent rotation and the cruciate ligaments constitute a primary mechanism in the production and control of rotation during anterior and posterior knee motion. Noyes and co-workers[121] and Butler and colleagues[21] have noted that when the cruciate ligaments are damaged, the axis of rotation is displaced within the medial compartment and may become located out of the joint entirely. This results in abnormal and excessive motion between the articular surfaces, with well-documented sequelae.

It has also been determined that the joint capsule has a significant role in restraining motion. For example, sectioning the posterolateral complex in cadaver specimens with ACL deficiencies results in increased internal rotation, whereas sectioning of the anterolateral capsule produces no increase in either internal or external rotation.[88] This finding has been supported by other reports.[85, 101] Although damage to the posterolateral corner does increase rotation Noyes and Sonstegard,[122] who studied anterolateral and anterior laxity in cadaver knees before and after sectioning of the ACL, suggested that primary laxity (whether translatory or rotatory motion) results from an approximately 100% increase in anteroposterior translation and only a 15% increase in rotation laxity.

With cruciate deficiencies, anterior or posterior displacement of the tibia on the femur must be controlled by the secondary static restraints, as well as by the primary dynamic restraints. Shoemaker and

Markolf[138] have reported that the internal muscular rotators of the knee can generate torque equal to the force necessary to rupture the ligaments under laboratory conditions. They postulated that the muscular rotators could actively resist disruption of the ligaments if they could generate enough torque in response to stress placed on the knee. Unfortunately, this is not the usual situation, and Noyes and associates[121] coined the term "functional stability" to refer to the ability of the neuromuscular components of the knee joint to support the ligamentous restraints to joint opening. When muscles and ligaments balance the external forces placed on the knee, the joint is stable. When an imbalance occurs, injury to the joint results in damage to such structures as the ligaments, menisci, and tendons.[18] This may also help explain why some individuals can perform asymptomatically after losing their ACL. It has been noted, however, that only minimal support exists from the secondary structures in deterring anterior or posterior movement following loss of the ACL or PCL.[21]

Muscle Activity

Much of the literature on this subject has addressed the quadriceps muscles because of their importance in the knee joint, but little information is available about the hamstrings because of their comparatively less significant role in knee control.[140] The hamstrings function to flex the knee and produce tibial rotation, the biceps femoris rotates the tibia externally, and the semimembranosus and semitendinosus rotate the tibia internally. Because of the hamstrings' insertion on the tibia, they can act as dynamic restraints in ACL-deficient knees. The neuromuscular development of the hamstrings is important in helping deter tibial translation. In the presence of anterolateral rotatory instability (ALRI) or anteromedial rotatory instability (AMRI), facilitation of enhanced neuromuscular control of the biceps femoris (ALRI) and of the semimembranosus and semitendinosus (AMRI), respectively, may help deter tibial excursion. Additionally, the popliteus muscle is responsible for tibial internal rotation when initial flexion occurs from knee extension, producing the unlocking of the screw-home mechanism.[92]

The quadriceps are considered the primary dynamic stabilizers of the knee and are responsible for knee extension. The role(s) of the quadriceps muscles in various ranges of knee extension and the effect of different positions on their activity have been studied. The isometric peak torque for the knee extensors has been recorded to be highest at 45° of flexion.[139] The influence of hip position on the rectus femoris while performing knee extension[23, 123] and a straight leg raise (SLR)[47] has also been investigated. Electromyography (EMG) results on the role of the rectus femoris in the sitting position conflict somewhat but it is evident that the rectus femoris and vastus muscles act simultaneously during supine knee extension.[23, 123] It does appear from EMG studies, however, that in the sitting position the rectus femoris functions only in the terminal phase of knee extension.[23, 47] Fisk and Wells[47] have also noted high levels of EMG activity in the rectus femoris during the initial range of the straight leg raise and throughout hip flexion with the knee flexed.

There is also much debate about the different roles of the quadriceps musculature in the various positions of range of motion, not unlike the confusion over the roles of the supraspinatus and deltoid at different ranges of motion when performing shoulder abduction. It has been generally accepted that the vastus medialis muscle increases activity during the terminal phases of knee extension, but several investigators have reported that EMG patterns of the three quadriceps muscles are similar throughout the entire range of knee extension, with none of the three muscles being predominantly responsible for extending the knee in any aspect of its range of motion.[15, 32, 71, 86, 87, 129]

The straight leg raise, isometric quadriceps contraction (quad set), and knee extension exercise are typical therapeutic exercises prescribed following knee injury or surgery. It appears that total quadriceps activity is greatest during isometric contraction[57] when compared with that during the straight leg raise or active knee extension exercise.[129] Furthermore, Knight and co-workers[81] have concluded that none of the three quadriceps muscles are as active during the straight leg raise as during knee extension at the same relative workload. This may be a result of active knee movement placing a greater load on the quadriceps femoris muscle.[6] Soderberg and Cook[141] have reported data from 40 normal subjects, in whom the straight leg raise was compared with quad sets. They noted an increase in rectus femoris activity with a straight leg raise and an increase in vastus medialis activity when performing a quad set.

The oblique fibers of the vastus medialis (VMO) have been studied[87, 132] in relation to their suggested ability to resist lateral displacement of the patella because of their position. The oblique fibers of the VMO insert at approximately 55° to the long axis of the femur and are responsible for maintaining proper patella tracking.[86, 87] The classic study by Lieb and Perry[87] evaluated the function of the VMO in the terminal phases of extension. They found that twice as much quadriceps force is required to accomplish the last 15° of extension, which is consistent with other results.[60, 143] The condition in which active range of knee extension is less than the passive range of knee extension is referred to as extension lag,[143] which had been traditionally thought to be a result of decreased VMO strength. Even when performing terminal extension[86, 87, 132] the VMO did not contribute any more in achieving full active extension than the other quadriceps muscles, but it did demonstrate increased activity in maintaining medial alignment of the patella. From these results it is postulated that the only selective function of the VMO is patellar alignment. Even though there is early and clinically recognizable atrophy of the vastus medialis, the prominence of the muscle and the thinness of the fascial covering have misled clinicians into believing that there is specific rather then general quadriceps atrophy.[86]

Patellofemoral Biomechanics

The patellofemoral joint is a major source of pain and dysfunction at the knee joint. The primary functions of the patella are to increase the efficiency of the quadriceps muscles and to provide anterior bony protection to the femur. Normal patellofemoral kinematics is based on the ability of the patella to resist mechanical loading and on the stabilization of the patella within the femoral groove.[19] This stability is based on bony geometry, ligamentous restraints, and active stability by muscles.[69] Patellar stability is maintained by both static and dynamic restraints. The osseous configuration of the patella and femoral groove and ligamentous structures act as static restraints to help retain its stability. Normally, the femoral groove sulcus should be between 130° and 145°, with the lateral ridge higher,[2, 108] and the center of the patella fits into this sulcus. However, varying shapes of the patellar and femoral grooves predispose individuals to patellofemoral dysfunctions.[158] The medial and lateral patellar retinacula, which also serve as static patellar restraints, resist lateral and medial subluxation of the patella, respectively. The medial and lateral patellofemoral ligaments also act as static stabilizers of the patella (Fig. 9–2).

The four quadriceps muscles serve as the major dynamic supports for the patella. They attach to the patella by way of the quadriceps tendon and then to the tibial tuberosity by way of the patellar tendon. Of these dynamic restraints, the VMO has been postulated to be primarily involved in patellofemoral problems. The VMO is not selectively re-

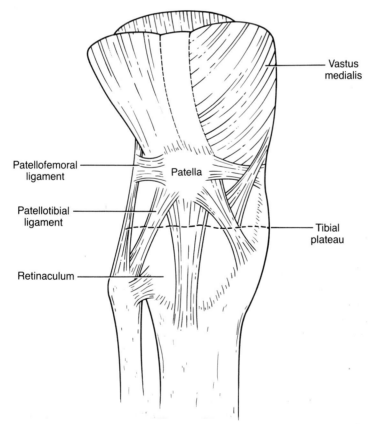

FIGURE 9–2 Static and dynamic supports of the patellofemoral joint. (From Woodall, W., and Welsh, J. (1990): A biomechanical basis for rehabilitation programs involving the patellofemoral joint. J. Orthop. Sports Phys. Ther., 11:536, © by the Orthopedic and Sports Physical Therapy Section of the APTA.)

sponsible for terminal knee extension, but provides the primary dynamic restraint in resisting the lateral forces that act on the patella.[49, 68, 86, 87, 127] Also, the pes anserine muscle group and biceps femoris dynamically affect patellar stability, because they control tibial internal and external rotation and can significantly influence patellar tracking.[72, 127]

Understanding patellofemoral biomechanics is important when prescribing knee exercises for a rehabilitation program. The connection between the tibiofemoral and patellofemoral joints must not be overlooked, nor should they be treated independently, because restriction of motion in one joint may result in restriction in the other. Knee extension is connected to superior patellar glide, anterior translation of the tibia, and external rotation of the knee.[18] This is referred to as the screw-home mechanism, which is a result of unequal motion of the medial and lateral compartments. Superior glide of the patella is a coupled motion with knee extension because of the tension applied to the patella by the quadriceps. When patellar glide is limited, by either muscular inhibition or adhesions, a lag in knee extension results.[9, 61, 114]

During flexion the opposite motion occurs between the femur and tibia and between the femur and patella. Flexion is associated with tibial internal rotation, posterior tibial translation, and inferior glide of the patella. During flexion, rotation of the tibia is initiated by the popliteus muscle.[11, 101, 130] If inferior glide of the patella is restricted by adhesions in the suprapatellar pouch, knee flexion is also limited.[18]

The patella must withstand large compressive and tensile loads caused by contraction of the quadriceps, especially under weight-bearing conditions. During daily activity the patellofemoral joint may be subjected to compressive loads of up to 10 times body weight.[18] Compression of the articular surfaces occurs when the patella contacts the femoral groove. In the normal patellofemoral joint, contact between the patellar undersurface and femoral groove first occurs at around 10° to 20° of flexion, and shifts from the distal margin at 20° to the most proximal margin at 120° of flexion (Fig. 9–3).[55, 56, 67] Contact joint pressure appears to be rather uniform between 20° and 90° of flexion. Past 90°, pressure appears to be higher along the medial patellar facet and may explain the increase in reported chondromalacia in the medial facet.[145, 158] With flexion past 125° very large forces are present over a very small articular area, creating large contact stress (Fig. 9–3).[55, 56, 67]

Of greater importance is the force per unit of area on the patella. In full extension the compressive forces on the patella are almost negligible but, as knee flexion increases, the patellofemoral joint reaction (PFJR) forces increase. With increasing flexion the contact area almost doubles as the knee flexion angle moves from 30 to 90°.[67] This serves to distribute an increasing PFJR force over a broader area, even though the total force across the joint is decreasing.[70] During extension against resistance the PFJR increases and the contact area decreases. Patellofemoral contact pressure appears to be highest at 60° and 90° of flexion; the maximum contact force has been extrapolated to be 6.5 times body weight at 90° of flexion.[67] These patellar forces appear to be about 20% higher in women than in men.[112] Also, increases or decreases in the Q angle can produce nonuniform pressure distribution

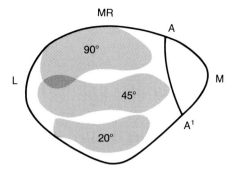

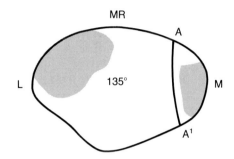

FIGURE 9–3 Patellofemoral contact pattern with knee flexion. (MR, median ridge; A-A[1], ridge separating medial and odd facets.) (From Goodfellow, J., Hungerford, D.S., and Zindel, M. (1976): Patellofemoral joint mechanics and pathology: 1. Functional anatomy of the patellofemoral joint. J. Bone Joint Surg. [Br.], 58:287–290.)

with higher peak stresses in some areas and relative unloading in others. Although the Q angle changes in relation to joint loading and flexion angle, it still must be considered as a potential causative factor in chondromalacia.

Forces between the patellar tendon and quadriceps muscle are not equal throughout the knee range of motion[134]—these forces are equal only at approximately 45°.[18] During terminal extension exercises, the force developed in the patellar tendon is greater than that of the quadriceps because of the mechanical advantage of the quadriceps, so this exercise may cause local irritation of the patellar tendon. It may be necessary for the athlete to avoid exercising within this range during certain stages of patellofemoral rehabilitation.[102] As the knee is flexed and extended through a full arc of motion the patella can grind against the femoral groove, causing irreversible damage to the patella's undersurface. This must be considered when designing a knee rehabilitation program whether or not knee pain and/or dysfunction is of patellofemoral origin.

OVERVIEW OF THE REHABILITATION PROGRAM

Rehabilitation following knee injury and/or surgery should concentrate on decreasing inflammation and swelling, early muscle turn-on, restoration of motion, protection of the patellofemoral joint, closed-chain rehabilitation, and restoration of proprioception. The initial inflammatory process should be treated with ice, compression, and elevation;

oral nonsteroidal anti-inflammatory drugs (NSAIDs) are also indicated following injury. Use of vasopneumatic compression devices and the active muscular pump through the initiation of therapeutic exercises aid in diminishing joint effusion and help promote early muscle turn-on. Ice before and after therapeutic exercise is recommended for pain and prophylactically after exercise for 4 to 6 weeks after the initial inflammation has subsided.

Early muscle turn-on of the quadriceps is of vital importance in preventing arthrofibrosis and promoting normal arthrokinematics. The reason for quadriceps shutdown was discussed in Chapter 2 but the fear of pain, joint effusion, and a neurologic feedback loop (H reflex) are the most plausible reasons for this phenomenon. The use of early electrical muscle stimulation (EMS) has little effect on deterring quadriceps atrophy, but does help facilitate quadriceps re-education.

The implementation of early knee joint motion following injury or surgery helps deter joint arthrofibrosis and promotes healing. The detrimental effects of immobilization were discussed in Chapter 2. Plaster casting of the knee following injury or surgery has been replaced by the use of hinged braces to provide for early protected motion. Loss of knee motion from any cause is a common occurrence that should be prevented. Loss of knee range of motion, particularly following ACL reconstruction, was common 5 or 6 years ago. Scar tissue was usually deposited in the intercondylar notch, resulting in notch impingement and causing loss of knee extension. Unfortunately, even though physicians and clinicians attempt to prevent it, loss of knee motion still occurs. Although some range of motion must be guarded initially (e.g., MCL injury, last 30°; PCL reconstruction, greater than 60° of flexion), early protected motion helps promote synovial fluid diffusion and orient collagen fibrils along lines of stress, helping to restore normal arthrokinematics.

Laubenthal and colleagues[84] have determined the amount of active knee motion necessary for performing activities of daily living, as follows:

83° knee flexion for stair climbing
93° knee flexion for sitting
106° knee flexion to tie shoes
65–70° knee flexion for normal gait

Initial range of motion can begin with supine heel slides (see App. A), in which athletes slide their heel toward their buttocks, as tolerated. Also, early tibiofemoral and patellofemoral mobilization are beneficial (Chap. 6) in restoring motion. Noyes and Mangine[119] have described a condition termed "patella infra," which can result from a combination of not restoring patellofemoral mobility, loss of tibiofemoral motion, and quadriceps shutdown. Inferior glide of the patella is necessary for knee flexion to occur; if inferior patellar glide is restricted (e.g., by adhesions), a loss of knee flexion results. Conversely, if superior patellar glide is diminished, a loss of knee extension occurs. Although heel slides are helpful in making the transition from flexion to extension and from extension to flexion, they do increase patellofemoral compression when compared with seated heel slides, knee flexion using under-the-chair rope-and-pulley (Fig. 9–4), active-assisted flexion (Fig. 9–5), or seated flexion with overpressure applied from the uninjured extremity. All these activities result in less patellofemoral pressure and are functionally more useful. These active-assisted exercises work well in restoring knee motion while athletes remain in touch with their pain threshold, thus reducing the chance of incurring greater knee injury or damage to a surgical repair.

The knee joint, along with its other lower extremity articulations (foot, ankle, and hip), functions ideally in a closed kinematic chain. The movements of sports and daily living usually involve opening and closing the lower extremity chain (e.g., running, jogging, walking). This synergy of joint motion is most readily detectable in activities such as rising from a chair or ascending stairs, which require the combination of knee and hip extension. The lower extremity joints generally function in a closed-chain relationship, with each joint affecting the other. It appears that only in weight rooms and therapeutic rehabilitation programs is an emphasis placed on open-chain activities, which are not sports-specific and subject the lower extremity joints to high compressive and shear forces. Over the last 5 years more emphasis has been

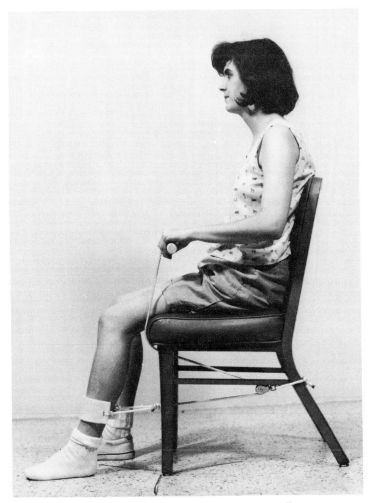

FIGURE 9–4   Knee flexion with rope-and-pulley.

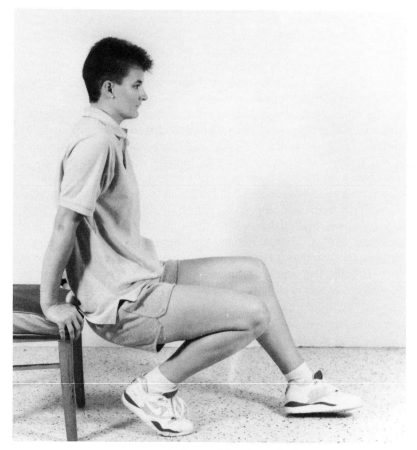

FIGURE 9–5   Active-assisted knee flexion.

placed on the use of closed kinematic chain exercises for the lower extremity. Closed-chain exercises help restore proprioception, muscle strength, and interdependency of lower extremity joints with each other, and are much safer, because the stress is applied through the entire kinematic chain. This particularly reduces patellofemoral shear and compressive forces at the knee joint.

Following most knee injuries or surgery closed-chain exercises can be implemented almost immediately, because the shear forces across the tibiofemoral joint are reduced. Most closed-chain exercises can advance in some form of functional progression, such as the minisquat exercise outlined in Table 9–2. Figures 9–6 through 9–19 illustrate closed-chain exercises that can be implemented throughout the various stages of knee rehabilitation.* Most of these can be progressed along a continuum of difficulty by increasing resistance, speed of movement, and, in some instances, by changing the athlete's visual feedback (e.g., from looking down at the floor, to looking straight ahead, to closing the eyes).

_____

* The ProFitter shown in Figures 9–15, 9–16, and 9–17 is manufactured by Fitter International, Calgary, Canada. The Slide Board shown in Figure 9–18 is available from Don Courson Enterprises, Birmingham, AL.

Text continued on page 287

TABLE 9–2   EXAMPLE OF CLOSED-CHAIN PROGRESSION OF THE MINISQUAT

Weight shifts with support
↓
Weight shifts without support
↓
Bilateral minisquats with support
↓
Bilateral minisquats without support
↓
Bilateral minisquats against wall
↓
Bilateral minisquats against wall with weights in hands
↓
One-legged minisquats with support
↓
One-legged minisquats without support
↓
One-legged minisquats against wall
↓
One-legged minisquats against wall with weight in hands
↓
Bilateral minisquats with tubing
↓
One-legged minisquats with tubing
↓
Gradually increase tubing strength and speed of movement

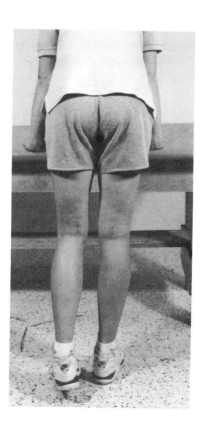

FIGURE 9–6   Weight shifts. Body weight is transferred from one extremity to the other.

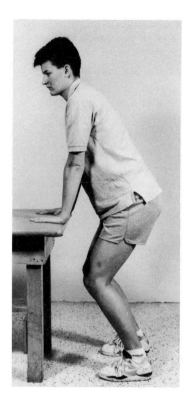

FIGURE 9-7 Bilateral minisquats with support.

FIGURE 9-8 Minisquats on one leg with support.

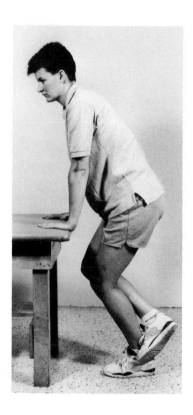

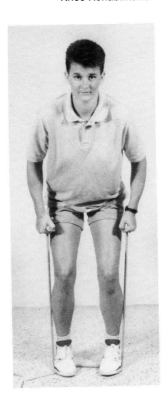

FIGURE 9–9 Bilateral minisquats with tubing. These can be progressed from slow to fast speeds with a progressive increase in tubing resistance.

FIGURE 9–10 Minisquats on one leg with tubing. These work on muscular strength and on proprioception, and can be progressed from slow to fast speeds.

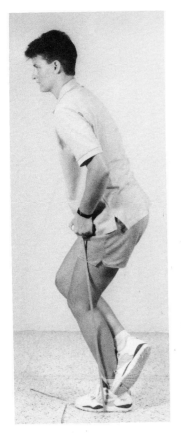

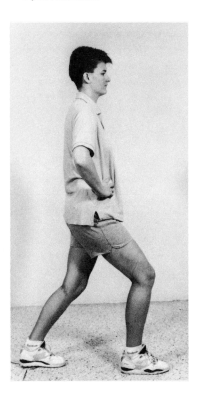

FIGURE 9–11 Lunges. These can progress to adding weight in hands.

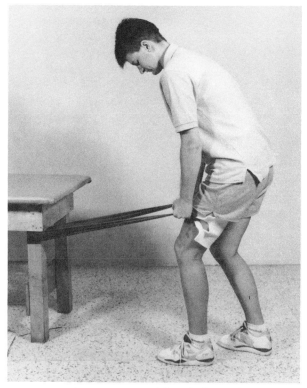

FIGURE 9–12 Don Tigney knee extension (closed-chain terminal knee extension).

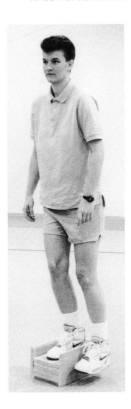

FIGURE 9–13 Lateral step-up. One-inch boards can be used to progress the height of this exercise.

FIGURE 9–14 Closed-chain running or lunges with tubing.

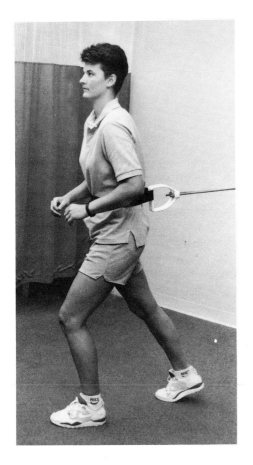

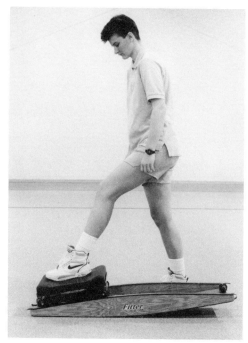

FIGURE 9–15   Closed-chain hip flexion and knee extension using the ProFitter. These can be gradually progressed in resistance and speed of movement.

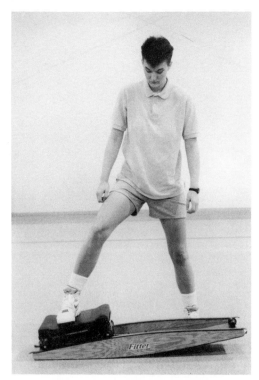

FIGURE 9–16   Closed-chain hip abduction using the ProFitter. These can be gradually progressed in resistance and speed of movement.

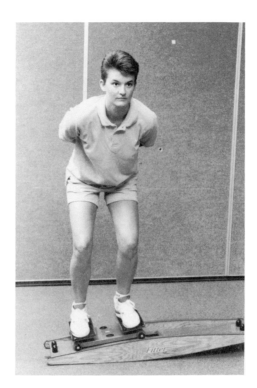

FIGURE 9–17   ProFitter used for developing muscular strength and proprioception.

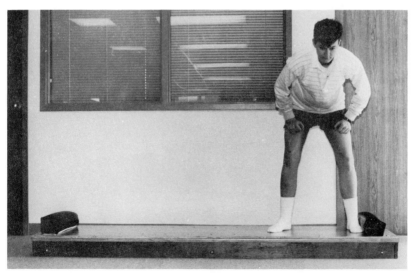

FIGURE 9–18   Slide Board. This can be used to develop muscular strength, proprioception, eccentric firing of the hamstring muscles, and cardiovascular conditioning.

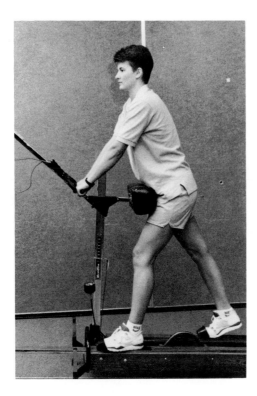

FIGURE 9–19 The NordicTrack. Closed-chain exercises for cardiovascular conditioning and knee extension.

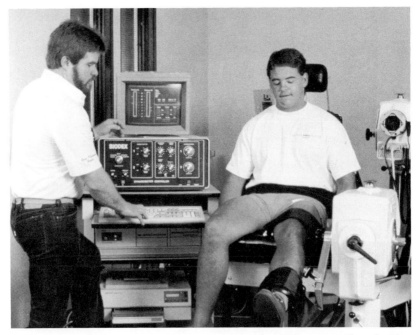

FIGURE 9–20 Isokinetic devices. These can be used at high contractile velocities to develop muscular strength and endurance. (Photo courtesy of Sports Medicine Update, Birmingham, AL; HealthSouth Sports Medicine.)

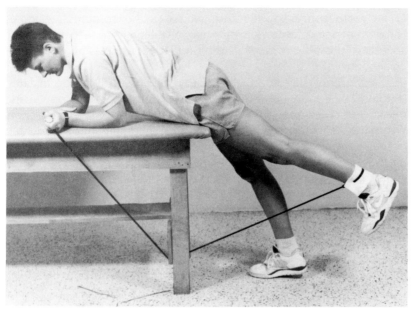

FIGURE 9–21   Surgical tubing. This can be used at various resistances and speeds.

Although closed-chain exercises are important in rehabilitation following a knee injury, open-chain exercises can also be used. Straight leg
raises in hip flexion, abduction, adduction, and extension are still used in
the early phases of rehabilitation. Appendix A presents some predominantly open-chain exercises, with instructions, and these can be used
for a home exercise program. Also, isokinetics can be used at higher
contractile velocities (Fig. 9–20). At the high contractile speeds it tends

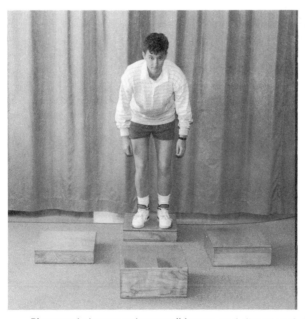

FIGURE 9–22   Plyometric jumps using small boxes and directional changes.

to be more sports-specific and decreases the compressive forces across the patellofemoral joint. Surgical tubing can be used at high speeds to promote muscular strength and endurance and neuromuscular control (Fig. 9–21).

In the later stages of rehabilitation plyometrics can be initiated (Figures 9–22 and 9–23). This helps develop the explosive power and muscle coordination necessary to resume sports participation. Plyometrics should also be progressed on a continuum of graduated difficulty. Depth jumps are not recommended, but small box jumps can be used with quick directional changes. Because of the increased eccentric contraction associated with plyometrics and the muscle microtrauma that is incurred, this type of exercise should be done only two or three times weekly. Plyometrics can also serve as a type of functional testing and can be used as part of the criteria for return to play.

Most closed-chain exercises also enhance proprioceptive function. It is well established that the mechanoreceptors that surround the joint are damaged with joint injury. The interrelationship between these

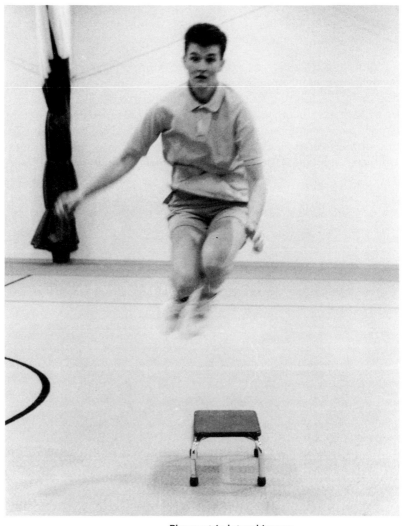

FIGURE 9–23 Plyometric lateral jumps.

mechanoreceptors and muscles forms the neuromuscular control necessary for normal joint movements. Return to activity before redevelopment of these mechanoreceptors can predispose that joint to additional injury. Kennedy and associates[77] have postulated that a loss of the ACL would result in reduced proprioceptive function and contribute to increasing instability over time through the loss of dynamic stabilizing reflexes. Schultz and co-workers[134] have demonstrated histologically the presence of mechanoreceptors in human cruciate ligaments, and hypothesized that they are active in the proprioceptive reflex arc that helps protect the knee from deformation beyond its anatomic limits. Barrack and colleagues[10] have investigated the effect of a deficient ACL on proprioception, and found that those with complete ACL disruptions and moderate to severe rotatory instability may experience a decline in knee proprioception.

Figures 9–24 through 9–28 outline various proprioceptive exer-

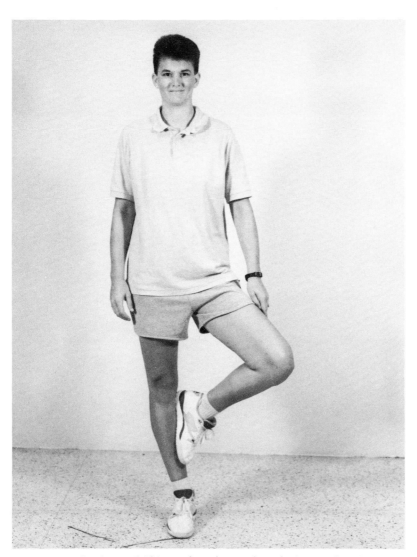

FIGURE 9–24   Stork stand. This can be advanced to playing catch with a ball.

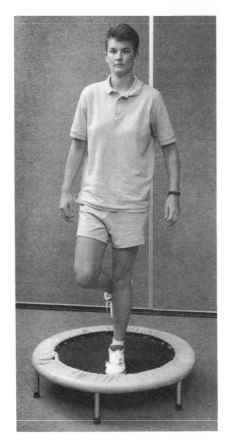

FIGURE 9-25 Stork stand on trampoline.

FIGURE 9-26 BAPS board on one leg with support.

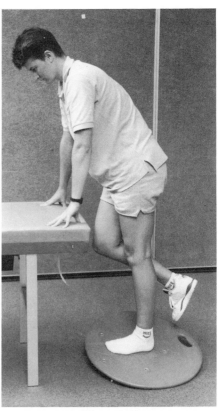

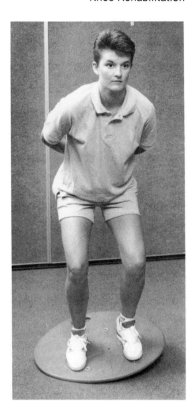

FIGURE 9-27 Bilateral BAPS board balancing.

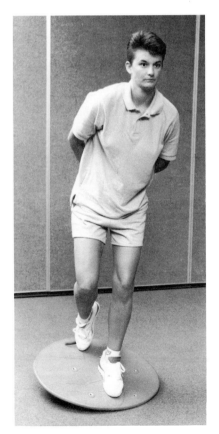

FIGURE 9-28 BAPS board on one leg without support.

cises that can be included in a knee rehabilitation program. There is a logical functional progression for proprioceptive exercises, as well as a motor learning component. Most individuals do better the day after a proprioceptive exercise, after having had time to think about it. With joint trauma there is still decreased proprioception, however, and after the learning effect, residual difficulty with proprioception exercises can be attributed to the joint's damaged mechanoreceptors. The more severe the injury, the greater the damage to joint mechanoreceptors and the longer it takes for this feedback mechanism to be restored.

Visual feedback is important in progressing proprioceptive exercises. In the early stages athletes may find that looking at the ground makes the exercise easier. They should then progress to looking straight ahead and then to eyes closed. Proprioceptive exercises can also progress from bilateral to unilateral on the injured leg and from using support to no support in the later stages of proprioceptive development.

Re-education of joint mechanoreceptors is very important in total rehabilitation of knee injuries, and is often overlooked. Proprioceptive exercises can be initiated early in rehabilitation and progressed along an increasing continuum of difficulty. These exercises can also be implemented into sports-specific skills (Figs. 9–29 and 9–30), and are closed-chain activities.

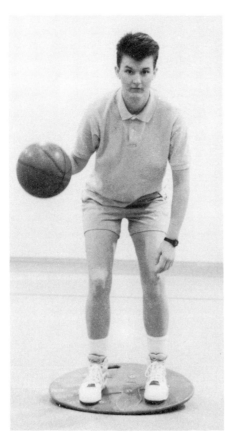

FIGURE 9–29   Bilateral BAPS board dribbling.

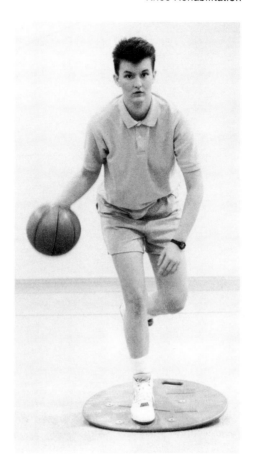

FIGURE 9–30 BAPS board dribbling on one leg.

Knee Extension Exercise

The full-arc knee extension exercise (90° to 0°) has long been used to increase quadriceps strength, during both therapeutic rehabilitation and conditioning programs. However, the efficacy of this exercise must be evaluated in regard to its consequences, specifically to the patellofemoral joint. As the knee moves from flexion to extension the patellar undersurface comes in direct contact with the underlying femoral groove, and the compressive forces generated during activity change with knee joint angle. The points on the patella that actually articulate with the femur change from distal to proximal as the knee goes from extension to flexion. Also, as flexion increases, there is a resultant reduction in patellar mobility. This can readily be observed by placing the knee in extension and moving the patella. Its mobility is evident with the knee in full extension but, as the knee flexes, the patella becomes less mobile, resulting in increased contact pressure between the patellar undersurface and femoral groove, which is greatest at 90° of flexion.[67, 112] The amount of patellar compression against the femur depends on the angle of knee flexion and on muscle tension; this can be calculated and is known as the patellofemoral joint reaction (PFJR) force (Fig. 9–31).

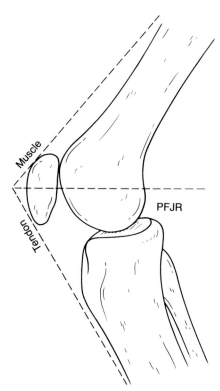

FIGURE 9–31   Schematic representation of patellofemoral joint reaction (PFJR) forces. (From Grana, W.A., and Kriegshauser, L.A. (1985): Scientific basis of extensor mechanism disorders. Clin. Sports Med., 4:251.)

Because the area of the patella in contact with the femur increases with knee flexion, the area over which forces are distributed essentially increases. This is an attempt to distribute the load over a broader area; but the opposite occurs during extension. Thus, at some point in the range of motion, compression exceeds the physiologic loading that occurs during weight-bearing. This appears to be around 52° short of full extension.[69]

Reilly and Martens[131] have studied joint reaction and quadriceps forces during straight leg raising and other activities. The lowest value for the PFJR force was found during walking, amounting to 0.5 times body weight. Stair climbing required a PFJR force of 3.3 times body weight, whereas the largest force (7.8 times body weight) was produced during deep knee bends to 130°. These values were determined with body weight acting as the main flexing force, and change considerably when free flexion and extension are considered. The crucial difference is not in the magnitude of the forces and moments but the fact that, in free extension, the flexing moment increases with a decreasing angle of knee flexion.[69] This means that the required quadriceps force increases with decreasing flexion, which is the reverse of flexion under body weight. In standing with the knee fully extended the quadriceps force is 0, with increasing force required with increasing knee flexion. With extension against resistance at 90° of flexion the quadriceps demand is 0, with increasing force required with increasing extension.

Reilly and Martens[131] have also calculated PFJR forces for knee extension against resistance with the subject sitting and the lower leg hanging free (Fig. 9–32). The PFJR force was initially 0 at 90°, increasing rapidly to a maximum of 1.4 times body weight at 36° of flexion and then decreasing rapidly to approximately 50% of body weight at full extension. However, in this situation, the quadriceps tension continues to increase to its maximum value at full extension. This explains why straight leg raising and short-arc knee extension exercises (20° to 0°) provide maximum stress to the quadriceps muscle while simultaneously producing minimum compression on the patellofemoral joint.[131]

Hungerford and Barry[69] have also determined PFJR forces for knee flexion under body weight and extension against 9-kg boot resistance. Extension with a 9-kg boot exceeds physiologic compression at 52° of flexion because the contact areas of the patella increase with increasing knee flexion, which distributes the increased PFJR force over a larger area to minimize contact stress. In extension against resistance, however, the increasing PFJR force is distributed over a smaller area and

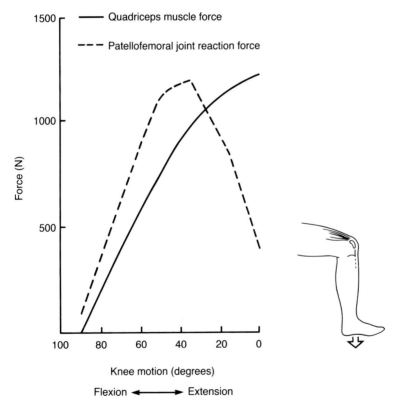

FIGURE 9–32   Knee extension forces in the patellofemoral joint and quadriceps exerted with a 9-kg boot, with the subject seated and the lower leg free. (From Reilly, D.T., and Martens, M. (1972): Experimental analysis of the quadriceps muscle force and patellofemoral joint reaction force for various activities. Acta Orthop. Scand., 43:126–137. © 1972 Munksgaard International Publishers Ltd., Copenhagen, Denmark.)

contact stress is increased. Therefore, patients with patellofemoral pain who do extension exercises against resistance from 90° of flexion experience increased pain, and other symptoms are exacerbated. Also, compressive forces between the quadriceps tendon and femoral intercondylar groove are present above a 60° knee angle.[112] These factors, together with changes in the size of the contact area of the patella on the femur, might explain why some exercises can produce significant forces at this joint.

Several investigators have reported safe ranges of motion in which injured patellofemoral joints can be exercised. Grood and associates[60] have found that quadriceps force increases little as the leg is extended from 50° to 15° and, in patients with patellofemoral chondrosis in whom a full range of joint motion is not desired, quadriceps exercises can be limited to this amount of extension without decreasing quadriceps force. Brownstein and co-workers[18] have recommended that the quadriceps be exercised initially using isometric and isotonic exercises in 90° to 60° of flexion, because stress on the patella is reduced in this range.

Reilly and Martens' data[131] suggest that, because peak force occurs approximately 40° from full knee extension, this point in the range of motion may be difficult for a patient with patellofemoral joint pathology. Force at this point decreases rapidly because, at this joint position, tension in the quadriceps and patellar tendon produces mostly shear in the joint rather then compressive forces.[69] Even though contact force decreases with extension, if contact area decreases at a faster rate there is a resultant increase in pressure. These biomechanical factors may help explain why many patellofemoral patients have no symptoms at 52° or greater but have severe pain at angles less than 52°. Hungerford and Lennox[70] have recommended avoidance of the nonphysiologic loading of the joint that is produced by such activities (e.g., extension exercises with weight from 90° of flexion, exercise machines that apply excessive resistance to the patellofemoral joint by loading the foot or ankle). Nisell and Ekholm[112] have suggested that a painful patellofemoral joint sensitive to high stress is better exercised at a straighter knee angle so that high compressive forces can be avoided.

Various recommendations have been made about safe angles for exercising the knee joint in flexion or extension without creating or contributing to patellofemoral chondromalacia or chondrosis. Full-arc knee extension should be avoided, even in normal knees, for fear of this exercise perpetuating patellofemoral pathology. In considering guidelines for exercising patellofemoral patients, Mangine[94] has suggested that the rehabilitation program be oriented around the area of crepitus. Often the patient is comfortable in the 90° to 45° range, which allows for a greater area of surface contact for dispersion of forces. This also correlates with greater quadriceps muscle activity in the lower ranges of motion. Exercising athletes into an area of crepitus should be avoided, because frequently this is the arthrosis area and adding weight only perpetuates the crepitus. Even use of the traditional open-chain terminal knee extension can sometimes be detrimental; it is preferable to perform this activity in the closed-chain position (Fig. 9–33).

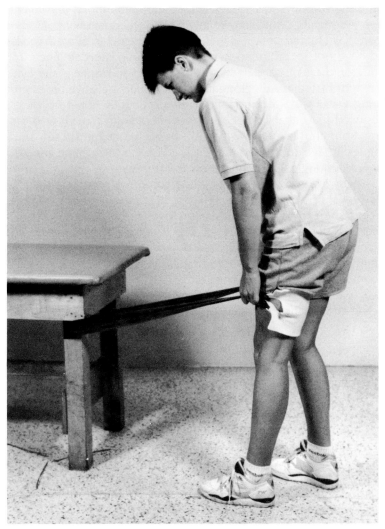

FIGURE 9-33   Don Tigney knee extension produces less patellofemoral compression than the traditional, open-chain terminal knee extension.

Stationary Cycling

The stationary bicycle has long been advocated. It has proven effective in restoring range of motion and muscle strength, particularly following knee injury or surgery, and is helpful for cardiovascular conditioning. The bike is generally used long before running can begin and subjects the knee to lower tibiofemoral forces than running. The athlete can strengthen the quadriceps and gastrocnemius using the bicycle.[106] With proper instruction athletes can be taught to bring into action the hamstrings, hip flexors, and anterior tibialis muscles.

Investigators have examined the compressive and shear forces around the tibiofemoral joint during cycling,[43] muscular function during cycling,[41] and the effects of varying seat height and pedal position on muscular forces around the knee.[106] The effect of different exercises on compressive and shear forces across the tibiofemoral joint has long been a concern, particularly following ACL reconstruction. Many surgeons have feared potential graft failures if these forces were too large, and have not recommended early therapeutic exercise. Shear forces acting on the ACL have been studied, however. Henning and Lynch[66] have reported that ACL elongation is approximately five times greater during walking on a normal floor than during stationary cycling and proposed that rehabilitation progress accordingly: crutch walking, cycling, normal walking, slow running, and fast running. Ericson and colleagues[46] have concluded that the load on the MCL of the knee is also very low during exercise on a bicycle ergometer.

Many investigators have studied compressive forces during various types of activity and estimated tibiofemoral joint compressive forces to be 2 to 4 times body weight (BW) during normal walking,[110] 4 times BW during stair climbing,[5] 3 to 7 times BW when rising from a normal chair,[35, 36] and 2.3 times BW when lifting a 12-kg burden.[33] A maximum tibiofemoral compressive force of almost 9 times BW was reported during isokinetic knee extension.[112, 113] Ericson and Nisell[33] have investigated tibiofemoral shear and compressive forces during cycling and reached a number of conclusions:

1. Tibiofemoral joint forces induced during standardized ergometer cycling are low compared with those induced during other daily activities, such as level walking, stair climbing, rising from a chair, and lifting.
2. Compressive force is reduced by a decrease in workload or an increase of saddle height
3. Stress on the ACL during cycling is lower and therefore cycling should be a beneficial exercise in early rehabilitation after ACL repair or reconstruction.
4. The ACL load is decreased by a reduction in workload or by using an anterior rather than posterior foot position.

Others have examined the effects of muscle force during cycle ergometry. Houtz and Fischer[66] reported that the tensor fasciae latae, sartorius, quadriceps femoris, and tibialis anterior muscles are considered the most important for the cycling motion. More recently, Ericson and associates[45] have quantified quadriceps activity during ergometer cycling and found that the vastus medialis and lateralis peak

TABLE 9-3 MEAN PEAK CONCENTRIC MUSCLE POWER OUTPUT DURING CYCLING

Muscles	Power (W)	Percentage of Total Work
Knee extension	110.1	39
Hip extension	74.4	27
Ankle plantar flexors	59.4	20
Knee flexors	30.0	10
Hip flexion	18.0	4

* Compiled from data in Ericson, M.O., Bratt, P., and Nisell, R., et al. (1986): Power output and work in different muscle groups during ergometer cycling. Eur. J. Appl. Physiol., 55:229.

TABLE 9–4 EFFECT OF BICYCLE SEAT HEIGHT AND PEDAL POSITION ON KNEE STRUCTURES

Seat Height and Pedal Position	Effect of Position on Knee Structures
Normal (high seat and no instruction in pedaling)	Increased gastrocnemius activity; no hamstring activity
Seat low, pedaling with ball of foot	Relies on patellofemoral force to stabilize the femoral tibial position
Low seat, pedaling with heel	Load transmitted to femur posteriorly, through ACL and meniscotibial ligament to tibia; the greater the posterior angle of the tibia, the greater the load applied to the ligaments
Seat height normal, pedaling with ball of foot	Increased knee extension; ball of foot increases gastrocnemius activity, which enhances the load applied to the ACL and meniscotibial ligaments; no hamstring activity
Normal seat height, pedaling with heel	No hamstring activity; no increased gastrocnemius activity; increased stress on ligaments
Low seat, pedaling with ball of foot using toe clips	Athlete instructed to pedal by pulling the pedal through at the bottom of the stroke, resulting in increased hamstring activity; this could provide some protection from stress applied to ACL and meniscotibial ligament

* Compiled from McLeod, W.D., and Blackburn, T.A. (1980): Biomechanics of knee rehabilitation with cycling. Am. J. Sports Med., 8:175–180.

activities are 54% and 50% of the maximum isometric EMG activity (% maximum EMG), respectively. Rectus femoris muscle activity determined in this study was lower (12% maximum EMG) than that of the vastus medialis and lateralis, probably because of its two-joint function. Ericson and associates[42] also analyzed the net mechanical muscular power output from stationary cycling (Table 9–3). It can be seen that the vastus muscles of the quadriceps benefit the most from stationary cycling, but other muscle groups also benefit.

McLeod and Blackburn[106] have studied variations of the inclination of the tibial plateau during cycling and its possible consequences on knee load (Table 9–4). They demonstrated that changing seat height and pedal positions can alter the forces placed on ligaments and other static restraints. They also noted that an insignificant load is transmitted throughout most of the crank angle by the quadriceps. It was concluded that ligaments can be protected from stress if the athlete is taught to pedal so that hamstring activity is enhanced while gastrocnemius activity is reduced. As ligament healing progresses this situation can be reversed, so that gastrocnemius activity is enhanced and hamstring activity reduced. This allows for controlled stresses to be applied to the ligaments and other connective tissues so that these structures can be strengthened gradually over the rehabilitation period.

The forces transmitted through the tibiofemoral joint are low, but what about the forces transmitted through the patellofemoral joint during ergometric cycling? Ericson and Nisell[44] have calculated force measurements on the patellofemoral joint and found that patellofemoral joint forces increase with increased workload or decreased saddle height. Different pedaling rates or foot positions do not significantly change these forces.

The vastus muscles benefit the most from stationary cycling, but other muscle groups are also exercised. In addition, there is a comparatively low load moment acting about the knee joint during cycling, as long as the following guidelines are observed (Fig. 9–34):

1. Seat high, knee flexed 15° to 30°
2. Low to moderate workload
3. Pedal with ball of the foot using toe clips and pull through at bottom of stroke

A number of conclusions have been drawn from the results of bicycle ergometer studies in regard to tibiofemoral compressive and shear forces and muscular activity:

1. An increased ergometer workload significantly increases compressive and shear forces across the patellofemoral joint.
2. Stress on the ACL and other knee ligaments is low, but can be further decreased in an anterior foot foot position.
3. Seat height should be high so that the knee lacks 15° to 30° of extension to decrease patellofemoral compressive forces.
4. Controlled stress can be applied to healing ligament restraints to promote collagen strengthening.

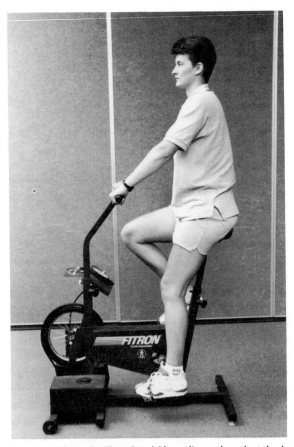

FIGURE 9–34   Stationary bicycle. This should be adjusted so that the knee is flexed 15° to 30° and the resistance is low to moderate.

5. Seat height and pedal position affect tibiofemoral compressive and shear forces.
6. The vastus muscles of the quadriceps muscle benefit the most, but other muscles of the lower extremity also benefit.

A high seat height and a low to moderate workload are recommended to decrease patellofemoral compressive forces, particularly when the stationary bike is used for conditioning or for athletes with patellofemoral pain. A seat height that is too high, however, results in rocking of the pelvis during pedaling.[106] Additionally, when implemented to restore knee range of motion, plantar flexing the ankle is a common response to help facilitate a revolution and should be considered "cheating." Although this ankle substitution may be used in early stages of restoring motion, it is not recommended in the later stages.

Studies tend to support the efficacy of implementing stationary cycling in early rehabilitation following knee surgery and/or injury. This excellent therapeutic rehabilitation modality can be used to control tibiofemoral forces, promote strengthening of collagen fibers, restore knee and ankle range of motion, enhance muscle strengthening and endurance, and improve cardiovascular conditioning.

Arthrometer Testing

Clinical tests for ligament instability are hard to quantify and difficult to reproduce. The physical examination allows for only a rough estimation of translation and rotation. Wroble and associates[160] evaluated 11 expert examiners in regard to grading anterior-posterior and internal-external rotation and varus-valgus displacement. Only 4 of 11 examiners (36%) estimated induced displacements in all three degrees of freedom within an acceptable range. There were large differences between starting flexion angles and the amount of displacement induced.

An objective method of testing provides quantitative and reproducible data. The first objective attempt to determine knee ligament laxity was made by Kennedy and Fowler,[78] who in 1971 used a clinic stress machine for in vivo measurements of anterior-posterior laxity using serial radiography after external forces had been applied to the tibia. Torzilli and colleagues[152] further refined this technique in 1978. Markolf and associates,[99] in 1978, presented a knee testing device that measured anterior-posterior forces versus displacement response curves; this was referred to as the UCLA instrumented clinical knee testing apparatus. In 1983 Daniel and co-workers[28] introduced the KT-1000,* which measures anterior-posterior laxity (Fig. 9–35). Since then other devices have been introduced to measure knee laxity in various planes, including the Genucom (Fig. 9–36),† the Knee Signature System (KSS),‡ and the Stryker knee laxity tester.§

---

* Available from Medmetric, San Diego, CA.
† Available from Faro Medical Technologies, Inc., Montreal.
‡ Available from Orthopaedic Systems, Hayward, CA.
§ Available from Stryker, Kalamazoo, MI.

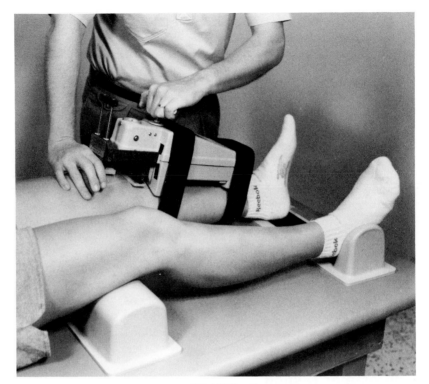

FIGURE 9–35   KT-1000 arthrometer.

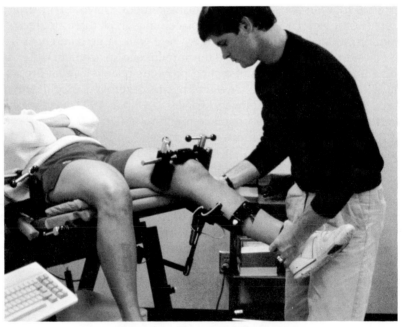

FIGURE 9–36   Genucom arthrometer.

Many investigations have been undertaken since these arthrometers have become available to evaluate their validity, and inter- and intrareliability and to make comparisons among devices.[4, 27, 29, 37, 63, 80, 107, 111, 124, 136, 160] It appears that knee ligament arthrometers can detect ACL disruption with a high degree of reliability.[4, 27, 124] Detection of PCL deficiency varies a little more, with the KT-1000 and Genucom appearing to perform best in this respect.[4] Varus-valgus laxity can be tested only by the Genucom, which appears to do so reliably.[37]

However, the ability of these arthrometers to reproduce reliable displacement readings within and among testers on the same and different days varies widely, and displacement forces as measured by different arthrometers is highly variable. Several investigators have calculated 90% confidence intervals.[4, 111, 159] Wroble[159] reported the following confidence intervals (90%) for normal knees in total anterior-posterior translations:

> KT-1000: $\pm$ 1.6 mm
> KSS: $\pm$ 2.7 mm
> Genucom: $\pm$ 3.4 mm

This is consistent with other research findings, and indicates that the KT-1000 has the lowest error in measurement.[112] It is also better than or equal to other arthrometers when considering interexaminer and intraexaminer reliability on the same and different days.[63, 159, 160] Hanten and Pace[63] have reported relatively high reliability coefficients of 0.85 for interexaminer and 0.83 for intraexaminer reliability. The KT-1000 is also the easiest to operate, is portable, and is the least expensive (Table 9–5).[160] Therefore, the KT-1000 appears to be the most often used arthrometer for clinical testing and research.[1, 19, 20, 50, 62, 93, 120, 137, 146, 150]

The KT-1000, Stryker, and KSS systems seem to be somewhat similar in displacement readings,[4, 117] whereas the Genucom produces higher absolute values than the other three devices.[107, 124, 160] Usually, a right-left knee difference of 2 to 3 mm is considered pathologic with most arthrometers.

Examiner experience is a large source of error and decreases reliability among and within examiners. Meticulous application and measuring techniques must be used to determine whether potential increased tibial translation is induced from ligament deficiency or examiner error. Error can also result from the patient or instrument itself.

TABLE 9–5   **COMPARISON OF THREE TYPES OF ARTHROMETERS**

	Reproducibility	Cost	Ease of Operation	Speed	Portability	Ease of Maintenance	Degrees of Freedom
KT-1000	+++	+	+++	+++	+++	++	1
KSS	++	++	++	++	++	+	4
Genucom	+	+++	+	+	−	+	6

* From Wroble, R.R. (1990): Practical rules for objective ligament assessment: KT-1000 and other devices. *In:* 1990 Advances on the Knee and Shoulder. Cincinnati, Cincinnati Sports Medicine and Deaconess Hospital.

Guidelines for the examiner have been compiled from various studies to enhance an arthrometer's accuracy:

1. Use total anterior-posterior translations. This eliminates the need to identify the neutral position of the knee, thereby eliminating this as a source of error.[159]
2. Report right-left differences with each test rather then individual knee measurements. This helps account for day-to-day changes, such as anxiety and patient relaxation. Also, single-knee measurements ignore simultaneously occurring changes in the contralateral knee that may appear during training, disuse, or rehabilitation.[160] All these are potential sources of error.
3. Repeat initial testing at least once to take into account the "learning effect."
4. Test at a 20-lb force level.
5. Carry out multiple examinations on different days.
6. Use meticulous examination technique.
7. Carefully assess patient relaxation.

If these guidelines are followed, the ability to reproduce tibial displacements with an arthrometer is greatly enhanced and the potential for the results' being caused by chance is diminished. The arthrometer can be used as a diagnostic instrument but may be more valuable as a rehabilitation tool. Some investigators use the arthrometer to determine advancement through an ACL rehabilitation program.[95] For instance, increased tibial translation early in rehabilitation results in a decrease in exercise intensity, modification of the rehabilitation program, and/or possible continuance of or regression back to crutch ambulation. If used wisely, the arthrometer can provide quantitative information about the surgical and rehabilitation techniques being employed. Also, if detected early by increased tibial translation, the arthrometer might help head off early graft and knee problems that might not be detected by physical examination.

REHABILITATION FOR SPECIFIC KNEE INJURIES

Ligament and Meniscal Injuries

Anterior Cruciate Ligament

The treatment of anterior cruciate ligament (ACL) injuries has been a subject of great debate. It is beyond our scope here to present the history of the treatment of ACL injuries, from clinical examination to surgical techniques to rehabilitation. Rather, the approach to ACL injuries is discussed in generic fashion, addressing the most common surgical techniques used today.

The need to reconstruct the ACL or treat ACL lesions conservatively has long been contested. Because of its unique features, the ACL does not lend itself to a simple, direct repair, as do other ligamentous sprains. On the other hand, conservative attempts at returning athletes to competition following an ACL injury have met with sporadic success. Noyes and colleagues[121] have carried out clinical evaluations of 84 individuals with documented ACL lesions using subjective and objective measures. They found that one-third of the population compensated, knew their limits, and did well; one-third compensated (although the condition was livable, it was aggravating); and one-third became worse and needed eventual surgery to correct their instability. They recommended[115] that, to have the best knee possible, competitive varsity or recreational athletes need surgical intervention, the light recreational athlete who is willing to limit sports may abstain from surgery, and the nonathlete who can easily limit activities may also defer surgery. Clinically, it appears that the competitive or varsity athlete does not perform well with a deficient ACL. ACL-deficient knees demonstrate abnormal joint kinematics during gait (walking and running)[89] and functional activities,[26] leading to early degenerative joint changes.[115]

Attempts have been made to identify factors that indicate who continues to function well without surgery and who warrants surgery following an ACL rupture.[7, 104] Clinical examination and isokinetic data

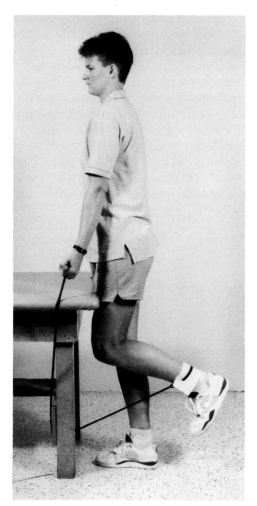

FIGURE 9–37 Hamstring curls with tubing. These can be progressed from slow to fast speeds when rehabilitating ACL-deficient knees.

are not conclusive in predicting functional return to activity following ACL disruption.[151, 154] Objective functional tests may be the best predictors of future success in those with an ACL-deficient knee,[8] but more studies are warranted.

Rehabilitation of the ACL-deficient knee should concentrate on development of neuromuscular control of the hamstrings, because these muscles become the primary secondary restraints for controlling anterior tibial excursion.[142] Shoemaker and Markolf[138] have documented in vivo that the dynamic tibial rotators can actively resist disruption of the ligaments if they can generate enough torque in response to stress placed on the knee. This is a direct function of neuromuscular control in the sports setting. Therefore, rehabilitation should concentrate on facilitating control of the hamstring muscles. Engle[38] and Engle and Canner[39, 40] have reported success in treating ACL-deficient knees with a program that emphasizes proprioceptive neuromuscular facilitation (PNF) techniques for the hamstrings. Also, the use of isokinetic units at high contractile velocities, surgical tubing (Fig. 9–37), the Slide Board (see Fig. 9–18), and the Inertia machine can all be used to emphasize hamstring strength, endurance, and control while helping to facilitate hamstring coordination to deter anterior tibial displacement during functional activities.

Tibial pad placement during isokinetic testing and exercise has been a concern in relation to the compressive and shear forces across the tibiofemoral joint, particularly the effects on the ACL. Isokinetic tibiofemoral compressive forces have been calculated to be almost 9 times body weight.[113] The tibiofemoral shear force becomes positive at 700 N or 1 body weight, indicating that high forces arise in the ACL when the knee is extended more than 60°. This anteriorly directed shear force is lowered considerably by locating the resistance pad in a proximal leg position.[113, 115] Johnson[73] has described a two-pad system (Fig. 9–38) that appears to reduce anterior tibial glide and may protect the ACL-deficient or ACL-reconstructed knee during isokinetic exer-

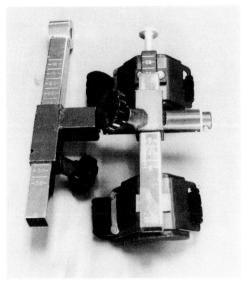

FIGURE 9–38 Johnson antishear device. This provides a dual-pad placement to reduce tibiofemoral shear.

cise. However, clinical observations show that patients tend to complain of irritation over the anterior incision from which the patellar tendon graft was harvested; a piece of foam used on the most proximal pad usually resolves this inconvenience. During ACL rehabilitation, whether deficient or reconstructed, a proximal pad placement or dual-pad system should be used to deter anterior tibial glide.

Table 9–6 outlines the protocol for rehabilitation of the acutely injured ACL-deficient knee. In those with chronic ACL lesions, the program can be accelerated. Initial concerns include controlled motion,

TABLE 9–6 REHABILITATION PROTOCOL FOR THE ANTERIOR CRUCIATE LIGAMENT–DEFICIENT KNEE

I. Rationale
  A. Immobilization to allow healing time for secondary restraints (4 weeks)
  B. Development of total leg strength
  C. De-emphasis on hamstring flexibility
  D. Proprioception
  E. Return to previous level of functional activity
II. Immediate postoperative phase
  A. Day 1
    1. Brace locked at 30°
    2. Touchdown weight-bearing with two crutches
    3. Sleep in brace 3 weeks
    4. Begin following exercises (all exercises performed wearing brace):
      a. Quad set
      b. Cocontractions
      c. Bent leg raises
      d. Ankle pumps
      e. Passive patellar mobilization to tolerance
    5. Electrical muscle stimulation (EMS)
  B. Days 2 to 14
    1. Brace, 90–30°
    2. Partial weight-bearing with two crutches.
    3. Add following exercises (perform in brace):
      a. Continue with above exercises
      b. Multiple angle isometric hamstring contractions
      c. Heel slides within brace restraints
      d. Straight leg raises (four planes)
      e. 90–45° knee extensions
      f. Standing hamstring curls
      g. Passive patellar mobilization
      h. Seated hip flexion
  C. Week 2 (do not push passive extension at this point)
    1. Continue brace at 90–30°
    2. Partial weight-bearing with two crutches
    3. May begin exercises without brace
    4. Begin progressive resistance exercises (PREs), if not already being done (0–10 lb)
    5. Continue EMS, if necessary
III. Intermediate phase
  A. Week 3
    1. Brace adjusted 90–0°
    2. May sleep without brace
    3. Partial weight-bearing with one crutch
    4. Continue PRE progression to 20 lb, as tolerated
    5. Replace bent leg raise with 6-inch straight leg raise

Table continued on following page

TABLE 9–6 REHABILITATION PROTOCOL FOR THE ANTERIOR CRUCIATE LIGAMENT–DEFICIENT KNEE *Continued*

6. Begin stationary bike
7. Begin nonaggressive passive extension
  B. Weeks 4 and 5
    1. KT-1000 test
    2. Discontinue brace (with exception of stressful situations and lateral step-ups)
    3. Add following exercises:
      a. 90–0° active extension with *no weight*
      b. Don Tigney knee extensions
      c. Heel raises
      d. Lateral step-ups
      e. 90–45° knee extensions
      f. Minisquats
      g. Slide board with gradual progression
      h. Tibial internal and external rotation with Thera-Band
      i. Calf raises, seated and standing
      j. Eccentric hamstring work
      k. Double leg press
      l. Retro (backward) walking on treadmill
      m. ALRI: external tibial rotation to isolate biceps femoris
      n. AMRI: internal tibial rotation to isolate semimembranosus and semitendinosus
    4. Pool program
    5. May begin submaximal isokinetic work, 90–45° at medium to high speeds, with gradual progression, as indicated, with monitoring
    6. Proprioception development. BAPS board, balance board, one-foot balance
  C. Weeks 6 and 7
    1. KT-1000 test
    2. Eccentric quad work
    3. Single leg press
    4. Begin retro (backward) running on flats and hills
    5. Maximal high-speed isokinetic work, 90–0° range of motion
    6. Increase proprioception and closed-chain exercises
    7. High-speed standing hamstring curls with tubing
IV. Advanced phase
  A. Weeks 8 to 12
    1. Isokinetic evaluation (week 12)
    2. Functional testing (week 12)
    3. Advancement to functional activities; begin running straight ahead (slow → fast → cutting)
    4. Fit for functional knee brace
    5. KT-1000 test
    6. Initiate plyometrics

particularly extension and patellofemoral precautions as rehabilitation progresses. In the late stages of rehabilitation, if anterolateral (ALRI) or anteromedial (AMRI) rotatory instability is present, surgical tubing can be used in tibial external rotation (Fig. 9–39) and internal rotation (Fig. 9–40), respectively, to help increase muscle strength and coordination, because these muscles are the primary resistors to controlling and deterring those rotatory movements.

The Slide Board* was first described by Bergfeld and Anderson[14] in the rehabilitation of the ACL (see Fig. 9–18). The Slide Board requires the athlete to mimic the activity of ice skating. In this position the hips

---

* Available from Don Courson Enterprises, Birmingham, AL.

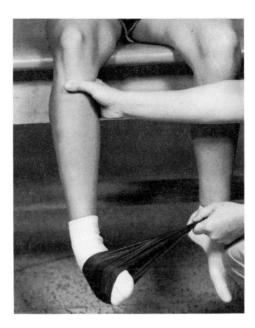

FIGURE 9–39 Tibial external rotation with tubing to isolate the biceps femoris muscle.

and knees are flexed in an attempt to avoid quadriceps contraction in the last few degrees of full extension, thus avoiding intense forces to the healing ACL. EMG studies have confirmed that the hamstring muscles fire in a decelerated fashion as the knee comes closer to full extension and the quadriceps is relatively inactive. The Slide Board also promotes proprioception and cardiovascular conditioning. In early lower extremity rehabilitation the Slide Board aids in restoring proprioception and it is used in the later stages for cardiovascular and muscular conditioning. The Slide Board should be made so that a

FIGURE 9–40 Tibial internal rotation with tubing to isolate the semitendinosus and semimembranosus.

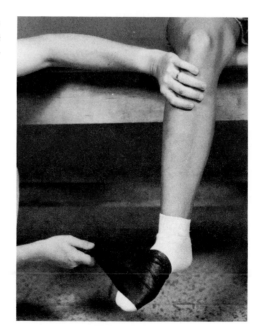

gradual progression over 9 to 12 feet can be attained. This allows for rehabilitation in ACL-reconstructed knees as early as 4 to 6 weeks, using submaximal short glides with a spotter. Although initially advocated for knee rehabilitation, the Slide Board is excellent for the rehabilitation of lower extremity injuries.

The use of backward (retro) walking and running can facilitate increased hamstring activity and reduce the stress to the knee joint while increasing knee extensor strength.[148] Initially, retrowalking can be used to facilitate knee extension during ambulation. As rehabilitation proceeds the athlete can retrowalk on the treadmill with a slight grade, progressing to running backward on flats and hills.

After satisfactory performance on isokinetic (80% to 90%) and functional testing, the ACL-deficient athlete may return to participation. The use of an ACL functional brace may also assist in reducing knee symptoms during sports participation.

The ACL can be reconstructed by an extra-articular, intra-articular, or combined surgical technique. The surgical procedure depends on the type and location of tear, patient age, level of activity of the patient, and patient motivational level.[157] Extra-articular procedures are designed to eliminate the pivot shift but cannot restore normal arthrokinematics through the axis of the normal ACL, which is an attempt to achieve functional control with a dynamic restraint(s). Extra-articular procedures consist of transposition of dynamic restraints or an iliotibial band tenodesis. Although once widely used, the success rate following this procedure in regard to retaining knee stability is low. These poor results are a result of stretching out of the tissues. Extra-articular procedures are now mostly used in adolescents with open epiphysis in whom bone tunnels cannot be drilled through the epiphysis for intra-articular graft placement, or as an augmentation of (or back-up to) an intra-articular graft.

Rehabilitation following an extra-articular procedure can progress according to the protocol outlined in Table 9–7. Initial concerns focus

TABLE 9–7   RECONSTRUCTION PROTOCOL FOR EXTRA-ARTICULAR ANTERIOR CRUCIATE LIGAMENT RECONSTRUCTION

I. Preoperative instruction
  A. Gait training → touchdown and partial weight-bearing
  B. Instruction in use of brace
  C. Instruction in exercise program and postoperative progression
  D. Stress importance of limited extension for 6 weeks to limit "stretching out" of repair and importance of wearing and sleeping in brace, as instructed
  E. Obtain baseline data, if tolerated: isokinetic testing, arthrometer testing, range of motion, circumference measurements
II. Immediate postoperative phase
  A. Day 1
    1. Brace set 90–30°
    2. Touchdown weight-bearing
    3. Continuous passive motion (CPM), 60–30°, as tolerated
    4. Begin following exercises, as tolerated:
      a. Quad sets
      b. Cocontractions
      c. Ankle pumps

Table continued on following page

TABLE 9–7 RECONSTRUCTION PROTOCOL FOR EXTRA-ARTICULAR ANTERIOR CRUCIATE LIGAMENT RECONSTRUCTION *Continued*

     d. Bent leg raises (active-assisted, if necessary)
  B. Day 2 to week 2
    1. Brace set 90–30°
    2. Continue partial weight-bearing ambulation with brace and crutches
    3. Home exercises twice daily in brace
    4. Shower after sutures have been removed and no drainage from wound is present
    5. CPM 90–30°, as tolerated
    6. May progress progressive resistance exercises (PREs) as tolerated with exercises in brace
    7. Add following exercises (in brace):
      a. Hip flexion
      b. Standing hamstring curls
      c. Heel slides (within confines of brace)
      d. Straight leg raises (four planes)
      e. Well-leg and upper body exercise
III. Intermediate phase
  A. Weeks 3 to 5
    1. KT-1000 test
    2. Brace 90–15°, range of motion
    3. Partial weight-bearing, progress from two to one crutch
    4. PRE, 1 to 10 lb
    5. Remove brace to progress flexion
    6. Begin stationary bike when range of motion is sufficient
    7. Begin proprioception training
  B. Weeks 6 and 7
    1. Full weight-bearing, discontinue brace
    2. Continue PRE, 10 to 20 lb
    3. Continue stationary bike
    4. May begin active swimming
    5. May perform exercises out of brace
    6. Add following exercises:
      a. Minisquats progressing to tubing
      b. Lateral step-ups
      c. Leg presses
      d. Don Tigney knee extensions
      e. 90–45° knee extensions
      f. Continue proprioception training
    7. KT-1000 test
  C. Week 8 to 2 months
    1. Begin the following exercises:
      a. Slide Board
      b. Eccentric hamstring curls
      c. Begin 90–45° knee extensions, submaximal effort, high speeds
IV. Advanced phase
  A. Month 3
    1. Begin submaximal isokinetics, high speeds, 90–0°, with gradual progression to maximum effort over next 4 weeks; use Johnson Anti-Shear or most proximal single pad placement
    2. KT-1000 test
    3. High-speed tubing exercises
  B. Month 4
    1. Isokinetic and KT-1000 tests
    2. Begin functional activities (e.g., straight-ahead running)
  C. Months 5 to 6
    1. Advance to full functional activities
    2. Isokinetic and KT-1000 tests
    3. Functional testing

on slow restoration of extension, because aggressive extension results in elongation of the tissues around the repair and early failure. Most adolescents who undergo an extra-articular repair return to surgery after their epiphyses close for an intra-articular procedure. Some surgeons use an intra-articular procedure when the epiphysis is open, drilling smaller holes through the tibia and routing the graft over the top of the femur.

Many types of tissue have been used for intra-articular repairs of the ACL, including autografts (tissue transferred from one part of a person's body to another) and allografts (human tissue), and prosthetic (synthetic) ligaments. Various types of autografts have different strength characteristics (Table 9–8). Currently, reconstructing the ACL is most commonly performed using the middle third of the patellar tendon with bone plugs as a free graft under arthroscopic guidance. This tissue provides a high tensile strength graft to compensate for the ACL. Amiel and colleagues,[3] using a rabbit model, showed that after being placed in this ACL environment the patellar tendon undergoes a "ligamentization" process. By 4 weeks the bone plugs have healed into the surrounding bone and by 8 weeks graft vascularization is well under way. The patellar tendon graft is at its weakest 4 to 6 weeks after surgery, with a gradual increase in strength from that point.

Historically, rehabilitation following ACL reconstruction using the patellar tendon has been concerned with minimizing stress on the graft. This usually entailed limitation of active extension past 30°, with an emphasis on hamstring strengthening and a de-emphasis on quadriceps strengthening. This philosophy was based in part on the work of Grood and associates,[60] who studied tibial translation following sectioning of the ACL. They found an increased anterior drawer with extension past 30° in the ACL-deficient knee, indicating that anterior cruciate repairs are loaded in this region. Furthermore, great importance was placed on the cocontraction of the quadriceps and hamstrings to deter anterior displacement and protect the graft. Investigators have ascertained that the anterior and posterior drawer force becomes 0 at approximately 45° and the posterior drawer force increases as the knee flexes past this point up to 90°, where it is greatest.[161] The hamstrings can exert a posterior drawer effect at any knee angle.[161] In 1989,

TABLE 9–8 **STRENGTH OF ANTERIOR CRUCIATE LIGAMENT (ACL) SUBSTITUTES**

Graft	% of ACL Strength
Patellar tendon	168
ACL	100
Semitendinosus	70
Gracilis	49
Iliotibial band	44
Fascia lata	36
Retinaculum	21

* Compiled from data in Noyes, F.R., Butler, D.L., and Grood, E.S., et al. (1984): Biomechanical analysis of human ligament repairs and reconstruction. J. Bone Joint Surg. [Am.], 66:344.

however, Draganich and co-workers[31] evaluated the knee extension exercise from 90° to 0° with variable amounts of weight attached at the ankle. Their study illustrated that the hamstrings function synergistically with the ACL to prevent anterior tibial displacement, which is produced by active contraction of the quadriceps in the terminal degrees of knee extension. The synergistic role of the hamstrings, along with growing appreciation for graft isometry (the same amount of tension is placed on the graft throughout knee flexion and extension), has eased the concerns of graft failure through early quadriceps exercises in the early stages of rehabilitation. Currently, as outlined in Table 9–9, unweighted terminal knee extensions can begin at about 4 weeks after surgery.

TABLE 9–9 REHABILITATION PROTOCOL FOR ANTERIOR CRUCIATE LIGAMENT RECONSTRUCTION USING THE PATELLAR TENDON GRAFT

I. Rehabilitation goals
  A. Minimize pain and swelling in the lower extremity
  B. Adhere to healing constraints of surgical procedure and protect other involved joints (especially patellofemoral) in the rehabilitation process
  C. Achieve good range of motion in the knee (0–90° prior to discharge from hospital)
  D. Maintain good patellar mobility
  E. Promote lower extremity muscle power
  F. Independence with activities, including postoperative exercise program, incision care, muscle stimulator use, brace application and wearing guidelines, ambulation with crutches on level surfaces and stairs
II. Preoperative instruction
  A. Gait training on flats and stairs
  B. Explanation of surgical procedure
  C. Review of rehabilitation protocol
  D. Stress importance of attaining and maintaining full passive extension as well as restoring full range of motion
  E. Obtain baseline measurements, as tolerated (e.g., circumference measurements, active and passive motion, arthrometer testing, isometric or isokinetic testing)
  F. Instruction in immediate postoperative exercises
III. Immediate postoperative phase
  A. Day 1 through week 1
    1. Brace: locked at 0° extension immediately postoperatively; sleep in brace for 4 weeks
    2. Crutch walking: two crutches, weight-bearing as tolerated (50% or less of body weight)
    3. Exercises:
      a. Ankle pumps
      b. Quad sets (with muscle stimulator)
      c. Patellar mobilization
      d. Straight leg raises (with muscle stimulator)
      e. Intermittent range of motion (bending)
      f. Multiangle quad isometrics (90° and 60°)
      g. Active knee extensions (90–40°)
      h. Minisquats (to 30°)
      i. Passive knee extension and hamstring stretching
      j. Standing weight shifts
    4. Muscle stimulator: EMS (electrical muscle stimulation) to be used 6 hours/day in physical therapy and in room
    5. Continuous passive motion (CPM): 0–90° as tolerated, at least 2 hours/day
    6. Ice and elevation
      a. Ice bags may be placed directly on skin, up to 20 minutes each hour

Table continued on following page

TABLE 9–9   REHABILITATION PROTOCOL FOR ANTERIOR CRUCIATE LIGAMENT RECONSTRUCTION USING THE PATELLAR TENDON GRAFT *Continued*

   b. Elevate leg on the elevation wedge as much as possible; while elevated, pump ankle up and down and use EMS to help decrease knee swelling

IV. Maximum protection phase
  A. Goals
    1. Absolute control of external forces and protection of graft
    2. Nourish articular cartilage
    3. Decrease fibrosis
    4. Stimulate collagen healing
    5. Decrease swelling
    6. Deter quad atrophy
  B. Weeks 2 and 3
    1. Goal: prepare patient for ambulation without crutches by end of second week
    2. Brace: locked at 0°, continue to perform self-range of motion
    3. Weight-bearing: as tolerated, 50% of body weight or greater
    4. Exercises:
      a. Multiangle isometrics: 90°, 60°, and 30°
      b. Straight leg raises (all four planes)
      c. Hamstring curls
      d. Knee extensions (90–40°)
      e. Minisquats
      f. Intermittent full range of motion (four or five times daily)
      g. Patellar mobilization
      h. Passive range of motion
      i. Calf stretching
      j. Proprioception training
      k. Well-leg exercises
    5. Swelling control: ice, compression, elevation
  C. Weeks 4 and 5
    1. Brace: locked at 0°, continue to perform active range-of-motion exercises
    2. Full weight-bearing; no crutches, one crutch if necessary
    3. KT-1000 test (20 lb)
    4. Exercises:
      a. Same as weeks 2 and 3
      b. Initiate eccentric quads, 40–100° of range of motion
      c. Passive range-of-motion exercises (0–120°)
      d. Pool walking
V. Controlled ambulation phase
  A. Goals: control forces during walking
  B. Brace: discontinue locked brace, brace open 0–125°
  C. Weeks 6 and 7
    1. Full weight-bearing without crutches, with brace
    2. Criteria for full weight-bearing:
      a. Active range-of-motion exercises, 0–115°
      b. Quad strength 70% of contralateral side, as determined by isometric test
      c. No change in KT-1000 test
      d. Decrease in effusion
    3. Range of motion, 0–125°, or greater
    4. Continue exercises of weeks 4 and 5 and add these:
      a. Swimming
      b. Stretching program
      c. Hamstring progressive resistance exercises (PREs)
    5. Increase closed kinetic chain rehabilitation
    6. Increase proprioception training
  D. Weeks 8 and 9
    1. Discontinue postoperative brace
    2. Exercise: continue PREs
    3. KT-1000 test

Table continued on following page

TABLE 9–9   REHABILITATION PROTOCOL FOR ANTERIOR CRUCIATE LIGAMENT RECONSTRUCTION USING THE PATELLAR TENDON GRAFT *Continued*

VI. Moderate protection phase (10 to 15 weeks)
  A. Goals
    1. Protect patellofemoral joint's articular cartilage
    2. Maximal strengthening for quads and lower extremity
  B. Week 12
    1. Begin isokinetics, 100–40° range of motion
    2. Continue minisquats with tubing
    3. Initiate lateral step-ups
    4. Initiate pool running (forward and backward)
    5. Emphasize eccentric quad work
    6. Bicycle for endurance (30 minutes)
    7. Begin walking program
    8. KT-1000 test
    9. Isometric strength test
    10. Proprioception test
  C. Week 14
    1. PREs for all lower extremity musculature
    2. Vigorous walking programs with functional brace
    3. Continue exercises outlined for week 12
VII. Light activity phase (3 to 4 months)
  A. Goals
    1. Development of strength, power, endurance
    2. Begin to prepare for return to functional activities
  B. Exercises
    1. Begin running program
    2. Straight line to figure-eights and then to cutting
    3. Agility drills
    4. Continue balance drills
    5. Continue midrange isokinetics (90–40°), intermittent speed
    6. Continue minisquats and lateral step-ups
    7. Continue high-speed isokinetics, full range of motion
  C. Tests
    1. Isokinetic tests (15 weeks)
    2. KT-1000 test (prior to running program)
    3. Functional tests (prior to running program)
  D. Initiate plyometric training (5 months)
  E. Criteria for running
    1. Isokinetic test interpretation satisfactory (70–80% of uninvolved side)
    2. KT-1000 test unchanged
    3. Functional test 70 percent of contralateral leg
VIII. Return to activity phase
  A. Advanced rehabilitation and return to competitive sports
    1. Achieve maximal strength and further enhance neuromuscular coordination and endurance
    2. All exercises accelerated
    3. KT-1000 test
    4. Isokinetic test prior to return to participation
  B. 6-month follow-up
    1. KT-1000 test
    2. Isokinetic test
    3. Functional test
  C. 12-month follow-up
    1. KT-1000 test
    2. Isokinetic test
    3. Functional test

Initial emphasis following ACL reconstruction is on promotion of patellar mobility through early mobilization (see Chap. 6), early muscle turn-on, and the achievement of full passive extension to anatomic zero. Fulfilling these criteria as soon as possible goes a long way in deterring the development of arthrofibrosis. Rehabilitation can proceed as outlined in Table 9–9 following ACL reconstruction using the middle third of the patellar tendon. During rehabilitation, patellofemoral kinematics must be monitored for pain and crepitus. This has often been a reported secondary complication of this surgery, probably resulting more from quadriceps atrophy than from the use of the middle third of the patellar tendon. This is the most common illustration of damage to the tibiofemoral joint affecting the patellofemoral joint, and patellofemoral precautions *must* be observed.

Allografts and prosthetic ligaments to compensate for ACL disruptions are now being used. Only a small number of surgeons use ACL allografts for ACL reconstructions,[116] mainly because of problems of tissue availability and the potential for transmission of disease, but early results are promising. Noyes[116] has reported the implantation of 57 ACL allografts from 1982 through 1986, with a 100% follow-up. There were no infections or rejections, and only one graft failure. Good to excellent results were reported in 86%. However, ACL allografts are still not used by most surgeons. Rehabilitation following allograft surgery is similar to that for the patellar tendon graft (Table 9–9).

Prosthetic ligaments have been used with only fair results in ACL reconstruction. The Gore-Tex prosthetic ligament* is the most well known and widely used, although other types have been used with varying degrees of success. Following an initial investigative study, the Gore-Tex ligament is currently approved by the FDA only for use in cases of previously failed autograft reconstructions and can be implanted only by those surgeons trained by the W.H. Gore Corporation in their implantation method. The advantage of using ACL prosthetic ligaments is that recovery is accelerated, because one does not have to wait for biologic healing and remodeling. Guidelines for rehabilitation following ACL reconstruction with a prosthetic ligament are presented in Table 9–10.

---

* Available from the W.H. Gore Corporation, Flagstaff, AZ.

TABLE 9–10   REHABILITATION PROTOCOL FOR SYNTHETIC LIGAMENT RECONSTRUCTION OF THE ANTERIOR CRUCIATE LIGAMENT

I. Preoperative instructions
  A. Gait training instruction: touchdown weight-bearing with crutches
  B. Instruct in immediate postoperative exercises and hospital course and familiarize patient with postoperative protocol through 9 months
II. Immediate postoperative phase
  A. Day 1
    1. Brace locked at 15°
    2. Begin touchdown weight-bearing, two crutches
    3. Continuous passive motion, 0–45°, as tolerated

Table continued on following page

TABLE 9–10   REHABILITATION PROTOCOL FOR SYNTHETIC LIGAMENT RECONSTRUCTION OF THE ANTERIOR CRUCIATE LIGAMENT *Continued*

    4. Exercises (in brace only):
      a. Quad sets
      b. Cocontractions
      c. Ankle pumps
      d. Straight leg raises
  B. Days 2 and 3
    1. Brace 0–90° as tolerated
    2. Progress partial weight-bearing, two crutches and brace
    3. CPM 0–90° as tolerated
    4. Exercises:
      a. Quad sets
      b. Cocontractions
      c. Ankle pumps
      d. Active flexion to 90°
      e. Straight leg raises
      f. 90–0° full knee extensions
      g. Terminal knee extensions
      h. Hip flexion
      i. Standing hamstring curls
      j. Hamstring stretching
      k. Weight shifts
      l. Patellar mobilization
    5. May use EMS, as needed, to assist with muscular recruitment
  C. Day 3 or 4—discharge instructions
    1. Brace, 90–0°
      a. Brace off to exercise and to bathe
      b. Sleep in brace for 2 weeks, then off at night
      c. After 2 weeks discontinue use of brace, except stressful activities
      d. After 4 weeks discontinue brace totally
    2. Continue two crutches, partial weight-bearing
    3. Exercises: continue exercises as outlined above three times daily; continue use of ice after exercise
    4. May shower after sutures have been removed; do not bathe until all drainage from wound has stopped
III. Intermediate postoperative phase
  A. Week 2
    1. Discontinue brace, except in stressful situations
    2. Progress partial weight-bearing with one crutch
    3. Exercises:
      a. Progress knee flexion, as tolerated
      b. Begin progressive resisted exercise (PRE), 1–5 lb
      c. Begin stationary bike with low resistance, as tolerated, 15–30 minutes daily
      d. Hip abduction, adduction, and extension
      e. Toe raises
      f. Proprioception exercises
      g. Minisquats
      h. Closed-chain exercises
    4. KT-1000 test
  B. Weeks 4 and 5
    1. Discontinue use of brace
    2. Progress to full weight-bearing off crutches
    3. Exercises:
      a. Progress biking 30–60 minutes daily
      b. Progress PRE, 5–10 lb
      c. Begin swimming program
      d. Slide Board
      e. Eccentric hamstring exercises
    4. KT-1000 test

Table continued on following page

TABLE 9–10   REHABILITATION PROTOCOL FOR SYNTHETIC LIGAMENT RECONSTRUCTION OF THE ANTERIOR CRUCIATE LIGAMENT *Continued*

C. Week 6
  1. Full weight-bearing
  2. Continue PRE, 10–20 lb
  3. Begin side step-ups
  4. Begin high-speed isokinetics
  5. KT-1000 test
  6. Increase closed-chain exercises
IV. Advanced phase
  A. Months 2 to 5
    1. KT-1000 test
    2. Advance functional activities
    3. Increase exercises:
      a. Eccentric quads
      b. Continue high-speed isokinetics
      c. Proprioception
      d. Walking program
    4. Isokinetic test (month 3)
  B. Months 6 to 9
    1. KT-1000 test
    2. Isokinetic test
    3. Advance to competitive sports

Posterior Cruciate Ligament

Posterior cruciate ligament (PCL) injuries are less common in the athletic and general population than ACL injuries. Thus, not as much research has been done on PCL injury, treatment, and rehabilitation as for ACL lesions. Whether to repair isolated PCL lesions is still debated. PCL lesions that involve posterolateral rotatory instability need to be surgically corrected. Athletes with isolated PCL ruptures can return to participation following rehabilitation (Table 9–11), with no instability symptoms. Degenerative medial compartment disease has been associated with PCL-deficient knees, however, as well as patellofemoral chondrosis resulting from the posteriorly sagging tibia.

Many tissues have been used to reconstruct and compensate for PCL deficiency, including the semitendinosus and medial head of the gastrocnemius,[48] middle third of the patellar tendon, and PCL allografts. The rehabilitation protocol outlined in Table 9–12 applies to using the free patellar tendon graft (PTG) with bone plugs under arthroscopic guidance (not unlike ACL reconstruction using the PTG). The main concern following PCL reconstruction is the limitation of flexion past 60° for about 6 to 8 weeks, because this stresses the graft and could result in failure. Also, hamstring exercises should not be performed because of the posterior drawer they produce.

Because PCL reconstruction is still in its developmental stage, most athletes are treated nonoperatively unless symptoms continue to persist (Table 9–11). If posterolateral instability is present, an early surgical procedure is indicated. Postoperatively, a long-leg hinged brace is used, initially set at 30° to 90° for 2 weeks and progressed to 0° to 90° at 6 weeks. Weight-bearing is partial for the first 6 to 8 weeks following

TABLE 9–11   REHABILITATION PROTOCOL FOR THE NONOPERATIVE POSTERIOR CRUCIATE LIGAMENT

I. Immediate phase
  A. Day 1 to week 4
    1. Brace: 0–60°
    2. Weight-bearing: partial weight-bearing with crutches for 2 weeks, 1 crutch for 2 weeks, then off crutches
    3. Initiate the following exercises as tolerated:
      a. Quad sets
      b. Ankle active range of motion
      c. Active flexion to 60°
      d. Terminal knee extensions with straight leg raises
      e. Hip flexions
      f. Hip abductions, adductions, and extensions
      g. Closed-chain exercises:
        1) Minisquats
        2) Don Tigney knee extensions
      h. Static weight loading
      i. Proprioception
    4. Remain in brace except while bathing and exercises
    5. Sleep in brace for 4 weeks
    6. Well-leg and upper body program
    7. PRE quads 60° flexion to full extension
    8. PRE, as tolerated with straight leg raises
II. Intermediate phase
  A. Weeks 4 and 5
    1. Brace 0° extension, 60° flexion
    2. Full weight-bearing
    3. Out of brace to progress flexion
    4. Out of brace to sleep
    5. Begin stationary bike
    6. Continue progressive resisted exercise (PRE) progression
    7. Increase closed-chain exercises
  B. Weeks 6 and 7
    1. Full weight-bearing
    2. Progress knee flexion
    3. Continue PRE with exercises
    4. Eccentric quads
    5. Continue to progress proprioceptive activities
  C. Weeks 8 to 11
    1. Brace, 0° extension
    2. Progress knee flexion
    3. Begin hamstring curls
    4. Initiate plyometrics
  D. Week 12 to month 5
    1. Continue exercises—progressive resistance, 10–15 lb
    2. Continue bike, proprioception, closed-chain exercises
    3. Begin high-speed isokinetics
III. Advanced phase
  A. Months 6 to 9: Begin functional activities, isokinetic test

**TABLE 9–12   REHABILITATION PROTOCOL FOR POSTERIOR
CRUCIATE LIGAMENT–PATELLAR TENDON
GRAFT RECONSTRUCTION**

I. Preoperative instruction
   A. Gait training on flats and stairs
   B. Explanation of surgical procedure
   C. Review of rehabilitation protocol
   D. Stress importance of attaining and maintaining full passive extension and
      limitation to 60° degrees of knee flexion for about 6 weeks
   E. Obtain baseline measurements, as tolerated (e.g., circumference
      measurements, active and passive motion, arthrometer testing, isometric or
      isokinetic testing)
   F. Instruction in immediate postoperative exercises
II. Immediate postoperative phase
   A. Day 1
      1. Brace: locked at 0° extension; sleep in brace 4 weeks
      2. Weight-bearing: two crutches, as tolerated (less than 50% of body weight)
      3. Exercises:
         a. Ankle pumps
         b. Quad sets
         c. Straight leg raises
      4. Muscle stimulation: electrical muscle stimulation (EMS) to quads
         (4 hours/day) during quad sets
      5. Continuous passive motion (CPM): 0–60° as tolerated
      6. Ice and elevation: ice 20 minutes each hour, elevate with knee in
         extension
   B. Days 2 to 5
      1. Brace: locked at 0° extension
      2. Weight-bearing: two crutches, as tolerated (50% of body weight)
      3. Range of motion (ROM): intermittent ROM out of brace four or five times
         daily (0–60°)
      4. Exercises
         a. Multiangle isometrics at 60°, 40°, and 20° of flexion (quads only)
         b. Intermittent ROM (four or five times daily)
         c. Patellar mobilization
         d. Ankle pumps
         e. Straight leg raises
         f. Hip abduction and adduction
         g. Continue quad sets
         h. Toe raises with knee in extension
      5. Muscle stimulation: EMS to quads (6 hours/day) during quad sets,
         multiangle isometrics, and straight leg raises
      6. CPM: 0–60°
      7. Ice and elevation: continue with ice and elevation 20 minutes each hour,
         elevate with knee in extension
III. Maximum protection phase (weeks 2 to 6)
   A. Goals:
      1. Absolute control of external forces to protect graft
      2. Nourish articular cartilage
      3. Decrease swelling
      4. Decrease fibrosis
      5. Deter quad atrophy
   B. Week 2
      1. Brace: locked at 0°
      2. Continue to perform intermittent ROM exercises
      3. Weight-bearing: as tolerated, 50% or greater
      4. KT-1000 test: performed with 15 lb maximum force

Table continued on following page

**TABLE 9–12 REHABILITATION PROTOCOL FOR POSTERIOR
CRUCIATE LIGAMENT–PATELLAR TENDON
GRAFT RECONSTRUCTION** *Continued*

    5. Exercises:
       a. Multiangle isometrics at 60°, 40°, and 20° of flexion
       b. Quad sets
       c. Knee extension, 60–0°
       d. Intermittent ROM, 0–60° (four or five times daily)
       e. Patellar mobilization
       f. Well-leg bicycling
       g. Proprioception training
    6. Continue electrical muscle stimulation to quads
    7. Continue ice and elevation
  C. Week 4
    1. Brace: continue locked at 0°; discontinue sleeping in brace
    2. Weight-bearing: as tolerated
    3. KT-1000 test
    4. Exercises:
       a. Continue all above exercises
       b. Intermediate ROM, 0–60°
       c. Initiate eccentric quads, 0–60°
  D. Week 6
    1. Goal: prepare for full weight-bearing with knee motion
    2. Brace: continue locked at 0°
    3. Weight-bearing: full weight-bearing
    4. KT-1000 test: performed at 20- and 30-lb maximum force
    5. Exercises:
       a. Weight-bearing shifts
       b. Minisquats (0–40°)
       c. Intermittent ROM 0–90°
       d. Knee extension 90–40°
       e. Pool walking
       f. Initiate stationary cycling
IV. Controlled ambulation phase (weeks 7 to 12)
  A. Goals:
    1. Control forces during ambulation
    2. Increase quad strength
  B. Week 7
    1. Brace: discontinue locked brace, open to 0–125°
    2. Criteria for full weight-bearing with knee motion:
       a. Active-assisted range of motion, 0–115°
       b. Quad strength, 70% of contralateral side (isometric test)
       c. No change in KT-1000 test
       d. Decrease joint effusion
    3. Ambulation: with functional knee brace
    4. Exercises:
       a. Continue all exercises outlined above
       b. Initiate hamstring curls (low weight)
       c. Initiate swimming
       d. Initiate vigorous stretching program
       e. Increase closed-chain rehabilitation
  C. Weeks 8 to 10
    1. Continue with all exercises
    2. KT-1000 test
  D. Week 12
    1. Discontinue ambulation with brace
    2. KT-1000 test
    3. Isometric test

Table continued on following page

TABLE 9–12   **REHABILITATION PROTOCOL FOR POSTERIOR CRUCIATE LIGAMENT–PATELLAR TENDON GRAFT RECONSTRUCTION** *Continued*

4. Exercises:
  a. Begin isokinetics (100–40°)
  b. Continue minisquats
  c. Initiate lateral step-ups
  d. Initiate pool running (forward only)
  e. Cycling for endurance (30 minutes)
  f. Begin walking program
V. Light activity phase (months 3 to 4)
 A. Goals:
   1. Development of strength, power, and endurance
   2. Begin to prepare for return to functional activities
 B. Exercises:
   1. Begin light running program
   2. Continue isokinetics (high speed, full ROM)
   3. Continue eccentrics
   4. Continue minisquats and lateral step-ups
   5. Continue closed-chain rehabilitation
   6. Continue endurance exercises
 C. Tests:
   1. Isokinetic test (week 15)
   2. KT-1000 test (prior to running program)
   3. Functional test—70% of contralateral leg
VI. Return to activity (months 5 to 6)
 A. Advance rehabilitation to competitive sports
 B. Goals: achieve maximal strength and further enhance neuromuscular coordination and endurance
 C. Exercises:
   1. Closed-chain rehabilitation
   2. High-speed isokinetics
   3. Running program
   4. Agility drills
   5. Balance drills
   6. Plyometrics initiated
VII. Follow-up
 A. 6 Months
   1. KT-1000 test
   2. Isokinetic test
   3. Functional test
 B. 12 Months
   1. KT-1000 test
   2. Isokinetic test
   3. Functional test

surgery, progressing to one crutch by week 8. Crutches are discontinued by week 10 and the brace is discontinued by week 12.

Medial Collateral Ligament

Although the MCL was once thought to be the most frequently injured ligament in the knee, studies of isolated MCL sprains are rarely carried out as a result of the attention given to the ACL. Such sprains can occur, but third-degree lesions are usually treated conservatively, not opera-

TABLE 9–13 REHABILITATION PROTOCOL FOR MEDIAL COLLATERAL LIGAMENT REPAIR

I. Immediate postoperative phase
  A. Day 1
    1. Brace locked at 30°
    2. Touchdown weight-bearing with two crutches
    3. Begin following exercises in brace:
      a. Quad sets
      b. Cocontractions
      c. Ankle pumps
      d. Bent leg raises
    4. Sleep in brace
  B. Days 3 to 6
    1. Brace adjusted to 90–15°
    2. Partial weight-bearing with two crutches
    3. Exercises in brace to be performed 2 or 3 times daily:
      a. Continue above exercises
      b. Active flexion to 90°
      c. Seated hip flexions
      d. 90–45° knee extensions
      e. Hip abductions and extensions
      f. Well-leg and upper body exercises
    4. Shower after sutures removed and no drainage from wound
    5. Brace off only to shower
II. Intermediate phase
  A. Weeks 1 to 4
    1. Full weight-bearing in brace, 90–15° range of motion (ROM)
    2. Out of brace for exercises, progress knee flexion
    3. Begin stationary cycling when ROM is sufficient
    4. Begin exercises:
      a. Continue with exercises out of brace (outlined above), progressing progressive resisted exercises (PREs) as tolerated
      b. Static weight loading
      c. Hamstring stretching
      d. Proprioception exercises
      e. 90–45° knee extensions
      f. Hip abductions
      g. Swimming program
  B. Weeks 5 to 8
    1. Continue PRE with exercises
    2. Progress to full active extension exercises:
      a. Increase proprioception exercises
      b. Closed-chain exercises:
        1) Minisquats
        2) Don Tigney knee extension
      c. Slide Board with gradual progression
      d. Double-leg press, progressing to single-leg press
      e. Continue cycling
      f. Begin high-speed isokinetics (week 8), full ROM
    3. Full weight-bearing
III. Advanced phase
  A. Months 2 to 6
    1. Eccentric work
    2. Continue progressing PRE
    3. High-speed tubing exercises
    5. Plyometrics
    6. Functional activities, including straight-ahead running
    7. Isokinetic test
    8. Functional testing

tively. Several studies[34, 51, 54, 153] have reported excellent results following nonsurgical treatment of grade III MCL sprains, with early motion. MCL sprains are often associated with ACL disruptions—the ACL is reconstructed and the MCL is left to heal on its own. In such cases rehabilitation follows the ACL rehabilitation guidelines (Table 9–9). Protocols for rehabilitation of MCL lesions are presented in Tables 9–13 and 9–14. Initial concern focuses on protection from valgus forces and gradual progression toward full extension to allow the MCL to reapproximate itself with scar tissue. Because full extension pulls the MCL taut, in injured MCL ligaments the torn ends may not reapproximate adequately and some residual valgus instability can occur.

TABLE 9–14   REHABILITATION PROTOCOL FOR GRADES I, II, AND III ISOLATED MEDIAL COLLATERAL LIGAMENT SPRAINS*

I. Maximum protection phase
  A. Goals:
    1. Early protected range of motion (ROM)
    2. Prevent quadriceps atrophy
    3. Decrease effusion and pain
  B. Day 1
    1. Ice, compression, elevation
    2. Knee hinged brace, nonpainful ROM, or knee immobilizer, if hinged brace not available
    3. Crutches (weight-bearing, as tolerated)
    4. Passive range of motion, active-assisted range of motion to maintain ROM
    5. Electrical muscle stimulation to quads (8 hours/day)
    6. Quad sets, 60 repetitions, three times daily
    7. Straight leg raises
  C. Day 2
    1. Straight leg raises
    2. Hamstring stretching
    3. Well-leg exercises
    4. Whirlpool for ROM (cold for first 3 or 4 days, then warm)
    5. High-voltage galvanic stimulation to control swelling
    6. Continue day 1 regimen
  D. Days 3 to 7
    1. Continue as above
    2. Crutches (weight-bearing, as tolerated)
    3. ROM, as tolerated
    4. Eccentric quad exercises
    5. Bicycle for ROM stimulus
    6. Multiangle isometrics with electrical stimulation
    7. Initiate hip abduction and extension
    8. Brace worn at night, during day, as needed
II. Moderate protection phase
  A. Goals:
    1. Full painless ROM
    2. Restore strength
    3. Ambulate without crutches
  B. Criteria for progression:
    1. No increase in instability
    2. No increase in swelling
    3. Minimal tenderness
    4. Passive ROM 10–100°
  C. Week 1

Table continued on following page

TABLE 9-14   REHABILITATION PROTOCOL FOR GRADES I, II, AND III ISOLATED MEDIAL COLLATERAL LIGAMENT SPRAINS* *Continued*

1. Continue strengthening program with progressive resisted exercise (PRE)
2. Continue electric muscle stimulation
3. Continue ROM exercises
4. Multiangle isometrics with electric stimulation
5. Discontinue crutches
6. Stationary bike for endurance
7. Pool exercises, running in water forward and backward
8. Full ROM exercises
9. Flexibility exercises, hamstrings, quads, iliotibial band
10. Proprioception training

D. Days 11 to 14
1. Continue as for week 1
2. PREs, emphasize quads, medial hamstrings, hip abduction
3. Initiate isokinetics, submaximal → maximal fast contractile velocities
4. Begin running program if full painless extension and flexion are present:
   a. Jog 1 mile if no pain or limp
   b. Then,
      1) 6 × 80 yards, 1/2 speed
      2) 6 × 80 yards, 3/4 speed
      3) 6 × 80 yards, full speed
      4) 6 × 80 yards, 1/2 speed cutting
      5) 6 × 80 yards, full-speed cutting
   c. Stop at any point if there is pain, limping, or undue fatigue. The next day the entire program must be started all over again until it can be finished in its entirety in one workout

III. Minimal protection phase
A. Goals: increase muscle strength and power
B. Criteria for progression:
   1. No instability
   2. No swelling or tenderness
   3. Full, painless ROM
C. Week 3
   1. Continue strengthening program; emphasize high-speed isokinetics, eccentric quads; isotonic hip adduction, medial hamstrings
   2. Isokinetic test
   3. Proprioception training
   4. Endurance exercises (e.g., stationary bike, 30–40 minutes; NordicTrack; swimming; Slide Board)

IV. Maintenance phase (weeks 4 to 8)
A. Return to competition
   1. Full ROM
   2. No tenderness over MCL
   3. No instability
   4. No effusion
   5. Muscle strength, 85% of contralateral side
   6. Quad strength = 60% of body weight
   7. Proprioceptive ability satisfactory
   8. Lateral knee brace if appropriate
B. Maintenance program: continue isotonic strengthening exercises, flexibility exercises, proprioception activities

Adapted from Clancy, W.J., et al. (1990): Medial collateral ligament of the knee. Part III: Treatment. Sports Med. Update, 5:8–9.

* This program may be accelerated for those with first-degree MCL sprains or it may be extended, depending on the severity of the injury. Any increase in pain, swelling, or loss of motion indicates that the program is progressing too fast.

Meniscal Injury

Meniscus lesions have been treated by total meniscectomy, partial meniscectomy and, most recently, by meniscal repair. Total meniscectomy, by arthrotomy, quickly alleviates the mechanical symptoms and short-term results have usually been good.[30] Long-term outcomes have been disappointing, however, because of the degenerative articular changes that occur in total meniscectomy knees.[74, 83, 105] Currently, the indications for total meniscectomy are rare.

Meniscus lesions are now repaired, or a partial meniscectomy is performed. The rationale behind partial meniscectomy is removal of the torn part of the meniscus. As much meniscus tissue as possible is retained in the hope that it will continue to perform, to some extent, the essential function of the meniscus.[30] Meniscus lesions are often associated with other intra-articular pathology, usually an ACL disruption. Some studies[74, 90] have reported very poor results in those patients with meniscectomy, but the ACL deficiency was not corrected. Patients continued to complain of increased knee symptoms, with progressive degenerative changes. The degree of degenerative change is directly proportional to the amount of meniscus removed.

Partial meniscectomy is now mainly performed using arthroscopy because of the reported decrease in morbidity. Most partial meniscectomies involve the inner two-thirds, because this aspect of the meniscus is avascular. Rehabilitation is generally uneventful and can be progressed as tolerated (Table 9–15). Most athletes can safely return to participation in 4 to 6 weeks after surgery.

Conversely, rehabilitation following meniscal repair is of longer duration, with return to participation at about 4 to 6 months after surgery. Meniscal repairs involve the peripheral third of the meniscus because of its vascularity. Although rehabilitation takes longer with a meniscal repair, many surgeons feel it is worthwhile because of the protection the meniscus affords the articular cartilage. Ten to 20% of meniscal lesions are reparable. In cases of ACL tears in which the meniscus lesion is reparable, it is recommended that the ACL also be reconstructed.

Rehabilitation following meniscal repair focuses on progression of motion and weight-bearing. Full weight-bearing is not allowed until 6 to 8 weeks after surgery. A gradual progression in weight-bearing could be as follows:

Weeks 2 to 3: partial weight-bearing—25% of body weight
Weeks 3 to 4: partial weight-bearing—50% of body weight
Weeks 5 to 6: partial weight-bearing—75% of body weight
Weeks 6 to 8: full weight-bearing

Range of motion is guarded for the first 3 weeks and protected from 0 to 20° of extension to 90° of flexion. By week 8 the athlete should have progressed to full weight-bearing, and full active range of motion, and should be well into the rehabilitation program. If a meniscal repair is performed with an ACL reconstruction rehabilitation proceeds following the ACL protocol, except for weight-bearing and knee motion limitations.

TABLE 9–15   REHABILITATION PROTOCOL FOR KNEE ARTHROSCOPY, MEDIAL/LATERAL MENISCECTOMY, AND LOOSE BODY REMOVAL

I. Immediate postoperative phase
  A. Day 1
    1. Partial weight-bearing on two crutches
    2. Begin following exercises:
      a. Quad sets with electrical muscle stimulation, if necessary
      b. Heel slides
      c. Standing hamstring curls
      d. Terminal knee extensions
      e. Seated hip flexions
      f. Hamstring stretching
      g. Ankle pumps
      h. Straight leg raises
      i. Minisquats
    3. Perform exercises twice daily
    4. Use ice before and after exercises for 20 minutes, and as needed
    5. Begin with 3 × 10, progress to 5 × 10 with exercises; progressive resisted exercise (PRE), as tolerated
  B. Days 2 to 5: Progress to partial weight-bearing with one crutch and full weight-bearing as tolerated
  C. Days 4 and 5
    1. Add following exercises:
      a. Straight leg raises (four planes)
      b. Proprioception exercises
      c. Increase closed-chain exercises:
        1) Stationary bike
        2) Minisquats with tubing
        3) Don Tigney knee extensions
      d. Swimming program
    2. Progress PRE with exercises, as tolerated
II. Intermediate phase
  A. Week 2
    1. Add following exercises:
      a. Static weight loading
      b. Lateral step-ups
      c. 90–45° knee extensions
      d. Double-leg presses progressing to single-leg presses
    2. Continue PRE progression
  B. Weeks 3 to 4
    1. Begin high-speed isokinetic work, full range of motion
    2. Begin Slide Board
    3. Increase proprioception and closed-chain exercises
    4. Eccentric quad work
    5. Begin functional activities
III. Advanced phase
  A. Weeks 5 to 8
    1. Isokinetic and functional testing (weeks 6–8)
    2. Plyometrics
    3. High-speed tubing exercises
    4. Begin interval running program, if indicated (see App. B.)
    5. Return to functional activities

Functional Knee Braces

Many authors[12, 16, 24, 25, 109] have investigated the effect of functional knee braces on deterring instability in those with ACL-deficient knees (Fig. 9–41). In vivo measurements have generally shown that braces reduce anterior tibial displacement at low loads, but the low forces used in laxity testing probably do not reveal the absolute excursions that result from higher physiologic loads.[24, 118] Markolf and colleagues[100] have stated that forces in excess of 200 N are required to produce an accurate measurement of absolute laxity. It is clinically evident, however, that some patients with a functional brace perform well, whereas others do not. The major subjective determinant in the success of a brace is a reduction in the number of "giving-way" episodes reported. Subjective improvements while wearing a brace have been hypothesized to be a result of heightened proprioception.[16, 25, 109] Tibone and associates[151] have found EMG evidence of a longer duration of medial hamstring muscle activity in the unbraced, ACL-deficient knees of subjects engaged in running. Those in the vastus medialis group showed an earlier onset during swing phase in the involved limb. This evidence of "out-of-phase" muscle activity, coupled with the observation of Cook and co-workers[25] that weaker patients perform much better in their braces, supports the increased proprioception

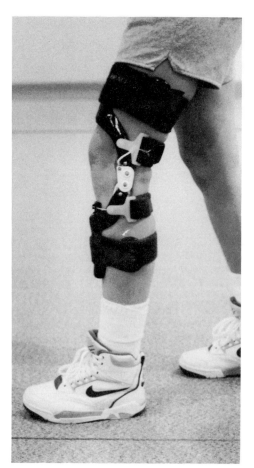

FIGURE 9–41   An example of an ACL functional brace.

theory, especially because braces do not prevent abnormal tibial displacement at physiologic force levels.

Bracing following ACL injury and/or reconstruction is an acceptable standard of care. Although bracing probably does not prevent tibial displacement at physiologic loads, evidence supporting its proprioception function continues to mount. Keeping this in mind, and being aware of the growing number of "off-the-shelf" functional braces on the market, physicians and clinicians must decide whether the custom-made brace is worth the extra cost to the athlete or patient if the protection offered is proprioceptive in nature.

Functional Testing

Physicians and clinicians often rely on isokinetic peak torque data and the time from injury or surgery to help determine when an athlete can return to play, but this is only a small part of the total picture. Objective test data that can be used in making a decision following knee injury or surgery include the results of knee arthrometer, isokinetic, proprioception, and functional testing.

Objective functional testing of the lower extremity aids in determining the functional capabilities of the knee joint during sports activities.[117] Functional tests can be used to determine functional limitations, which cannot be determined through muscle testing alone. This is evidenced by a report from Tibone and colleagues,[151] who examined functional abilities in ACL-deficient individuals. They reported isokinetic peak torque data for quadriceps and hamstrings of 86% and 96%, respectively, but this was not sufficient to eliminate the subjective need for ACL reconstruction.

Several functional tests have been used to assess functional performance objectively following ACL injury. Tegner and associates[147] have used the one-legged hop, figure-eight running, running up and down a spiral staircase, and running up and down a slope to evaluate functional knee integrity. They found that those athletes with ACL injuries perform significantly less well than uninjured players.

Barber and co-workers[8] have evaluated the effectiveness of five hopping, jumping, and cutting-type tests (shuttle runs) in determining lower extremity functional limitations in those with ACL-deficient knees, including one-legged hop for distance, one-legged vertical jump, one-legged timed hop test, and two types of shuttle runs. The shuttle runs and vertical jump test did not detect functional limitations reliably. In the one-legged hop test 50% of patients performed normally but all reported giving-way episodes, indicating a lack of sensitivity of these tests in defining functional limitations. Also, their data showed that 60% of the ACL-deficient knees performed abnormally on at least one out of two tests in the combined test analysis. Therefore, the authors[8] recommended that clinicians use two one-legged hop tests as a screening procedure to determine lower limb function, in addition to subjective complaints of giving-way. Individuals who score abnormally on the two functional tests have a significant functional limitation for sports activities. Those who score normally may still have giving-way episodes under uncontrolled sports situations.

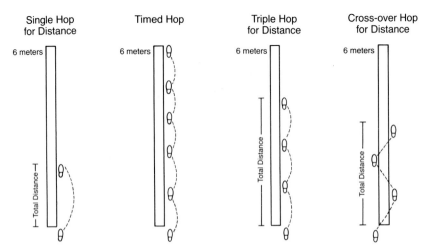

FIGURE 9–42   Four tests for appraising functional stability. (From Noyes, F.R. (in press): Abnormal lower limb symmetry determined by function hop tests after anterior cruciate ligament rupture. Am. J. Sports Med.)

Noyes[117] and Mangine[96] have reported four tests for appraising functional stability (Fig. 9–42): (1) one-legged hop for distance; (2) one-legged hop for time; (3) one-legged triple hop for distance; and (4) one-legged crossover hop for distance. From their results, the one-legged hop for distance and the one-legged crossover hop for distance appear to be the most reliable in determining functional stability.[96] Mangine[96] has noted that the one-legged hop for distance may be normal, but the one-legged crossover hop for distance may be abnormal if the posterolateral knee complex is involved.

Functional testing allows the athlete to be tested in a closed kinematic chain environment, rather than the traditional open kinematic chain isokinetic testing. It is hoped that the combined data from arthrometer, isokinetic, and functional testing can be used to extrapolate how an individual will perform on the field and thus reduce the chance for reinjury.

Patellofemoral Dysfunction

Anterior knee pain can emanate from patellofemoral dysfunction, which can be traumatic or insidious in onset. General anterior knee pain is a common complaint in athletes, and, if no significant clinical findings are noted, the cause of the pain may be overlooked. The need for a *complete lower extremity evaluation* in athletes who present without serious trauma, but who may be suffering from an overuse phenomenon, cannot be overemphasized.[133] Proper functioning of the quadriceps musculature is paramount in deterring patellofemoral dysfunction. Because of the close relationship between the patellofemoral and tibiofemoral joints, disability in one can affect the other. Conversely, rehabilitation involving one joint must consider the other; often, tibiofemoral rehabilitation does not take into account the patellofemoral joint, and this can result in perpetuating an underlying patellofemoral problem.

Patellofemoral pain can originate from mechanical malalignment, the static and/or dynamic stabilization system, or mechanical load placed across the joint as a result of various activities.[133] Mechanical malalignment can result from a patellar dislocation or subluxation as a result of the mechanical pull of the quadriceps. Quadriceps contraction results in a natural pull of the patella laterally, which is referred to as the law of valgus. This predisposes the patella to dislocation or subluxation. If this is associated with one or a combination of various factors (e.g., large Q angle, abnormally tight lateral static structures such as the lateral retinaculum, atrophy and/or weakness in the vastus medialis oblique, from trauma or general weakness, or foot pronation), it becomes evident why patellofemoral problems are so common. Patellofemoral dysfunction that goes unchecked can lead to permanent patellar articular cartilage damage (patellar chondrosis). Most patellofemoral pathologies can be classified as patellar subluxation or dislocation, extensor mechanism malalignment, lateral patellar compression syndrome, or patellofemoral chondrosis (chondromalacia patellae).[64] Clinically, it appears that patellofemoral dysfunction is more common in females than in males.

Rehabilitation of patellofemoral dysfunction should concentrate on closed-chain exercises (see Figs. 9–6 through 9–19). Care must be taken not to cause large forces to be transmitted through the patella during exercise (see Patellofemoral Kinematics and Knee Extension Exercise in this chapter). The athlete should not exercise through pain or crepitus. Those athletes who complain of anterior knee pain that may be of patellofemoral origin should initially be treated conservatively. Many of these individuals respond to control of the inflammation process, quadriceps muscle strengthening, and avoidance of harmful activities until the rehabilitation process is complete.

Isometrics and straight leg raises are initially recommended until muscle function has been restored. These exercises are usually tolerated best and increase patellofemoral compression the least. Closed-chain exercises are highly recommended and should be the mainstay of the program because of the lower patellofemoral compression produced by these exercises. Restoration of proprioception is vital when attempting to re-establish neuromuscular control. Those with acute conditions (patellar subluxators) may find use of the BAPS board difficult at certain angles. As rehabilitation progresses, high-speed, straight-leg tubing exercises are indicated to help facilitate muscle control (Fig. 9–43). Also, retrowalking may be beneficial before straight-ahead walking or jogging is initiated, because knee forces decrease with backward activities. Straight-ahead running can begin when isokinetic testing results on the injured side are 70% to 80% of those on the uninjured side. Anterior knee pain has been reportedly reduced with an eccentric quadriceps program,[13] and this can be included in the functional progression. Table 9–16 outlines a conservative treatment plan for a subluxating patella and/or patellofemoral syndrome.

Several authors have reported other techniques that may be beneficial in the treatment of lateral compression syndrome and subluxating patellas. Kramer[82] has reported success with a manual lateral retinaculum stretching regimen in conjunction with the traditional patellofemoral program. It was noted that in the patellar malalignment syndrome

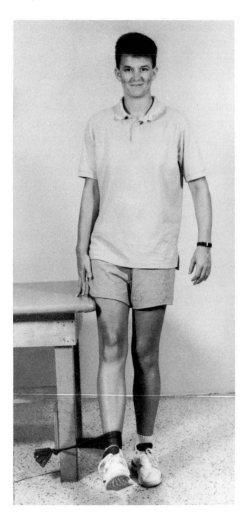

FIGURE 9–43 Hip flexion and extension with tubing. These can be performed at high speeds with the knee straight. Because the knee is extended, patellofemoral compression forces are low.

there is excessive pressure on the lateral aspect of the patellofemoral joint, with resultant damage to the articular cartilage. By stretching the lateral tissues and reducing the lateral pressure, cartilage metabolism is facilitated. Kramer has proposed two types of manual maneuvers: (1) medial patellar glide with the knee extended, held 1 minute to stretch the lateral retinaculum; and (2) patellar compression with tracking.[8] With the athlete sitting and the knee flexed to 90°, the patella is compressed against the patellofemoral articular surface and tracked medially by the clinician as the athlete extends the knee.

McConnell[103] has reported a 96% success rate with a patellofemoral treatment regimen. This not only emphasizes closed-chain exercises but corrects the glide, tilt, and rotation components of the patella. Initially, quadriceps isometrics are performed at varying angles until pain is incurred. If pain can be alleviated by manually gliding the patella medially and then performing isometric quad contractions at the angle at which pain was incurred, then the individual probably can respond well to the treatment regimen. After an evaluation, tape is used to correct patellar orientation. The tilt component is corrected by pull-

TABLE 9–16   REHABILITATION PROTOCOL FOR SUBLUXATING PATELLA AND PATELLOFEMORAL SYNDROME

I. Rationale
A. Restore patellofemoral arthrokinematics
B. Decrease patellofemoral crepitus and pain
C. Do not exercise through patellofemoral crepitus; continually monitor during exercise and modify exercises as crepitus indicates
D. Emphasize on closed-chain and proprioceptive exercises
II. Initial phase
A. Day 1 to week 2
1. Ice and elevation to control inflammation, pain, swelling
2. Electrical muscle stimulation to facilitate quad recruitment, if necessary
3. Initiate following exercises, as tolerated:
a. Static weight loading
b. Don Tigney knee extensions
c. Straight leg raises (four planes)
d. 90–45° or 90–30° knee extensions, if crepitus allows
e. Stationary bike (seat high, low to moderate tension)
f. Hamstring stretching
g. Minisquats
h. Proprioception exercises (BAPS board)
4. Progress progressive resisted exercises, as tolerated
5. Fit with patella tracking brace for patella subluxators or McConnell taping technique; depending on symptoms, patient may need to wear brace with daily activities and/or exercise, or only with functional activities
6. Instruct patient to avoid squatting and stairs as much as possible until symptoms have been resolved
III. Intermediate phase
A. Weeks 2 to 4
1. Continue stationary bike
2. Begin Thera-Band in standing hip flexion and extension; increase speed as tolerated
3. Double-leg presses progressed to single-leg presses
4. Minisquats with tubing
5. Increase proprioception and closed-chain exercises
B. Weeks 4 to 6
1. Begin lateral step-ups
2. Increase speed with tubing exercises
3. May begin high-speed isokinetics as crepitus allows
4. Begin plyometrics, as tolerated
5. Begin functional activities and drills
IV. Advanced phase
A. Weeks 6 to 8
1. Isokinetic test, if needed
2. Functional testing
3. Increase plyometric program
4. Return to functional activities, as tolerated

ing the tape from the midline of the patella medially (Fig. 9–44). This lifts the lateral border and provides a passive stretch to the lateral structures, which is important if the deep lateral retinacular fibers are tight. The medial glide is corrected by pulling the patella medially (Fig. 9–45); most individuals require this correction. Finally, the rotation component is corrected either by taping from the middle inferior patellar pole upward and medially or from the middle superior pole downward and medially. The superior and inferior poles of the patella should

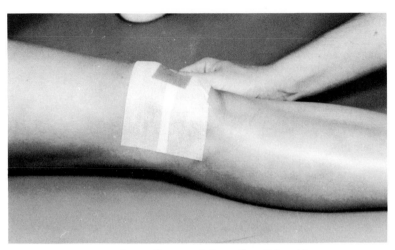

FIGURE 9–44   Controlling medial patellar glide with tape.

be in line with the longitudinal axis of the femur. The athlete performs the rehabilitation program with the tape in place. Additionally, many patellar subluxation braces are on the market and have proven beneficial.[65, 75, 126]

As noted, it is of the utmost importance that the entire lower extremity be evaluated. It is suggestive that pronated feet and patellofemoral pain are associated.[149, 155] If this is the case, orthotic correction is necessary. After 1 or 2 weeks of orthotic use the symptoms should resolve. Pain from pronated feet is postulated to be a result of excessive lower leg rotation.

If conservative care fails, surgery is indicated. One of the most common procedures is a lateral retinaculum release in which the lateral retinaculum is cut, thus freeing the patella laterally. This procedure can be done arthroscopically or open. The major complication is a large hemarthrosis caused by cutting of the lateral geniculate artery. Initial concern involves decreasing the large effusion through compression

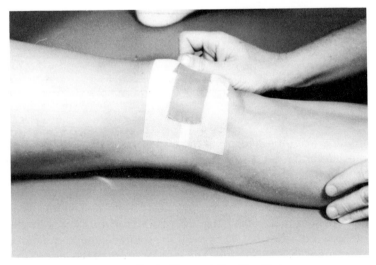

FIGURE 9–45   Controlling patellar tilt with tape.

dressing, vasopneumatic compression, and the muscular pump. Table 9–17 outlines the rehabilitation protocol following a lateral retinaculum release.

Sometimes a distal realignment is performed, which involves transferring the patellar tendon and tibial tubercle to decrease the Q angle. The main concern with this procedure is progression of knee motion

---

TABLE 9–17 REHABILITATION PROTOCOL FOR LATERAL RETINACULUM RELEASE

I. Initial postoperative phase
  A. Day 1
    1. Partial weight-bearing with two crutches
    2. Straight leg immobilizer
    3. Exercises in immobilizer twice daily:
      a. Quad sets with EMS, if necessary
      b. Straight leg raises (four planes)
      c. Ankle pumps
      d. Hamstring stretching
      e. Passive patella mobilization
    4. Use modalities to decrease effusion (e.g., compression dressing, vasopneumatic compression)
  B. Days 2 to 7
    1. Goal: progression of exercises to 5 sets of 10 repetitions
    2. Full weight-bearing progressed in immobilizer, as tolerated
    3. Continue with above exercises in immobilizer
  C. Weeks 1 and 2
    1. Begin exercises out of immobilizer
    2. Progress weight-bearing, as tolerated
    3. Fit with lateral patella tracking brace as pain and swelling allow
    4. Exercises:
      a. Supine heel slides
      b. Seated heel slides
      c. Don Tigney knee extensions
      d. Standing hamstring curls
      e. Stationary cycling
      f. Seated hip flexions
      g. Minisquats
      h. Proprioception exercises
    5. Progress PRE, as tolerated
II. Intermediate phase
  A. Weeks 3 and 4
    1. Full weight-bearing out of immobilizer (by week 3)
    2. Progress biking, as tolerated
    3. Begin Slide Board, NordicTrack, StairMaster
    4. Standing hip flexion and extension with tubing; gradually increase speed of movement
  B. Weeks 4 to 6
    1. Isokinetic high-speed work, full range of motion
    2. Increase closed-chain and proprioception exercises
    3. Begin plyometrics
III. Advanced phase
  A. Weeks 6 to 10
    1. Discontinue use of lateral patella tracking brace
    2. Gradual return to functional activities; may begin running program and agility drills when isokinetic test is 70–80% uninvolved extremity
    3. Isokinetic test
    4. Functional testing
    5. Begin plyometrics

**TABLE 9–18   PROGRESSION OF KNEE MOTION AND
WEIGHT-BEARING AFTER DISTAL REALIGNMENT**

Week	Knee Motion	Weight-Bearing
1–3	Brace, 0–60°	Nonweight-bearing
3–4	Brace, 0–90°	Partial weight-bearing
4–6	Progress active range of motion	Progress weight-bearing
6–8	Discontinue brace	Discontinue crutches

and weight-bearing (Table 9–18). A progressive running program can begin at about weeks 16 to 20, with progression to full activity by 6 months after surgery.

Patellofemoral pain should initially be treated conservatively, with emphasis on closed-chain rehabilitation. Successful conservative treatment includes restoring muscle function (strength), particularly to the vastus medialis, decreasing lateral compressive forces, and protecting the patellofemoral joint from compressive forces during rehabilitation. In those athletes with pronated feet, orthotics are indicated to decrease lower leg rotation and help reduce symptoms.

Rehabilitation of the lower extremity should emphasize closed-chain exercises along an increasing continuum of difficulty. Early controlled motion, muscle turn-on, restoration of joint arthrokinematics, and understanding the relationship of the tibiofemoral to the patellofemoral joint help deter arthrofibrosis following knee injury or surgery. Normal knee joint kinematics must be understood so that a safe rehabilitation program that emphasizes restoration of joint motion, muscle strength, power, and endurance, and proprioception can be developed. Functional testing and other objective measurements, such as arthrometer and isokinetic testing, should be used to help determine when an athlete can return to competition.

References

1. Aglietti, P., Buzzi, R., and Bassi, P.O. (1988): Arthroscopic partial meniscectomy in the anterior cruciate-deficient knee. Am. J. Sports Med., 16:597–602.
2. Aglietti, P., and Ceralli, G. (1979): Chondromalacia and recurrent subluxation of the patella: A study of malalignment with some indications for radiography. Ital. J. Orthop. Traumatol., 5:187–190.
3. Amiel, D., Kleiner, J.B., and Akeson, W.H. (1986): The natural history of the anterior cruciate ligament autograft of patellar tendon origin. Am. J. Sports Med., 14:449–462.
4. Anderson, A.F., and Lipscomb, A.B. (1989): Preoperative instrumented testing of anterior and posterior knee laxity. Am. J. Sports Med., 17:387–392.
5. Andriacchi, T.P., Anderson, G.B.J., and Ferlier, R.W., et al. (1980): A study of lower-limb mechanics during stair-climbing. J. Bone Joint Surg. [Am.], 62:749–757.
6. Antich, T.J., and Brewster, C.E. (1986): Modification of quadriceps femoris muscle exercises during knee rehabilitation. Phys. Ther., 66:1246–1251.
7. Arnold, J.A., Coker, T.P., and Heaton, L.M., et al. (1979): Natural history of anterior cruciate tears. Am. J. Sports Med., 7:305–3313.
8. Barber, S.D., Noyes, F.R., and Mangine, R.B., et al. (1990): Quantitative assessment of functional limitations in normal and anterior cruciate ligament-deficient knee. Clin. Orthop., 255:204–214.

9. Barnett, C.H., and Richardson, A. (1953): The postural function of the popliteus muscle. Ann. Phys. Med., 1:177.

10. Barrack, R.L., Skinner, H.B., and Buckley, S.L. (1989): Proprioception in the anterior cruciate-deficient knee. Am. J. Sports Med., 17:1–6.

11. Basmajian, J.V., and Lovejoy, J.F. (1971): Functions of the popliteus muscle in man: A multi-factorial electromyographic analysis. J. Bone Joint Surg. [Am.], 53:557.

12. Beck, C., Drez, D., and Young, J., et al. (1986): Instrumented testing of functional knee braces. Am. J. Sports Med., 14:253–256.

13. Bennett, J.G., and Stauber, W.T. (1986): Evaluation and treatment of anterior knee pain using eccentric exercise. Med. Sci. Sports Exerc., 18:526–530.

14. Bergfeld, J.A., and Anderson, T.E. (1984): Achieving mobility, strength, and function of the injured knee. In: Hunter, L.Y., Funk, F.J. (eds.): Rehabilitation of the Injured Knee. St. Louis, C.V. Mosby.

15. Bos, R.R., and Bloser, T.G. (1970): An electromyographic study of vastus medialis and vastus lateralis during selected isometric exercises. Med. Sci. Sports, 2:218–223.

16. Branch, T., Hunter, R., and Reynolds, P. (1988): Controlling anterior tibial displacement under static load: A comparison of two braces. Orthopedics, 11:1249–1252.

17. Brantigan, O.C., and Voshell, A.F. (1941): The mechanics of the ligaments and menisci of the knee joint. J. Bone Joint Surg., 23:44–66.

18. Brownstein, B., Mangine, R.E., Noyes, F.R., and Kryger, S. (1988): Anatomy and biomechanics. In: Mangine, R.E. (ed.): Physical Therapy of the Knee. New York, Churchill Livingstone.

19. Burks, R., Daniel, D., and Losse, G. (1984): The effect of continuous passive motion on anterior cruciate ligament reconstruction stability. Am. J. Sports Med., 12:323–327.

20. Burks, R.T., and Leland, R. (1988): Determination of graft tension before fixation in anterior cruciate ligament reconstruction. J. Arthrosc. Rel. Surg., 4:260–266.

21. Butler, D.L., Noyes, F.R., and Grood, E.S. (1980): Ligamentous restraints to anterior-posterior drawer in the human knee. J. Bone Joint Surg. [Am.], 62:259–270.

22. Cabaud, H.E. (1983): Biomechanics of the anterior cruciate ligament. Clin. Orthop., 172:26–31.

23. Close, J.R. (1964): Motor Function in the Lower Extremity: Analyses by Electronic Instrumentation. Springfield, IL, Charles C Thomas.

24. Colville, M.R., Lee, C.L., and Ciullo, J.V. (1986): The Lenox Hill brace. An evaluation of effectiveness in treating knee instability. Am. J. Sports Med., 14:257–261.

25. Cook, F.F., Tibone, J.E., and Redfern, F.C. (1989): A dynamic analysis of a functional brace for anterior cruciate ligament insufficiency. Am. J. Sports Med., 17:519–524.

26. Czerniecki, J.M., Lippert, F., and Olerud, J.E. (1988): A biomechanical evaluation of tibiofemoral rotation in anterior cruciate-deficient knees during walking and running. Am. J. Sports Med., 16:327–333.

27. Daniel, D.M., Malcom, L.L., and Losse, G., et al. (1985): Instrumented measurement of anterior laxity of the knee. J. Bone Joint Surg. [Am.], 67:720–726.

28. Daniel, D.M., Stone, M.L., and Malcom, L., et al. (1983): Instrumented measurement of ACL disruption. Orthop. Res. Soc., 8:12.

29. Daniel, D.M., Stone, M.L., Sachs, R., and Malcom, L. (1985): Instrumented measurement of anterior knee laxity in patients with acute anterior cruciate ligament disruption. Am. J. Sports Med., 13:401–407.

30. DeHaven, K.E. (1985): Rationale for meniscus repair or excision. Clin. Sports Med., 4:267–273.

31. Draganich, L.F., Jaeger, R.J., and Kralj, A.R. (1989): Coactivation of the hamstrings and quadriceps during extension of the knee. J. Bone Joint Surg. [Am.], 71:1075–1081.

32. Duarte-Cintra, A., and Furlani, J. (1981): Electromyographic study of quadriceps femoris in man. Electromyogr. Clin. Neurophysiol., 21:539–554.

33. Ekholm, J., Nisell, R., and Arborelius, U.P., et al. (1984): Load on knee joint structures and muscular activity during living. Scand. J. Rehabil. Med., 16:1–9.

34. Ellasasser, J.C., Reynolds, F.C., and Omohundro, J.R. (1974): The non-operative treatment of collateral ligament injuries of the knee in professional football players. J. Bone Joint Surg. [Am.], 56:1185–1190.

35. Ellis, M.I., Seedhom, B.B., and Amis, A.A., et al. (1979): Forces in the knee joint whilst rising from normal and motorized chairs. N. Engl. J. Med., 8:33–40.
36. Ellis, M.I., Seedhom, B.B., and Wright, V. (1984): Forces in the knee joint whilst rising from seated positions. J. Biomed. Eng., 6:113–120.
37. Emery, M., Moffroid, M., and Boerman, J., et al. (1989): Reliability of force/displacement measures in a clinical device designed to measure ligamentous laxity at the knee. J. Orthop. Sports Phys. Ther., 10:441–447.
38. Engle, R.P. (1988): Hamstring facilitation in anterior instability of the knee. Athletic Training, 23:226–228, 285.
39. Engle, R.P., and Canner, G.G. (1989): Proprioceptive neuromuscular facilitation (PNF) and modified procedures for anterior cruciate ligament (ACL) instability. J. Orthop. Sports Phys. Ther., 11:230–236.
40. Engle, R.P., and Canner, G.C. (1989): Rehabilitation of symptomatic anterolateral knee instability. J. Orthop. Sports Phys. Ther., 11:237–244.
41. Ericson, M.O. (1988): Muscular function during ergometer cycling. Scand. J. Rehabil. Med., 20:35–41.
42. Ericson, M.O., Bratt, P., and Nisell, R., et al. (1986): Power output and work in different muscle groups during ergometer cycling. Eur. J. Appl. Physiol., 55:229.
43. Ericson, M.O., and Nisell, R. (1986): Tibiofemoral joint forces during ergometer cycling. Am. J. Sports Med., 14:285–290.
44. Ericson, M.O., and Nisell, R. (1987): Patellofemoral joint forces during ergometer cycling. Phys. Ther., 67:1365–1369.
45. Ericson, M.O., Nisell, R., Arborelius, U.P., and Ekholm, J. (1985): Muscular activity during ergometer cycling. Scand. J. Rehabil. Med., 17:53.
46. Ericson, M.O., Nisell, R., and Ekholm, J. (1984): Varus and valgus loads on the knee joint during ergometer cycling. Scand. J. Sports Sci., 6:39–45.
47. Fisk, R., and Wells, J. (1980): The quadriceps complex in bipedal man. J. Am. Osteopath. Assoc., 80:291–294.
48. Fleming, R.E., Blatz, D.J., and McCorroll, J.R. (1981): Posterior problems in the knee. Am. J. Sports Med., 9:107–113.
49. Fowler, P.J. (1984): Functional anatomy of the knee. In: Hunter, L.Y., and Funk, F.J., (eds.): Rehabilitation of the Injured Knee. St. Louis, C.V. Mosby.
50. Fox, J.M., Sherman, O.H., and Markolf, K. (1985): Arthroscopic anterior cruciate ligament repair: Preliminary results in instrumented testing for anterior stability. J. Arthrosc. Rel. Surgery, 1:175–181.
51. Frank, C, Akeson, W.H., and Woo, S.L.-Y., et al. (1984): Physiology and therapeutic value of passive joint motion. Clin. Orthop., 185:113.
52. Fukubayashi, T., and Kurosawa, H. (1980): The contact area and pressure distribution pattern of the knee. Acta Orthop. Scand., 51:871–879.
53. Fukubayashi, T., Torzilli, P.A., Sherman, M.F., and Warren, R.F. (1982): An in vitro biomechanical evaluation of anterior-posterior motion of the knee. J. Bone Joint Surg. [Am.], 64:258–264.
54. Goldstein, W.M., and Barmada, R. (1984): Early mobilization of rabbit medial collateral ligament repairs: Biomechanic and histologic study. Arch. Phys. Med. Rehabil., 65:239–242.
55. Goodfellow, J., Hungerford, D.S., and Woods, C. (1976): Patello-femoral joint mechanics and pathology. J. Bone Joint Surg. [Br.], 58:291–299.
56. Goodfellow, J., Hungerford, D.S., and Zindel, M. (1976): Patellofemoral joint mechanics and pathology: 1. Functional anatomy of the patello-femoral joint. J. Bone Joint Surg. [Br.], 58:287–290.
57. Gough, J.V., and Ladley, G. (1971): An investigation into the effectiveness of various forms of quadriceps exercises. Physiotherapy, 57:356–361.
58. Girgis, F.G., Marshall, J.L., and Al-Monajem, A.R.S. (1975): The cruciate ligaments of the knee joint: Anatomical, functional, and experimental analysis. Clin. Orthop., 106:216–231.
59. Grood, E.S., Noyes, F.R., Butler, D.L., and Suntay, W.J. (1981): Ligamentous and capsular restraints preventing straight medial and lateral laxity in intact human cadaver knees. J. Bone Joint Surg. [Am.], 63:1257–1269.
60. Grood, E.S., Suntay, W.J., Noyes, F.R., and Butler, D. (1984): Biomechanics of the knee-extension exercise. J. Bone Joint Surg. [Am.], 66:725–733.
61. Hallen, L.F., and Lindahl, O. (1966): The "screw-home" movement of the knee joint. Acta Orthop. Scand., 37:97.

62. Hanley, S.T., and Warren, R.F. (1987): Arthroscopic meniscectomy in the anterior cruciate ligament-deficient knee. J. Arthrosc. Rel. Res., 3:159–165.

63. Hanten, W.P., and Pace, M.B. (1987): Reliability of measuring anterior laxity of the knee joint using a knee ligament arthrometer. Phys. Ther., 67:357–359.

64. Heckmann, T.P. (1988): Conservative versus postsurgical patellar rehabilitation. In: Mangine, R. (ed.): Physical Therapy of the Knee. New York, Churchill Livingstone.

65. Henning, C., and Lynch, M. (1985): Current concepts of meniscal function and pathology. Clin. Sports Med., 4:259.

66. Houtz, S.J., and Fischer, F.J. (1959): An analysis of muscle action and joint excursion during exercise on a stationary bicycle. J. Bone Joint Surg. [Am.], 41:123.

67. Huberti, H.H., and Hayes, W.C. (1984): Patellofemoral contact pressure. J. Bone Joint Surg. [Am.], 55:715–724.

68. Hungerford, D.S. (1983): Patellar subluxation and excessive lateral pressure as a cause of fibrillation. In: Pickett, J.C., and Radin, E.L. (eds.): Chondromalacia of the Patella. Baltimore, Williams & Wilkins, pp.24–42.

69. Hungerford, D.S., and Barry, M. (1979): Biomechanics of the patellofemoral joint. Clin. Orthop., 144:9–15.

70. Hungerford, D.S., and Lennox, D.W. (1983): Rehabilitation of the knee in disorders of the patellofemoral joint: Relevant biomechanics. Orthop. Clin. North Am., 14:397–402.

71. Jackson, R.T., and Merrifield, H.H. (1972): Electromyographic assessment of quadriceps muscle group during knee extension with weighted boot. Med. Sci. Sports, 4:116–119.

72. James, S.L. (1979): Chondromalacia of the patella in the adolescent. In: Kennedy, J.C. (ed.): The Injured Adolescent Knee. Baltimore, Williams & Wilkins, pp. 205–251.

73. Johnson, D. (1982): Controlling anterior shear during isokinetic knee extension exercise. J. Orthop. Sports Phys. Ther., 4(1):23–31.

74. Johnson, R.J., Kettelkamp, D.B., and Clack, W., et al. (1974): Factors affecting late results after meniscectomy. J. Bone Joint Surg. [Am.], 56:719–729.

75. Kannus, P., and Jarvinen, M. (1987): Conservatively treated tears of the anterior cruciate ligament. J. Bone Joint Surg. [Am.], 69:1007.

76. Kapandji, I.A. (1970): The Physiology of the Joints, Vol. 2. New York, Churchill Livingstone.

77. Kennedy, J.C., Alexander, I.J., and Hayes, K.C. (1982): Nerve supply of the human knee and its functional importance. Am. J. Sports Med., 10:329–335.

78. Kennedy, J.C., and Fowler, P.M. (1971): Medial and anterior instability of the knee. An anatomical and clinical study using stress machines. J. Bone Joint Surg. [Am.], 53:1257.

79. Kennedy, J.C., Hawkins, R.J., and Willis, R.B. (1977): Strain gauge analysis of knee ligaments. Clin. Orthop., 129:225–229.

80. King, J.B., and Kumar, S.J. (1989): The Stryker knee arthrometer in clinical practice. Am. J. Sports Med., 17:649–650.

81. Knight, K.L., Martin, J.A., and Londeree, B.R. (1979): EMG comparison of quadriceps femoris activity during knee extension and straight leg raises. Am. J. Phys. Med., 58:57–69.

82. Kramer, P.G. (1986): Patella malalignment syndrome: Rationale to reduce excessive lateral pressure. J. Orthop. Sports Phys. Ther., 8:301–309.

83. Krause, W.R., Pope, M.H., and Johnson, R.J., et al. (1976): Mechanical changes in the knee after meniscectomy. J. Bone Joint Surg. [Am.], 58:599–604.

84. Laubenthal, K.N., Smidt, G.I., and Kettelkamp, D.B. (1972): A quantitative analysis of knee motion during activities of daily living. Phys. Ther., 52:34–42.

85. Levy, I.M., Torzilli, P.A., and Warren, R.F. (1982): The effect of medial meniscectomy on anterior-posterior motion of the knee. J. Bone Joint Surg. [Am.], 64:883–888.

86. Lieb, F.J., and Perry, J. (1968): Quadriceps function: An anatomical and mechanical study using amputated limbs. J. Bone Joint Surg. [Am.], 50:1535–1548.

87. Lieb, F.J., and Perry, J. (1971): Quadriceps function—an electromyographic study under isometric conditions. J. Bone Joint Surg. [Am.], 53:749–758.

88. Lipke, J.M., Janecke, C.J., and Nelson, C.L., et al. (1981): The role of incompetence of the anterior cruciate and lateral ligaments in anterolateral and anteromedial instability. J. Bone Joint Surg. [Am.], 63:954–960.

89. Limbird, T.J., Shiavi, R., Frazer, M., and Borra, H. (1988): EMG profiles of knee joint

musculature during walking: Changes induced by anterior cruciate ligament deficiency. J. Orthop. Res., 6:630–638.

90. Lynch, M.A., Henning, C.E., and Glick, K.R. (1983): Knee joint surface changes. Long-term follow-up meniscus tear treatment in stable anterior cruciate ligament reconstructions. Clin. Orthop., 172:148–153.

91. Lysholm, J., Nordin, M., Ekstrand, J., and Gillquist, J. (1984): The effect of a patella brace on performance in a knee extension strength test in patients with patellar pain. Am. J. Sports Med., 12:110–112.

92. MacConnail, M.A. (1953): The movement of bone and joints. 5. The significance of shape. J. Bone Joint Surg., 35:290.

93. Malcom, L.L., Daniel, D.M., Stone, M.L., and Sachs, R. (1985): The measurement of anterior knee laxity after ACL reconstructive surgery. Clin. Orthop., 196:35–41.

94. Mangine, R. (1989): Knee flexion-extension exercise. In: 1989 Advances on the Knee and Shoulder. Cincinnati, Cincinnati Sports Medicine and Deaconess Hospital.

95. Mangine, R. (1990): Post-surgical management following PCL surgery. In: 1990 Advances on the Knee and Shoulder. Cincinnati, Cincinnati Sports Medicine and Deaconess Hospital.

96. Mangine, R. (1990): Rules for management, functional testing, braces. In: 1990 Advances on the Knee and Shoulder. Cincinnati, Cincinnati Sports Medicine and Deaconess Hospital.

97. Mangine, R., and Price, S. (1988): Innovative approaches to surgery and rehabilitation. In: Mangine, R. (ed.): Physical Therapy of the Knee. New York, Churchill Livingstone.

98. Markolf, K.L., Bargar, W.L., Shoemaker, S.C., and Amstutz, H.C. (1981): The role of joint load in knee stability. J. Bone Joint Surg. [Am.], 63:570–585.

99. Markolf, K.L., Graff-Radford, A., and Amstutz, H.C. (1978): In vivo knee stability: A quantitative assessment using instrumented clinical testing apparatus. J. Bone Joint Surg. [Am.], 60:664.

100. Markolf, K.L., Kochan, A., and Amstutz, H. (1984): Measurement of knee stiffness and laxity in patients with documented absence of the anterior cruciate ligament. J. Bone Joint Surg. [Am.], 66:242.

101. Markolf, K.L., Mensch, J.S., and Amstutz, H.C. (1976): Stiffness and laxity of the knee—the contributions of the supporting structures. J. Bone Joint Surg. [Am.], 58, 583.

102. Marshall, J., Girgis, F.G., and Zelko, R.R. (1972): The biceps femoris tendon and its functional significance. J. Bone Joint Surg. [Am.], 54:1444.

103. McConnell, J. (1986): The management of chondromalacia patellae: A long-term solution. Aust. J. Physiother., 32:215–223.

104. McDaniel, W.J., and Dameron, T.B. (1980): Untreated ruptures of the anterior cruciate ligament. J. Bone Joint Surg. [Am.], 62:696–705.

105. McGinty, J.B., Guess, L.F., and Marvin, R.A. (1977): Partial or total meniscectomy. A comparative analysis. J. Bone Joint Surg. [Am.], 59:763–766.

106. McLeod, W.D., and Blackburn, T.A. (1980): Biomechanics of knee rehabilitation with cycling. Am. J. Sports Med., 8:175–180.

107. McQuade, K.J., Sidles, J.A., and Larson, R.V. (1989): Reliability of the Genucom knee laxity system. Clin. Orthop., 245:216–219.

108. Merchant, A.C., Mercer, R.L. Jacobsen, R.H.J., and Cool, C.R. (1974): Roentgenographic analysis of patellofemoral congruence. J. Bone Joint Surg. [Am.], 56:1391–1398.

109. Mishra, D.V., Daniel, D.M., and Stone, M.L. (1989): The use of functional knee braces in the control of pathologic anterior knee laxity. Clin. Orthop., 241:213–220.

110. Morrison, J.B. (1968): Bioengineering analysis of force actions transmitted by the knee joint. Biomed. Eng., 3:164–170.

111. Neuschwander, D.C., Drez, D., Paine, R.M., and Young, J.C. (1990): Comparison of anterior laxity measurements in anterior cruciate-deficient knees with two instrumented testing devices. Orthopaedics, 13:299–302.

112. Nisell, R., and Ekholm, J. (1985): Patellar forces during knee extension. Scand. J. Rehabil. Med., 17:63–74.

113. Nisell, R., Ericson, M.O., Nemeth, G., and Ekholm, J. (1989): Tibiofemoral joint forces during isokinetic knee extension. Am. J. Sports Med., 17:49–54.

114. Nissan, M. (1980): Review of some basic assumptions of knee biomechanics. J. Biomech., 13:175.

115. Noyes, F.R. (1989): Rules for surgical indications in ACL surgery. *In:* 1989 Advances on the Knee and Shoulder. Cincinnati, Cincinnati Sports Medicine and Deaconess Hospital.

116. Noyes, F.R. (1990): ACL allografts surgical results 1981–1990. *In:* 1990 Advances on the Knee and Shoulder. Cincinnati, Cincinnati Sports Medicine and Deaconess Hospital.

117. Noyes, F.R. (1990): Objective functional testing. *In:* Noyes, F.R. (ed.): The Noyes Knee Rating System. Cincinnati, Cincinnati Sports Medicine Research and Education Foundation.

118. Noyes, F.R., Grood, E.S., Butler, D.L., and Malek, M. (1980): Clinical laxity tests and functional stability of the knee: Biomechanical concepts. Clin. Orthop., 146:84.

119. Noyes, F.R., and Mangine, R. (1990): Patella infra syndrome and management of quad shutdown. *In:* 1990 Advances on the Knee and Shoulder. Cincinnati, Cincinnati Sports Medicine and Deaconess Hospital.

120. Noyes, F.R., Mangine, R.E., and Barber, S. (1987): Early knee motion after open and arthroscopic anterior cruciate ligament reconstruction. Am. J. Sports Med., 15:149–160.

121. Noyes, F.R., Matthews, D.S., Mooar, P.A., and Grood, E.S. (1983): The symptomatic anterior cruciate-deficient knee. Part II: The results of rehabilitation, activity modification, and counseling on functional disability. J. Bone Joint Surg. [Am.], 65:163–174.

122. Noyes, F.R., and Sonstegard, D.A. (1973): Biomechanical function of the pes anserinus at the knee and the effect of its transplantation. J. Bone Joint Surg. [Am.], 55:1225–1241.

123. Okamoto, T. (1969): Electromyographic study of the function of muscle rectus femoris. Res. J. Phys. Educ., 12:175–182.

124. Oliver, J.H., and Coughlin, L.P. (1987): Objective knee evaluation using the Genucom Knee Analysis System. Am. J. Sports Med., 15:571–578.

125. Otis, J.C., and Gould, J.D. (1986): The effect of external load on torque production by knee extensors. J. Bone Joint Surg. [Am.], 65:65–70.

126. Palumbo, P.M. (1981): Dynamic patellar brace: A new orthosis in the management of patellofemoral disorder. Am. J. Sports Med., 9:45–49.

127. Paulos, L., Rusche, K., Johnson, C., and Noyes, F. (1980): Patellar malalignment: A treatment rationale. Phys. Ther., 60:1624–1632.

128. Pizali, R.L., Seering, W.P., Nagel, D.A., and Schurman, D.J. (1980): The function of the primary ligaments of the knee in anterior-posterior and medial-lateral motions. J. Biomech., 13:777–784.

129. Pocock, G.S. (1963): Electromyographic study of the quadriceps during resistive exercise. J. Am. Phys. Ther. Assoc., 43:427–434.

130. Reider, B, Marshall, J.L., and Ring, B. (1981): Patellar tracking. Clin. Orthop., 157:143.

131. Reilly, D.T., and Martens, M. (1972): Experimental analysis of the quadriceps muscle force and patellofemoral joint reaction force for various activities. Acta Orthop. Scand., 43:126–137.

132. Reynolds, L., Levin, T.A., Medeiros, J.M., et al. (1983): EMG activity of the vastus medialis oblique and the vastus lateralis in their role in patellar alignment. Am. J. Phys. Med., 62:61–70.

133. Rusche, K., and Mangine, R. (1988): Pathomechanics of injury to the patellofemoral and tibiofemoral joint. *In:* Mangine, R. (ed.): Physical Therapy of the Knee. New York, Churchill Livingstone.

134. Schultz, R.A., Miller, D.C., Kerr, C.S., and Micheli, L. (1984): Mechanoreceptors in human cruciate ligaments. J. Bone Joint Surg. [Am.], 66:1072–1076.

135. Seebacher, J.R., Inglis, A.E., Marshall, J.L., and Warren, R.F. (1982): The structure of the posterolateral aspect of the knee. J. Bone Joint Surg. [Am.], 64:536–541.

136. Sherman, O.H., Markolf, K.L., and Ferkel, R.D. (1987): Measurement of anterior laxity in normal and anterior cruciate-absent knees with two instrumented test devices. Clin. Orthop., 215:156–161.

137. Shields, C.L., Silva, I., Yee, L., and Brewster, C. (1987): Evaluation of residual instability after arthroscopic meniscectomy in anterior cruciate-deficient knees. Am. J. Sports Med., 15:129–131.

138. Shoemaker, S.C., and Markolf, K.L. (1982): In vivo rotatory knee stability. Ligamentous and muscular contributions. J. Bone Joint Surg. [Am.], 64:208.

139. Smidt, G.L. (1973): Biomechanical analysis of knee flexion and extension. J. Biomech., 6:79–92.

140. Soderberg, G.L. (1986): Kinesiology. Application to Pathological Motion. Baltimore, Williams & Wilkins.

141. Soderberg, G.L., and Cook, T.M. (1983): An electromyographic analysis of quadriceps femoris muscle setting and straight leg raising. Phys. Ther., 63:1434–1438.

142. Solomonow, M., Baratta, R., and Zhou, B.H., et al. (1987): The synergistic action of the anterior cruciate ligament and thigh muscles in maintaining joint stability. Am. J. Sports Med., 15:207–213.

143. Sprague, R.B. (1982): Factors related to extension lag at the knee joint. J. Orthop. Sports Phys. Ther., 3:178–181.

144. Steindler, A. (1955): Kinesiology of the Human Body under Normal and Pathological Conditions. Springfield, IL, Charles C Thomas.

145. Stougard, J. (1978): Chondromalacia of the patella. Physical signs in relation to operative findings. Acta Orthop. Scand., 46:685–694.

146. Straub, T., and Hunter, R.E. (1988): Acute anterior cruciate ligament repair. Clin. Orthop., 227:238–250.

147. Tegner, Y., Lysholm, J., Lysholm, M., and Gillquist, J. (1986): A performance test to monitor rehabilitation and evaluate anterior cruciate ligament injuries. Am. J. Sports Med., 14:156–159.

148. Threlkeld, A.J., Horn, T.S., and Wojtowicz, G.M., et al. (1989): Kinematics, ground reaction force, and muscle balance produced by backward running. Orthop. Sports Phys. Ther., 11:56–63.

149. Tiberio, D. (1987): The effect of excessive subtalar joint pronation on patellofemoral mechanics: A theoretical model. J. Orthop. Sports Phys. Ther., 9:160–165.

150. Tibone, J.E., and Antich, T.J. (1988): A biomechanical analysis of anterior cruciate ligament reconstruction with the patellar tendon. Am. J. Sports Med., 16:332–333.

151. Tibone, J.E., Antich, T.J., and Fanton, G.S., et al. (1986): Functional analysis of anterior cruciate ligament instability. Am. J. Sports Med., 14:276–284.

152. Torzilli, P.A., Greenberg, R.L., and Install, J. (1981): An in vivo biomechanical evaluation of anterior-posterior motion of the knee. Roentgenographic measurement technique, stress machine, and stable population. J. Bone Joint Surg. [Am.], 63:960.

153. Vailas, A.C., Tipton, C.M., and Matthes, R.D., et al. (1981): Physical activity and its influence on the repair process of medial collateral ligaments. Conn. Tissue Res., 9:225–231.

154. Walla, D.J., Albright, J.P., and McAuley, E., et al. (1985): Hamstring control and the unstable ligament-deficient knee. Am. J. Sports Med., 13:34–39.

155. Wallace, L. (1988): Foot pronation and knee pain. In: Mangine, R. (ed.): Physical Therapy of the Knee. New York, Churchill Livingstone.

156. Wang, C.J., Walker, P.S., and Wolf, B. (1973): The effects of flexion and rotation on the length patterns of the ligaments of the knee. J. Biomech., 6:587–596.

157. Warren, R.F. (1983): Primary repair of the anterior cruciate ligament. Clin. Orthop., 172:38.

158. Wiberg, G. (1941): Roentgenographic and anatomic studies on the femoropatellar joint. With special reference to chondromalacia patella. Acta Orthop. Scand., 12:319–410.

159. Wroble, R.R. (1990): Practical rules for objective ligament assessment: KT-1000 and other devices. In: 1990 Advances on the Knee and Shoulder. Cincinnati, Cincinnati Sports Medicine and Deaconess Hospital.

160. Wroble, R.R., Van Ginkel, L.A., and Grood, E.S., et al. (1990): In: Noyes, F.R. (ed.): The Noyes Knee Rating System. Cincinnati, Cincinnati Sports Medicine Research and Education Foundation.

161. Yasuda, K., and Sasaki, T. (1985): Exercise after anterior cruciate ligament reconstruction: The force exerted on the tibia by separate isometric contractions of the quadriceps or the hamstrings. Clin. Orthop. Rel. Res., 220:275–283.

CHAPTER 10

◆

Hamstring, Quadriceps, and Groin Rehabilitation

James B. Gallaspy, M.Ed., A.T.,C.

The quadriceps, hamstrings, adductor group, sartorius, and tensor fasciae latae constitute the thigh muscles, and are subject to extreme forces as they propel the body under various degrees of resistance.[16] Muscle strains are the most common injury to the hamstrings and adductors, whereas contusions rank first in the quadriceps area.[3] Strains involving the quadriceps occur less frequently than hamstring strains because of the great strength and size of the quadriceps muscle.[8] Strains involve injury to the muscle, tendon, musculotendinous junction, or tendon-bone attachment. They can result from muscle imbalance, poor flexibility, overstretching, violent muscle contraction against heavy resistance, idiosyncrasy of nerve innervation, or leg length discrepancy.[2-4, 8, 11, 14]

Strains are graded by their degree of severity. Each is determined by the amount of muscle or tendon damage and is labeled as mild, moderate, or severe (or first, second, or third degree). Athletes suffering a muscle strain present with the signs and symptoms shown in Table 10–1.

The goals in treating muscle strains are to reduce pain, restore muscle function, and deter the likelihood of reinjury. Restoration of muscle length is important in reinjury prevention, because a shortened muscle is more susceptible to strains.[1, 4, 15]

Initial treatment of strains and contusions consists of ice, compression, elevation, and rest, along with the use of nonsteroidal anti-inflammatory drugs (NSAIDs) to decrease inflammation.[3, 7, 8] Additional modalities such as pulsed ultrasound to decrease hematoma formation, without the adverse affects of increasing tissue temperature (as with continuous ultrasound in the early stages of healing), and electrical stimulation to decrease pain and inflammation can be beneficial.[18] The use of deep water pool exercises is excellent during the early phases of the rehabilitation program (see Chap. 13). An elastic wrap (e.g., Tubi-Grip*) or other supporting orthosis should be used in the early stages of

---

* Available from SePro, Montgomeryville, PA.

TABLE 10–1   **SIGNS AND SYMPTOMS OF MUSCLE STRAINS**

Severity	Symptoms	Signs
Mild (first degree)	Local pain, mild pain on passive stretch and active contraction of the involved muscle; minor disability	Mild spasm, swelling, ecchymosis; local tenderness; minor loss of function and strength
Moderate (second degree)	Local pain; moderate pain on passive stretch and active contraction of the involved muscle; moderate disability	Moderate spasm, swelling, ecchymosis; local tenderness; impaired muscle function and strength
Severe (third degree)	Severe pain; disability	Severe spasm; swelling, ecchymosis; hematoma; tenderness, loss of muscle function; palpable defect may be present

treatment to provide compression and should be continued throughout the rehabilitation program to support the thigh.

The restoration of muscle length precedes muscle strengthening unless the injured muscle length is equal to or greater than that of the uninjured muscle.[5] The decision to begin restoring muscle length depends on the athlete's response to stretching. If intense or moderate pain develops in the injured muscle before the athlete perceives a stretch, the injured muscle is not ready for stretching.[5] Once the athlete can feel the muscle stretch before or with pain, stretching may begin. In mild to moderate strains, stretching can begin within 2 to 7 days of injury. Muscle strengthening can begin when the muscle can tolerate strengthening with light resistance that is pain-free. The rehabilitation program should include active and passive stretching, proprioceptive neuromuscular facilitation (PNF) stretching and strengthening techniques, and isometric, isotonic, and isokinetic strengthening exercises.

If low-grade muscle spasm is present the use of cryostretching, as described by Knight,[12] may be beneficial. This technique consists of cold applications and the PNF technique of hold–relax, and can be summarized as follows*:

1. Ice—until numb (20 minutes maximum)
2. Exercise
   a. First exercise bout (65 seconds total)
      (1) Static stretch (20 seconds)
      (2) Isometric contraction (5 seconds)
      (3) Static stretch (10 seconds)
      (4) Isometric contraction (5 seconds)
      (5) Static stretch (10 seconds)

---

* From Knight, K.L. (1985): Cryotherapy: Theory, Technique, and Physiology. Chattanooga, Chattanooga Corp., pp. 63 and 66.

    (6) Isometric contraction (5 seconds)
    (7) Static stretch (10 seconds)
  b. Rest (20 seconds)
  c. Second exercise bout (65 seconds, total; same as first exercise
      bout)
3. Renumb with ice application (3 to 5 minutes)
4. Exercise—two bouts and rest as in step 2, above
5. Renumb with 3 to 5 minutes of ice application
6. Exercise—two bouts and rest as in step 2, above

Although similar to cryokinetics in that exercise is performed while the body part is numbed, it is different in regard to the number of exercise sets and the exercise itself.[12] During cryostretch the affected muscle is alternately stretched statically and contracted isometrically.[12]

Knight[12] has also proposed a neuromuscular training session prior to the first initial exercise session; this may be done prior to or immediately after ice application, but before the first exercise bout. The purpose of this session is to help the athlete "get the feel" of contracting the proper muscle group. Sometimes, without this session, the athlete contracts both the agonist and antagonist muscle groups when asked to contract the spasmed muscle. During the neuromuscular training session the clinician moves the appropriate body part in a direction that elongates the muscle in spasm. The athlete is then asked to return the body part to the anatomic position, which requires contracting the affected muscle. This is repeated three to four times, always within a comfortable range of motion.

The stretchings consist of 65-second exercise bouts, with a static stretch interspersed with three isometric contractions of about 5 seconds each, as outlined above. The exercise is begun by stretching the affected muscle until pain or tightness is incurred; the athlete backs off just a little until the pain disappears and holds the limb in that position for 20 seconds. The athlete then begins a slow contraction of the spasmed muscle, building up to a maximal muscle contraction. A second stretch is held for 10 seconds, followed by a second isometric contraction of about 5 seconds. The athlete moves forward again so that tightness or slight pain is felt in the traumatized area and a 10-second stretch is repeated. Finally, the body part is rested in the anatomic position for 20 seconds and the 65-second exercise bout is repeated as outlined above. Second and third renumbing sequences are also carried out.

Once muscle spasm begins to abate (often within 2 or 3 days) a combination of cryostretching and cryokinetics can be implemented, as follows*:

1. Ice for 15 to 20 minutes, or until numb
2. Cryostretch exercise
3. Renumb
4. Cryokinetic exercise
5. Renumb

---

* From Knight, K.L. (1985): Cryotherapy: Theory, Technique, and Physiology. Chattanooga, Chattanooga Corp., pp. 63 and 66.

6. Cryokinetic exercise
7. Renumb
8. Cryokinetic exercise
9. Renumb
10. Cryostretch exercise

Cryokinetic excercise should begin with manual, resisted muscle contractions through a full range of motion and progress to isotonic, isokinetic, and functional drills. The use of cryostretch and cryokinetic techniques should not be overlooked in the early phases of rehabilitation to return muscular strength and endurance to their preinjury level sooner. Progressive resistance exercises can begin when tolerated, with an emphasis on eccentric exercises.[3, 7, 8]

HAMSTRING REHABILITATION

Hamstring strain is one of the most common and frustrating injuries that an athlete can incur; it also can recur frequently.[8, 10, 11, 16, 19] The biceps femoris laterally and the semitendinosus and semimembranosus medially comprise the hamstring muscle group. These muscles function in knee flexion, hip extension, and internal and external rotation of the tibia, and antagonistically resist knee extension.[6, 21] The semimembranosus also dynamically reinforces the posterior and medial knee capsular structures, retracts the medial meniscus posteriorly, and supports the anterior cruciate ligament to prevent anterior tibial translation.[21] The tendons of insertion of the semitendinosus, sartorius, and gracilis form the pes anserinus, which inserts on the proximomedial aspect of the tibia.[21] Cumulatively, the hamstrings support the anterior cruciate ligament to help deter anterior excursion of the tibia on the femur and to assist the medial capsule and medial collateral ligament.[6] The hamstrings perform an important role in walking and assume an extensor action with foot strike.[10, 21] During running, the hamstrings are active longer during the swing and early stance phases of gait.[10]

Hamstring injuries usually occur during sprinting or high-speed exercises (e.g., a sprinter leaving the blocks, the lead leg of a hurdler, a jumper's takeoff leg).[10, 14] Hamstring strains can have various causes: (1) a sudden change from a stabilizing flexor to an active extensor, combined with muscle imbalance between the quadriceps and hamstrings; (2) poor flexibility; (3) faulty posture; and (4) leg length discrepancy. These are all potential mechanisms for hamstring injuries.[2, 3, 8, 11, 14] The short head of the biceps femoris is most often injured; it is believed to contract simultaneously with the quadriceps muscle as a result of an idiosyncrasy in nerve innervation, thus contributing to the high injury rate of this hamstring muscle.[3, 6, 11, 15] It has been suggested that hamstring strength should be 60 to 70% that of the antagonist quadriceps to help prevent hamstring injuries.[1, 3, 14]

The clinician should perform active, passive, and resistive knee flexion and hip extension tests to determine injury severity. Usually, the amount of knee extension the athlete can achieve while prone indicates injury severity. Once severity has been ascertained treatment can proceed as follows:

1. Initial phase
   a. RICE (rest, ice, compression, elevation)
   b. Compressionette for effusion
   c. Modalities
      (1) Pulsed ultrasound
      (2) Electrical stimulation
      (3) Ice, postexercise
   d. Cryostretch and cryokinetics with the following exercises:
      (1) Hamstring setting
      (2) Cocontractions
      (3) Heel slides (seated and supine)
      (4) Active hamstring curls
      (5) Active hip extensions
      (6) Active gluteal extensions
      (7) Single-leg hamstring stretches (nonaggressive)
      (8) Heel slides (seated and supine)
   e. Aquatic therapy
   f. Active range of motion (AROM), as tolerated
2. Intermediate phase
   a. Stationary bike, StairMaster
   b. Modalities
      (1) Continuous ultrasound
      (2) Moist heat
   c. Hamstring stretching
      (1) Single-leg hamstring stretch
      (2) Straddle groin and hamstring stretch
      (3) Side straddle and hamstring stretch
      (4) Supine assisted hamstring stretch
   d. Progressive resistance exercise (PRE) with the following:
      (1) Hamstring curls
      (2) Hip extension
      (3) Gluteal extensions
      (4) Hip adduction and abduction
      (5) Straight leg raises
   e. Proprioceptive exercises
   f. Prophylactic cryotherapy
   g. Increased pool program
   h. PNF patterns
   i. Functional activity progression to begin:
      (1) Forward and backward walking or jogging (use neoprene sleeve for support)
3. Advanced phase
   a. High-speed isokinetic (neutral and prone)
   b. Eccentric hamstring curls
   c. Functional drills
      (1) Jogging/running (forward and backward)
      (2) Jogging/running (uphill, backward)
      (3) Slide Board
      (4) Lateral drills
   d. High-speed surgical tubing exercises in hip flexion, extension, abduction and adduction, knee flexion, mini-squats
   e. Protective wrapping

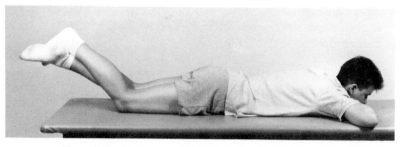

FIGURE 10–1 Use of the prone position and the uninvolved leg to promote hamstring elasticity. This can be used in conjunction with cryotherapy techniques.

In the acute stage emphasis is on reducing inflammation, pain, and spasm through the use of appropriate modalities. Depending on injury severity, about day 2 to 4 postinjury athletes can begin a stretching program within their pain-free range. Initially, the injured extremity can be stretched in the prone position using the uninvolved extremity to control the amount of hamstring stretch achieved (Fig. 10–1). As pain decreases and elasticity increases, a more aggressive stretching program can be implemented (Figs. 10–2 and 10–3). The exercise session should be terminated with cryotherapy and a traction weight used above the knee to facilitate lengthening of the spasmed hamstring muscle (Fig. 10–4).

Later in the rehabilitation process isokinetic equipment can be used at higher speeds because of the high percentage of type II or fast twitch muscle fibers located in the hamstrings.[10, 21] The hamstrings can

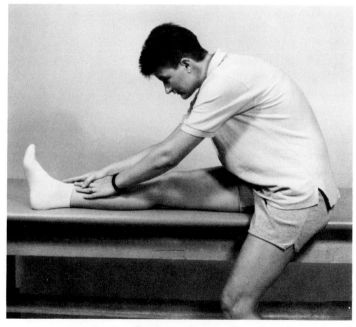

FIGURE 10–2   Single-leg hamstring stretch.

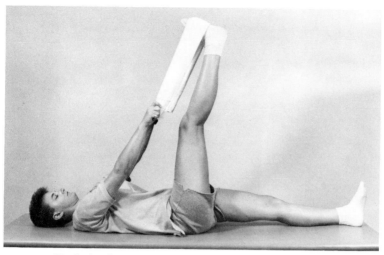

FIGURE 10–3   Single-leg hamstring stretch with towel. The uninvolved leg is kept flat on the table.

be isolated isokinetically to a greater degree by having the athlete lie prone (Fig. 10–5A) or by having the athlete lean forward while in the traditional seated position (Fig. 10–5B). Isokinetic equipment can also be used to obtain data that can aid in determining when the athlete has reached the optimal hamstring-to-quadriceps ratio for deterring injury.

The athlete can also use surgical tubing (Fig. 10–6) for high-speed resistance exercise to fatigue in hip flexion, extension, abduction, adduction, and knee flexion (hamstring curls) or can use the Inertia machine in the above planes, if available.

The athlete may return to unlimited participation, wearing a neoprene sleeve for support and proprioception, when the following criteria are met:

1. Hamstring flexibility is equal bilaterally.
2. Muscular strength, power, endurance, and time to peak torque, as measured by an isokinetic dynamometer, are 85 to 90% of those of the contralateral limb.

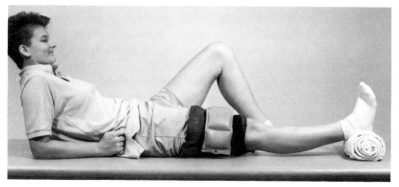

FIGURE 10–4   Use of a traction weight with cryotherapy postexercise to facilitate the return of hamstring length.

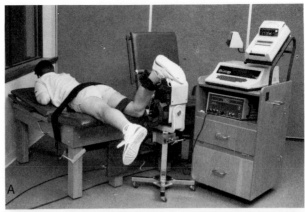

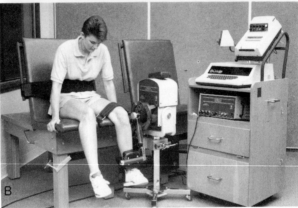

FIGURE 10–5 The athlete can accentuate hamstring muscle activity by lying prone (*A*), or leaning forward while in the traditional position (*B*).

3. Hamstring strength is 60 to 70% that of the quadriceps.
4. No symptoms are noted with functional activities.

QUADRICEPS REHABILITATION

Quadriceps injuries are a common occurrence in sports. The quadriceps muscle is subject to both strains and contusions, with the latter having a higher incidence.[2, 3] The quadriceps is composed of the rectus femoris, vastus medialis, vastus lateralis, and vastus intermedius muscles. Its static role is to prevent knee buckling while standing, and its dynamic function is to extend the knee forcefully, as in running or jumping exercises. The rectus femoris is a biarticular muscle, functioning in knee extension and hip flexion. The tensor fasciae latae and the sartorius are also considered part of the anterior thigh.

Contusions

The quadriceps is constantly exposed to direct contact in various vigorous sports such as football, soccer, and basketball.[2, 3] A quadriceps

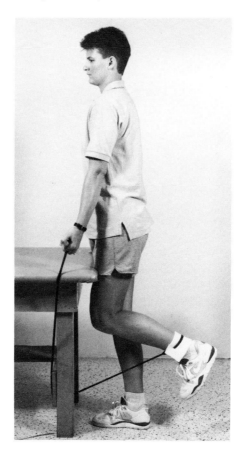

FIGURE 10-6 Hamstring curls with surgical tubing can be performed at varying rates of speed to fatigue to help increase muscle endurance.

contusion can vary from a mild bruise to a large, deep hematoma that may take months to heal.[2] The mechanism of injury is usually a direct blow to the relaxed thigh, compressing the muscle against the femur. The anterior or anterolateral aspect of the quadriceps is most often involved, because the medial aspect is protected by the athlete's contralateral leg.[14, 16, 19] A quadriceps contusion displays standard signs and symptoms of other muscle injuries, but the symptoms are less localized than those in a more subcutaneous area.[16] The athlete may exhibit local pain, stiffness, pain on passive stretching, disability that varies with the site and extent of injury, tenderness, ecchymosis, hematoma formation, and loss of active extension.[2-4, 14, 16, 19] Injury severity can usually be determined by the degree of limitation of active knee flexion.

Moderate to severe quadriceps contusions should be treated nonaggressively to prevent the development of myositis ossificans, and exercise is progressed according to the athlete's tolerance. Some authors[3, 8] have advocated the use of cryotherapy with simultaneous prolonged knee flexion at 20-minute intervals to help deter the transitory loss of knee flexion that usually accompanies a quadriceps contusion. The degree of active knee flexion is determined by the athlete's pain tolerance. Such modalities as massage, heat, and forced stretching of the muscle during the acute phase are contraindicated.[2, 16, 19, 20]

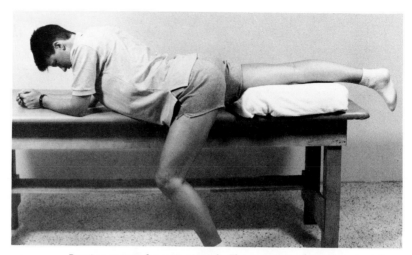

FIGURE 10–7   Passive rectus femoris stretch. The amount of passive stretch can be modified by the amount of the hip extension, which is based on the athlete's tolerance to stretch. It can be used in conjunction with cryotherapy techniques.

Quadriceps setting can be performed and electrical muscle stimulation can be used to help deter muscle atrophy and to increase quadriceps re-education if they cause no pain.[3, 19] Also, passive range-of-motion devices can be useful in the early stages of injury. Figures 10–7 to 10–14 depict stretching exercises that can be used at various stages of the healing process to increase the elasticity of the quadriceps muscle.

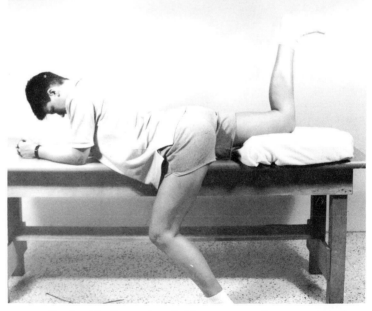

FIGURE 10–8   Passive hip flexor stretch. The amount of passive stretch can be modified by the amount of hip extension, which is based on the athlete's tolerance to stretch. It can be used in conjunction with cryotherapy techniques.

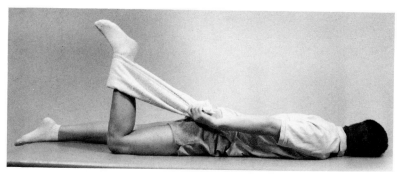

FIGURE 10–9 Single-leg quadriceps stretch. A towel is used to stretch the quadriceps muscle gradually. In the later stages of rehabilitation the PNF technique of contract—relax can be used to facilitate the range of motion.

The following protocol outlines the progression of rehabilitation following quadriceps injury:

1. Initial phase
    a. RICE
    b. Modalities
        (1) Pulsed ultrasound
        (2) Electrical muscle stimulation
        (3) Ice postexercise
    c. Compressionette for effusion
    d. AROM, as tolerated

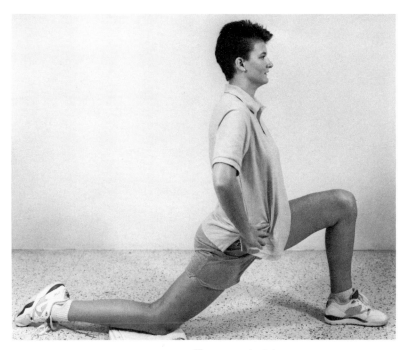

FIGURE 10–10 Iliopsoas stretch.

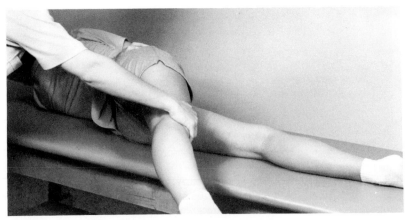

FIGURE 10–11   Manual iliopsoas stretch. This can later be adapted into the PNF technique of contract—relax, or other PNF patterns.

   e. Cryostretch and cryokinetics with the following exercises:
      (1) Active straight leg raises
      (2) Active terminal knee extensions
      (3) Active hip flexion
      (4) Heel slides (seated and supine)
      (5) Quadriceps sets
      (6) Cocontractions
   f. Aquatic therapy
2. Intermediate phase
   a. Stationary cycling
   b. Modalities

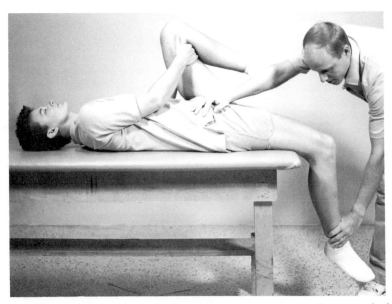

FIGURE 10–12   Manual rectus femoris stretch. This can be used to stretch the rectus femoris muscle and can also be used as a test to determine its length.

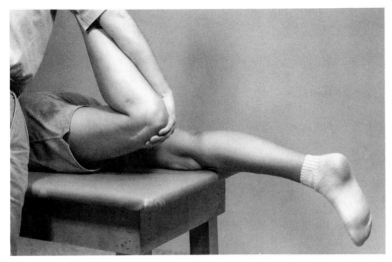

FIGURE 10–13 Manual hip flexor stretch. This can be adapted into the PNF contract–relax technique to increase the range of motion.

FIGURE 10–14 Single-leg standing quadriceps stretch. The athlete can also pull the hip into extension to accentuate the stretch.

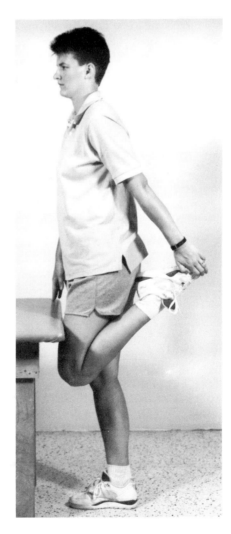

(1) Continuous ultrasound
(2) Moist heat
c. Increase in aquatic program
d. Quadriceps stretching
e. Concentric 90° to 45° knee extensions
f. PNF patterns
g. Proprioception exercises
h. PRE with exercises initiated in initial phase
i. Active assisted flexion
j Closed-chain exercises:
(1) Terminal knee extensions with Thera-Band
(2) Lateral step-ups
3. Advanced phase
a. High-speed isokinetic exercises (neutral and supine)
b. Functional drills
c. Eccentric 90° to 0° knee extensions
d. High-speed surgical tubing in hip flexion, extension, abduction, adduction, and minisquats
e. Protective wrapping

In contusions, if the hematoma is not readily resolved, the clinician should suspect the development of myositis ossificans. Third-degree injuries need protective rest—that is, cryotherapy, isometric exercise, and gentle active range of motion, as tolerated, before aggressive rehabilitation can begin. With severe thigh contusions, the use of massage, heat, and forced stretching or running is contraindicated in the early phases of healing.

The athlete may return to unlimited participation when the following criteria are met:

1. Quadriceps flexibility is equal bilaterally.
2. Muscular strength, power, endurance, and time to peak torque, as measured by an isokinetic dynamometer, are 85% to 90% of those of the contralateral limb.
3. Minimal or no tenderness is present in the quadriceps.
4. No symptoms are noted with functional activities at full speed.
5. The traumatized area should be protected. Use of a pad made of Orthoplast,* with a raised section over the injured area, is recommended.

Strains

Quadriceps strains usually involve the rectus femoris muscle.[8, 19] Strains to this area occur less frequently than hamstring strains because of the great strength, size, and flexibility of the quadriceps muscle group.[8] The mechanism of injury is usually a result of insufficient warm-up, poor stretching, tight quadriceps, bilateral quadriceps imbalance, or a short leg.[19] Signs and symptoms vary with injury severity but are characterized by pain down the entire length of the rectus femoris and tender-

---

* Available from Johnson & Johnson, New Brunswick, NJ.

ness in the area of the strain. The athlete exhibits pain on active quadriceps contraction and passive stretching. If the muscle is ruptured swelling may initially mask a muscle defect, but a permanent bulge in the thigh is present as the swelling subsides.[8, 19]

Rehabilitation for a quadriceps strain is similar to that for strains of other muscles. The severity of injury determines when active rehabilitation may begin, and all exercises should be performed within a pain-free range of motion. Static stretching is begun as tolerated (Figs. 10–7 to 10–9) along with passive range-of-motion exercises. Progression should be made to active range-of-motion and resistive exercises with emphasis on knee extension and hip flexion.

In the late phases of rehabilitation isokinetic equipment can be used, at higher speeds, with the athlete in the supine position to accentuate the quadriceps muscle (Fig. 10–15A) or in the traditional seated position (Fig. 10–15B).

Additionally, surgical tubing can be used for exercising in the planes of hip flexion, extension, adduction, abduction, and knee extension at high contractile speeds to fatigue for endurance (Fig. 10–16).

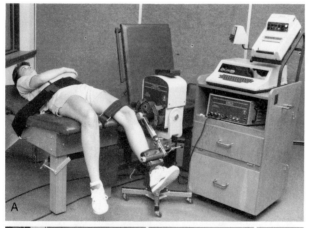

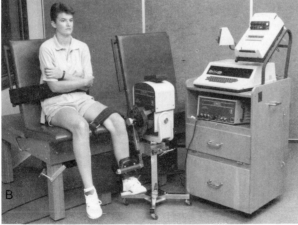

FIGURE 10–15 The athlete can accentuate quadriceps activity by lying supine (A) and by exercising in the traditional seated position (B).

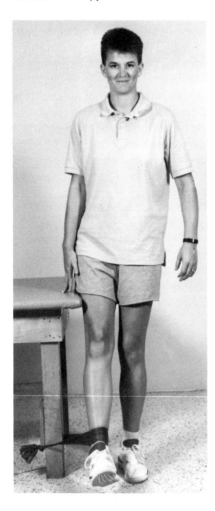

FIGURE 10–16 Hip flexion–extension using Thera-Band at varying speeds. The knee is straight and the athlete performs hip flexion–extension at varying rates of speed. In the final stages of rehabilitation the athlete performs this exercise as fast as possible to fatigue, but not at the expense of good mechanics.

The quadriceps rehabilitation protocol outlined above can be used as a guideline for quadriceps strains. Although designed for quadriceps contusions, the program can be accelerated to accommodate quadriceps strains, because usually this injury can be rehabilitated more quickly than a quadriceps contusion.

The athlete may return to unlimited participation, wearing a neoprene sleeve for support and proprioception, when the following criteria are met:

1. Muscular strength, power, endurance, and time to peak torque, as measured by an isokinetic dynamometer, are 85 to 90% of those of the contralateral limb.
2. Quadriceps flexibility is equal bilaterally.
3. No symptoms are noted with functional activities at full speed.

GROIN REHABILITATION

The groin is the depressed region that lies between the thigh and abdominal area. The muscles of this region include the adductor group, rectus femoris, and iliopsoas. The adductor group is composed of the adductor longus, adductor brevis, adductor magnus, pectineus, and gracilis. These muscles adduct the thigh and flex and externally and internally rotate the hip.[21] The adductors function dynamically to adduct the thigh and serve as hip flexors and extensors, depending on their anterior or posterior relationship to the hips' flexion–extension axis. During walking and running, contraction of the adductors contributes to the forward and backward swing motion of the leg. The static effect of these muscles is to stabilize the trunk by constantly adjusting the position of the pelvis. Twisting the pelvis is prevented by the adduction and internal-external rotating components of the adductor group.[21]

Groin strains can result from any forced adduction, overextension, twisting, running, or jumping with external rotation.[2, 3, 8, 16, 17] This stretching usually occurs when the muscular unit is overloaded during the eccentric phase of muscular contraction.[9, 13, 22] The athlete complains of a sudden, sharp pain located along the ischiopubic ramus, lesser trochanter, or the adductor's musculotendinous junction.[7, 16] The athlete complains of pain on passive abduction and resistive adduction. The pain may begin at the origin of the traumatized muscle and radiate along the medial aspect of the thigh into the rectus abdominis area.[20]

The injury should be assessed by administering active, passive, and resistive tests in hip flexion, extension, adduction, abduction, and internal and external rotation, and in knee extension.[3] The use of a hip spica with the hip internally rotated may help to alleviate some of the pain and discomfort experienced with activities of daily living and during the rehabilitation program (Fig. 10–17). Lateral movements and abduction with external rotation should be avoided until symptoms subside. The following protocol outlines a rehabilitation program for groin strains.

1. Initial phase
   a. RICE
   b. Modalities

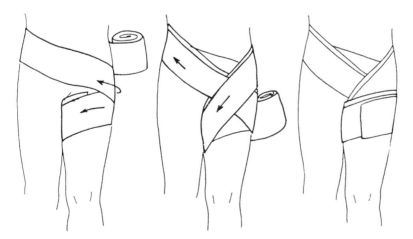

FIGURE 10–17   Hip spica. With the leg internally rotated to relax the adductor muscles, a 6-inch extra-long elastic bandage is used to help support the groin area. (From Arnheim, D. (1989): Modern Principles of Athletic Training, 7th ed. St. Louis, C.V. Mosby, p. 341.)

    (1) Pulsed ultrasound
    (2) Electrical stimulation
    (3) Ice postexercise
  c. Cryostretch and cryokinetics with the following exercises:
    (1) Active hip abduction
    (2) Active straight leg raise
    (3) Active hip flexion
    (4) Isometric hip adduction
  d. Hip active range of motion
  e. Aquatic therapy
  f. Stationary cycling
2. Intermediate phase
  a. Modalities
    (1) Continuous ultrasound
    (2) Moist heat
  b. Proprioceptive exercises
  c. PRE with active exercises initiated in initial phase
  d. Active adduction
  e. Groin stretching
    (1) Straddle groin and hamstring stretch
    (2) Side straddle groin and hamstring stretch
    (3) Groin stretch
    (4) Wall groin stretch
  f. Increase of aquatic program
  g. Prophylactic cryotherapy
  h. PNF patterns
  i. Stationary cycling
3. Advanced phase
  a. Concentric and eccentric hip abduction, adduction
  b. High-speed exercises using surgical tubing in hip abduction, adduction, flexion, extension
  c. Functional drills
    (1) Running
    (2) Carioca
    (3) Cutting
    (4) Lateral movements
    (5) Slide Board, if available
  d. Protective wrapping—hip spica

The athlete may return to unlimited participation when the following criteria are met:

1. Muscular strength is equal bilaterally, as determined by manual muscle testing.
2. Full, pain-free hip range of motion is present.
3. The athlete can perform the sports-specific functional activities required, asymptomatically, at full speed.

Most injuries to the thigh region usually result in trauma to the soft tissue, particularly muscle. Although fractures can occur to this area, they are not as prevalent as muscle strains and contusions. Strains are most often produced indirectly though poor muscle flexibility, abnormal agonist- or antagonist-to-strength ratio, or eccentric muscle contraction. Contusions are generally incurred more in contact sports and result from a direct blow to the soft tissue.

Soft tissue injuries of the thigh are treated initially with emphasis on decreasing pain, spasm, and inflammation of the traumatized region. Early range-of-motion and stretching exercises can be instituted as tolerated, except for quadriceps contusions, where the potential for myositis ossificans exists. Early aggressive motion, stretching, heat, and massage to quadriceps contusions are contraindicated.

As muscle elasticity is restored and inflammation subsides, the athlete can begin active PRE exercises, as tolerated. Later stages of rehabilitation should concentrate on high functional speed and eccentric exercise. Isokinetic machines can be used at higher speeds, and surgical tubing can be used for exercises at varying speeds to aid in reconditioning the type II muscle fibers. The athlete should also perform sports-specific functional activities at 50%, 75%, and then full speed. This allows the clinician to judge how the athlete performs in the sport. The athlete should be able to perform these functional activities asymptomatically before returning to participation. Once the athlete returns to competition, the area should be supported or protected with an appropriate orthosis. Most muscular strains to this region can be prevented through an adequate stretching and warm-up program before participation.

APPLICATION

Hamstring and Groin Exercises

1. Hamstring Stretch.   The athlete lies on a table and an object is placed under the foot to apply a gentle stretch of the hamstring. The quadriceps should be relaxed.

2. Straddle Groin and Hamstring Stretch.   The athlete sits on the floor with the legs spread and the back straight (Fig. 10–18). The athlete then leans forward until a stretch is felt, holds for 10 seconds, relaxes, and repeats the exercise.

3. Side Straddle Groin and Hamstring Stretch.   The athlete sits on the floor with the legs spread and the back straight (Fig. 10–19). The athlete leans to the left and tries to grasp as far down the leg as possible, holding 10 seconds, and then relaxing and repeating on the opposite side.

4. Supine Assisted Hamstring Stretch.   With the help of a partner or towel, the athlete raises the leg until a stretch is felt in the hamstring, holds for 10 seconds, relaxes, and then repeats the exercise (see Fig. 10–3). PNF contract–relax can also be performed easily in this position.

5. Single Hamstring Stretch.   The athlete straightens the supported leg with the other leg off to the side (Fig. 10–20) and slowly leans forward until a stretch is felt in the back of the hamstring. This is held for 10 seconds and then the athlete relaxes and repeats the exercise. The stretch is performed with the chin up and the back straight, and without bouncing.

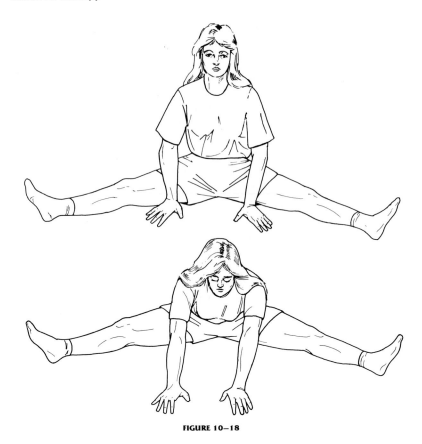

FIGURE 10—18

6. Groin Stretch. In the sitting position, with the back straight, the athlete bends the knees, places the feet together, and pulls the feet toward the groin (Fig. 10–21). The elbows are placed on the knees and pressed down. This is held for 10 seconds followed by the athlete's relaxing and repeating the exercise.

7. Wall Groin Stretch. The athlete lies on the back with the buttocks and legs against the wall. The legs are spread enough so that a stretch is

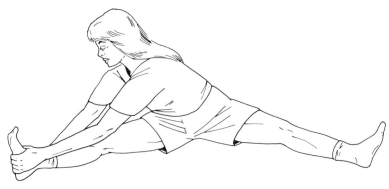

FIGURE 10—19

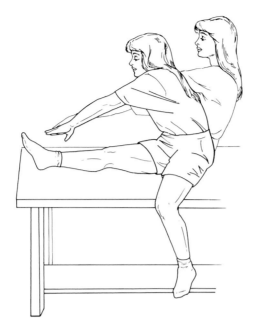

FIGURE 10–20

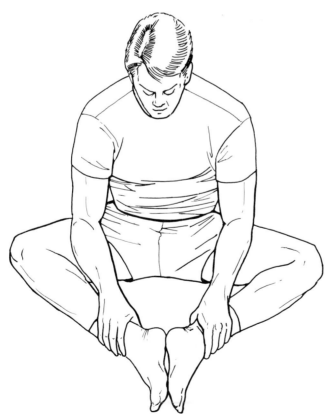

FIGURE 10–21

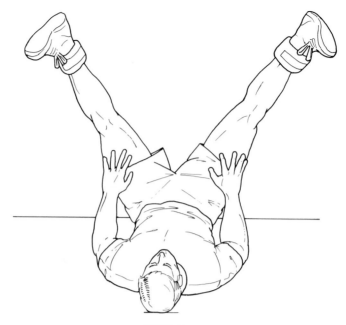

FIGURE 10—22

felt in the groin region (Fig. 10—22). A small amount of weight can be used around the ankles to increase the stretch and allow it to be more passive. This is held for 10 seconds. The athlete then relaxes and repeats the exercise.

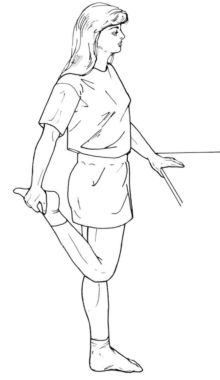

FIGURE 10—23

Quadriceps Exercise

8. Standing Quadriceps Stretch.   The athlete holds on with one arm for balance, grasps the foot of the injured extremity with the hand, and brings the heel to the buttocks (Fig. 10–23). While standing up straight, the athlete slowly extends the leg, maintaining the hold on the foot, and holds for 10 seconds. A stretch should be felt in the quadriceps. The athlete then relaxes and repeats the exercise.

References

1. Agre, J.C. (1985): Hamstring injuries: Proposed etiological factors, prevention, and treatment. Sports Med., 2:21–33.
2. American Academy of Orthopaedic Surgeons (1984): Athletic Training and Sports Medicine. Chicago, American Academy of Orthopaedic Surgeons.
3. Arnheim, D.H. (1989): Modern Principles of Athletic Training, 7th ed. St. Louis, C.V. Mosby, pp. 621–626, 637–639.
4. Booher, J.M., and Thibodeau, G.A. (1989): Athletic Injury Assessment, 2nd ed. St. Louis, C.V. Mosby, pp. 170–172.
5. Cibulka, M.T. (1989): Rehabilitation of the pelvis, hip, and thigh. Clin. Sports Med., 8:777–803.
6. Distefano, V. (1978): Functional anatomy and biomechanics of the knee. Athletic Training, 13(3):113–118.
7. Estwanik, J.J., Sloane, B., and Rosenberg, M.A. (1990): Groin strain and other possible causes of groin pain. Physician Sports Med., 18(2):54–65.
8. Fahey, T.D. (1986): Athletic Training: Principles and Practice. Palo Alto, CA, Mayfield, pp. 77, 340–343.
9. Gardner, L. (1977): Hip abductors and adductors in rehabilitation. Physician Sports Med., 5(11):103–104.
10. Garrett, W.E., Califf, J.C., and Gassett, F.H. (1984): Histochemical correlates of hamstring injuries. Am. J. Sports Med., 12(2):98–103.
11. Heiser, T.M., Weber, J., Sullivan, G., et al. (1984): Prophylaxis and management of hamstring muscle injuries in intercollegiate football. Am. J. Sports Med., 12(5):368–370.
12. Knight, K.L. (1985): Cryotherapy: Theory, Technique, and Physiology. Chattanooga, Chattanooga Corp., pp. 63–66.
13. Knight, K.L. (1985): Strengthening hip abductors and adductors. Physician Sports Med., 13(7):161.
14. Kuland, D.N. (1982): The Injured Athlete. Philadelphia, J.B. Lippincott, pp. 356–358.
15. Liemohn, W. (1978): Factors related to hamstring strains. J. Sports Med. Phys. Fitness, 18:71–75.
16. O'Donoghue, D.H. (1984): Treatment of Injuries to Athletes, 4th ed. Philadelphia, W.B. Saunders, pp. 433–442.
17. Peterson, L., and Renstrom, P. (1986): Sports Injuries. Chicago, Year Book Medical Publishers, pp. 440–443.
18. Prentice, W.E. (1990): Therapeutic Modalities in Sports Medicine. St. Louis, C.V. Mosby, pp. 24, 132.
19. Roy, S., and Irvin, R. (1983): Sports Medicine: Prevention, Evaluation, Management, and Rehabilitation. Englewood Cliffs, NJ, Prentice-Hall, pp. 299–305
20. Torg, J.S., Vegso, J.J., and Torg, E. (1987): Rehabilitation of Athletic Injuries. Chicago, Year Book Medical Publishers, pp. 97–101, 110–115.
21. Weineck, J. (1986): Functional Anatomy in Sports. Chicago, Year Book Medical Publishers, pp. 102–115.
22. Zarins, B., and Ciullo, J.V. (1983): Acute muscle and tendon injuries in athletes. Clin. Sports Med., 2(1):167–182.

CHAPTER 11

◆

Shoulder Rehabilitation

Gary L. Harrelson, M.S., A.T.,C.

Most shoulder injuries are a result of throwing or a blow to the shoulder region. The volatile action of throwing results in high stresses applied to the shoulder and elbow. Most of these injuries are a result of a chronic overuse mechanism. Tullos and King[80] have reported that 50% of all baseball players experience sufficient shoulder or elbow joint symptoms that keep them from throwing for varying periods of time in their careers. The synchronous kinematics of throwing can be influenced by glenohumeral and scapulothoracic motions, connective tissue flexibility, and muscle balance and symmetry. The shoulder region is further predisposed to injury, because its tremendous mobility comes at the price of poor glenohumeral stability.

JOINT ARTHROLOGY

The shoulder region is composed of three synovial joints, the glenohumeral, acromioclavicular, and sternoclavicular, and two physiologic joints, the scapulothoracic joint and the coracoacromial arch. These joints, along with the ligaments (Fig. 11–1), musculotendinous cuff, and major muscle movers in the area, must work as one entity to produce the various ranges of motion possible in the shoulder joint. Dysfunction of one of these joints and/or structures can result in injury.

Sternoclavicular Joint

The sternoclavicular joint has a joint capsule, three major ligaments, and a joint disc. The joint is stabilized anteriorly and posteriorly by the sternoclavicular ligament, which serves to check anterior and posterior movements of the clavicle head. The costoclavicular ligament functions as the principal stabilizer of the sternoclavicular joint, acting as the shoulder axis for elevation–depression and protraction–retraction,[66] serving to stabilize the clavicle against the pull of the sternocleidomas-

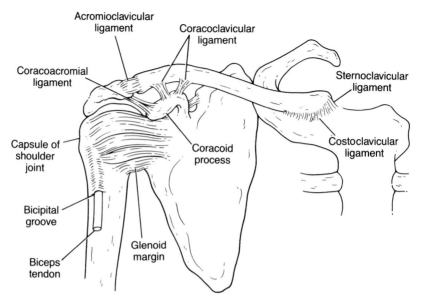

FIGURE 11–1   Ligamentous structures of the shoulder girdle. (From O'Donaghue, D.H. (1984): Treatment of Injuries to Athletes, 4th ed. Philadelphia, W.B. Saunders, p. 119.)

toid muscle, and checking proximal elevation of the clavicle.[16] The proximal end of the clavicle is separated from the manubrium by an intra-articular meniscus, which helps absorb forces transmitted along the clavicle from its lateral end and aids in checking the tendency of the clavicle to dislocate medially on the manubrium.[66] This tendency toward dislocation is a result of the incongruency of the articular surfaces.

Acromioclavicular Joint

The acromioclavicular joint consists of two major ligaments and a joint meniscus, which is sometimes absent. Joint integrity is maintained by surrounding ligaments rather than by the bony configuration. The primary functions of the acromioclavicular joint are maintaining the relationship between the clavicle and scapula in the early stages of upper limb elevation and allowing the scapula additional range of rotation on the thorax in the later stages of limb elevation.[66]

Integrity of the acromioclavicular joint is maintained by the inferior and superior acromioclavicular ligaments. The coracoclavicular ligament is the primary acromioclavicular joint stabilizer, however, and is divided into a lateral portion, the trapezoid, and a medial portion, the conoid. A fall on an outstretched arm tends to translate the scapula medially, and the small acromioclavicular joint alone cannot prevent scapular motion without resulting in joint dislocation. As the scapula and its coracoid process attempt to move medially, the trapezoid ligament tightens, transferring the force of impact to the clavicle and, ultimately, to the strong sternoclavicular joint.[66] The coracoclavicular ligament is also responsible for producing the longitudinal rotation of the clavicle necessary for full range of motion in elevation of the upper extremity.

Glenohumeral Joint

The glenohumeral joint is more mobile and less stable than the acetabulofemoral joint. It is composed of the large head of the humerus and the shallow glenoid fossa. The glenohumeral joint capsule has a volume twice as great as that of the humeral head,[12] which allows for slightly more than 1 inch of humeral head distraction from the glenoid fossa.[16, 25] The joint capsule is relatively thin and rather lax, contributing to the joint's mobility and lack of stability. Ligament restraints can be considered no more than a mere thickening of the joint capsule. Because of the joint's intrinsic weaknesses, it is susceptible to both degenerative changes and derangement.

Some joint stability is provided by a fibrocartilaginous rim, called the glenoid labrum, which surrounds the glenoid fossa. The labrum blends posteriorly with the tendon of the long head of the biceps brachii and anteriorly with the inferior glenohumeral ligament. It also enhances the glenoid fossa's total available articular surface. Anterior glenohumeral stability is provided by the glenohumeral ligament, which is a redundancy in the anterior joint capsule. With the arm dependent at the side, the loose capsule is taut superiorly and slack inferiorly.[66]

The glenohumeral ligament is composed of three portions, superior, middle, and inferior parts, which form a Z on the anterior capsule; each portion becomes taut in and provides a check to certain motions of the humerus, with all portions becoming taut on external rotation.[66] The middle and inferior aspects are particularly important in deterring humeral head subluxation in abduction and external rotation.[81] The musculotendinous cuff also helps reinforce the joint capsule.[47, 76] Further anterior support is supplied by the subscapularis, especially when the arm is positioned next to the body.[81] Posterior stabilization is provided by the teres minor and infraspinatus, with the supraspinatus assisting in additional superior support.[76] Inferiorly there are no muscular or capsular ligament restraints, making it the weakest area.

The glenohumeral joint is capable of three combined movements: flexion–extension, abduction–adduction, and internal–external rotation. With the arm at the side, internal and external rotation may be limited to as little as 50°; abducting the humerus to 90° frees the arc of rotation to 120°.[78] Restricted motion of the shoulder is a result of bony restraints based on the rotation of the limb. For example, if the humerus is maintained in internal rotation, it cannot abduct beyond 90° because of impingement of the greater tubercle on the acromion. With the humerus in full external rotation, however, the greater tubercle passes behind the acromion process and abduction can continue. With bony limitations eliminated by external rotation of the humerus, the checks of motion become capsular and muscular. Glenohumeral joint elevation depends on the state of rotation of the bones.

Finally, the subacromion and subdeltoid bursae are located in the glenohumeral joint. These bursae separate the supraspinatus tendon and humeral head below from the acromioclavicular joint and deltoid muscle above.[66] The bursa allows the tendons of the supraspinatus and long head of the biceps brachii to glide smoothly under the acromion process.

Scapulothoracic Joint

The scapulothoracic joint is not a true anatomic joint because it has none of the usual joint characteristics, such as a joint capsule. It is a free-floating physiologic joint, however, without any ligamentous restraints, except where it pivots about the acromioclavicular joint.[23] According to Steindler,[78] the primary force holding the scapula to the thorax is atmospheric pressure. The ultimate function of scapular motion is to orient the glenoid fossa for optimal contact with the maneuvering arm and to provide a stable base for the controlled rolling and sliding of the humeral head's articular surface.[66]

Coracoacromial Arch

The coracoacromial arch, or subacromial space, is also considered a physiologic joint.[48] It provides protection against direct trauma to the subacromial structures and prevents the humeral head from dislocating superiorly. It is bordered by the acromion process superiorly, coracoid process anteromedially, acromioclavicular joint superiorly, and the rotator cuff and greater tuberosity of the humeral head inferiorly.[23] The coracohumeral ligament, which serves as a "roof" over the greater tubercle of the humerus, rotator cuff tendons, portions of the biceps tendon, and subdeltoid bursa, further decreases the available space. Approximately a 1-cm space separates the humeral head and acromion undersurface; this space can decrease further in the presence of inflamed or swollen soft tissues. Soft tissue structures, such as the supraspinatus and infraspinatus tendons, lying between the two unyielding joint borders, are at risk for impingement or compressive injuries in the presence of abnormal glenohumeral joint mechanics or trauma.

Shoulder Elevation

Most glenohumeral motion occurs around the scapular plane, which is approximately 30 to 45° anterior to the frontal plane.[68] Codman[18] first reported that abduction of the humerus to 180° overhead requires that the clavicle, scapula, and humerus move through essentially their full range of motion in a specific pattern of interaction. When internally rotated the humerus can abduct on the scapula 90° before the greater tubercle butts up against the acromion. If the humerus is fully rotated externally, however, the greater tubercle and accompanying cuff tendons "clear" the acromion, coracoacromion ligament, and/or superior edge of the glenoid fossa,[47, 52, 75] and another 30° of abduction can be

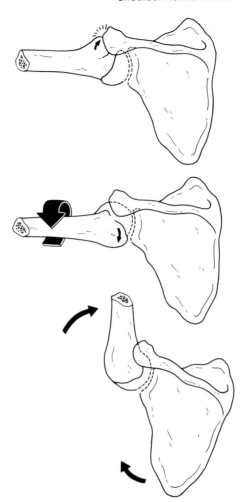

FIGURE 11–2 Clearing of the greater tubercle from under the acromion to gain full abduction at the glenohumeral joint. (From Gould, J.A. (1990): Orthopaedic and Sports Physical Therapy, 2nd ed. St. Louis, C.V. Mosby, p. 488.)

obtained (Fig. 11–2). Thus, the glenohumeral joint contributes 90 to 120° to shoulder abduction.[16, 40, 52] The remaining 60° are supplied by scapular elevation. This combined motion between the scapula and humerus is known as scapulohumeral rhythm. During the first 30° of glenohumeral abduction the contribution of scapular elevation is negligible and is not coordinated with the movement of the humerus.[40, 52] This is referred to as the setting phase, during which the scapula is seeking a position of stability in relationship to the humerus.[40] The purpose of scapular rotation is twofold:[66] (1) to achieve a ratio of motion for maintaining the glenoid fossa in an optimal position to receive the head of the humerus, thus increasing range of motion; and (2) to ensure that the accompanying motion of the scapula permits muscles acting on the humerus to maintain a satisfactory length–tension relationship. Following the initial 30° of humeral elevation, scapular motion becomes better coordinated. Toward the end range of humeral elevation, however, the scapula provides more of the motion and the humerus less.[39, 47] It is generally agreed that, in gross terms, every 1° of scapular motion is accompanied by 2° of humeral elevation.

Scapulohumeral rhythm is considered to be a ratio of 1 : 2.[40] If scapular movement is prevented, only 120° of passive abduction and 90° of active motion are possible.[52]

Clavicular motion at both the acromioclavicular and sternoclavicular joints is essential for full shoulder abduction. Inman and Saunders[39] have demonstrated that, for full abduction of the arm to occur, the clavicle must rotate 50° posteriorly. Surgical pinning of the clavicle to the coracoid process, which has been performed in some complete acromioclavicular ligament tears, dramatically limits shoulder abduction.

Glenohumeral elevation in abduction is the primary function of the deltoid and supraspinatus muscles. The contribution of the deltoid and supraspinatus to shoulder abduction has been investigated extensively. It was commonly assumed that abduction of the arm is initiated by the supraspinatus and continued by the deltoid.[34] Using selective nerve blocks to deactivate the deltoid and supraspinatus muscles, respectively, studies have shown that complete abduction still occurs with a 50% loss in power when one or the other is deactivated.[20, 21] Simultaneous nerve blocks of both these muscles result in the inability to raise the arm.[20] Thus, each muscle can elevate the arm independently, but with a resultant loss of about 50% of normal power.[6]

Additionally, the other three rotator cuff muscles—teres minor,

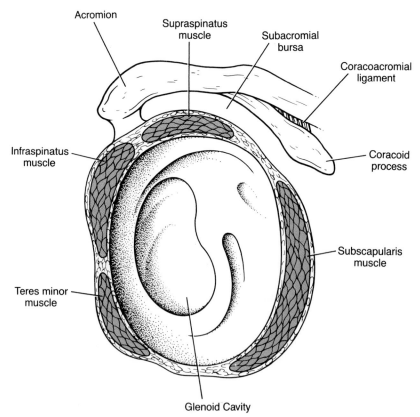

FIGURE 11–3   Anatomic view of the glenoid cavity with its surrounding structures. (From Hill, J.A. (1988): Rotator cuff injuries. Sports Med. Update, 3:5.)

infraspinatus, and subscapularis—are active to some degree throughout the abduction range of motion.[40] These three cuff muscles work as a functional unit to depress the humeral head by an inferior pull to counteract the superior pull of the deltoid.[40, 47]

Musculotendinous Cuff

The supraspinatus, infraspinatus, teres minor, and subscapularis muscles comprise the musculotendinous or rotator cuff (Fig. 11–3). Collectively, each tendon blends with and reinforces the glenohumeral capsule and all contribute significantly to the dynamic stability of the glenohumeral joint.[66] The rotator cuff muscles could be considered the fine tuners of the glenohumeral joint and shoulder girdle, whereas the latissimus dorsi, deltoid, and pectoralis muscles are the powerful rotators and abductors.[37] All the rotator cuff muscles contribute to some degree to glenohumeral abduction; the supraspinatus and the deltoid are the primary abductors. The supraspinatus also functions to compress the glenohumeral joint and acts as a vertical steerer for the humeral head.[24, 75] The supraspinatus can also stabilize the glenohumeral joint with the assistance of gravity.[53]

The infraspinatus, teres minor, and subscapularis muscles also aid in abduction. The infraspinatus is considered the next most active rotator cuff muscle, after the supraspinatus.[39, 43, 45] Selective nerve blocks have shown that the supraspinatus and infraspinatus are responsible for 90% of the external rotation strength.[36] The teres minor also contributes to external rotation of the glenohumeral joint. The subscapularis is the primary internal rotator, with abduction activity peaking around 90°.[5]

THROWING MECHANISM

Throwing is an integral part of many sports, but different techniques are required, depending on the endeavor. High-speed photography has allowed investigators to slow down the pitching act and examine the arthrokinematics involved (Fig. 11–4). The throwing act, as performed by the baseball pitcher, is a series of complex and synchronized movements involving the upper and lower extremities. As described by McLeod,[57] the throwing mechanism can be divided into five phases (Fig. 11–5): (1) wind-up, (2) cocking, (3) acceleration, (4) release and deceleration, and (5) follow-through. Injuries to the shoulder joint usually occur during the acceleration and deceleration phases of throwing.

Wind-up

The wind-up is a slow-motion phase that prepares the pitcher for correct body posture and balance and leads into the cocking phase (see Fig. 11–5). It can last from 0.5 to 1.0 second.[82] It is characterized by shifting of the shoulder away from the direction of the pitch, with the opposite leg becoming cocked quite high and the baseball being re-

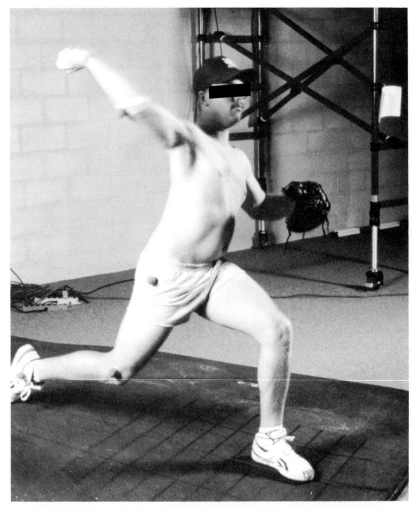

FIGURE 11–4   High-speed photography allows investigators to slow down the pitching act and examine the arthokinematics involved. (Photo courtesy of Sports Medicine Update, Birmingham, AL. HealthSouth Rehabilitation.)

moved from the glove.[57] It is also during this phase that the head of the humerus can wear and roughen from leverage on the posterior glenoid labrum, and the tendon of the long head of the biceps brachii stretches.[49]

Cocking

During the cocking phase (see Fig. 11–5) the shoulder is abducted to approximately 90°, externally rotated 90° or more, and horizontally abducted to approximately 30°.[57, 82] This is primarily accomplished by the deltoid and fine-tuned by the rotator cuff muscles, which pull the humeral head into the glenohumeral joint.[15] This places the anterior joint capsule and internal rotators, which are used to accelerate the ball, on maximum tension. Also, the opposite leg is kicked forward and

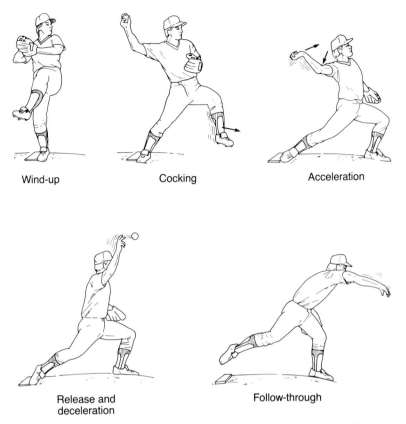

Wind-up   Cocking   Acceleration

Release and   Follow-through
deceleration

FIGURE 11-5   Dynamic phases of pitching. (From Walsh, D.A. (1989): Shoulder evaluation of the throwing athlete. Sports Med. Update, 4:24.)

placed directly in front of the body. Kinetic energy begins to be transferred from the lower extremities and trunk to the arm and hand, where the ball is held.[82] Anterior shoulder pain usually presents itself in this phase and is associated with rotator cuff irritation and subluxation of the humeral head or the long head of the biceps brachii.[49]

Acceleration

The acceleration phase (see Fig. 11-5) begins with deceleration of the forward movement of the chest and shoulder and ends prior to ball release.[58] This phase lasts an average of 50 milliseconds, approximately 2% of the duration of the pitching act.[67, 82] Muscles that once were on stretch in the cocking phase become the accelerators in a concentric act.[82] The body is brought forward, with the arm following behind. The energy developed by the body moving forward is transferred to the throwing arm to accelerate the humerus.[82] This energy is enhanced by contraction of the internal rotators (primarily the subscapularis) as the humerus is rotated internally from its previously externally rotated position, and brings acceleration of the ball to delivery speed.[57] During this phase a maximum internal rotation or angular velocity of about 9,189°/second and an average velocity of 6,180°/second can be produced.[15, 67] Rotatory torque at the shoulder can start at approximately 14,000 inch-pounds and builds up to approximately 27,000 inch-pounds of kinetic energy at ball release.[15]

During the acceleration phase some deceleration force is used to stop horizontal adduction of the humerus as the elbow is brought closer to the pitcher's side.[57] This is accomplished by the three posterior rotator cuff muscles—the supraspinatus, infraspinatus, and teres minor. Injuries that may be perpetuated during the acceleration phase include impingement syndrome, bursitis, tendinitis, synovitis, fractures, strains, and tendon ruptures.[82] Additionally, the forces produced by the accelerator muscles may pull the humeral head forward over the glenoid labrum, particularly in the presence of a lax anterior capsule, causing a lesion.

Release and Deceleration

In the release and deceleration phase the ball is released and the shoulder and arm decelerate (see Fig. 11–5). Generally, deceleration forces are approximately twice as great as acceleration forces but act for a shorter period of time (approximately 40 milliseconds).[11, 57] Initially, in the deceleration phase, the humerus has a relatively high rate of internal rotation and the elbow is rapidly extending.[57] There are great forces applied to the posterior rotator cuff muscles; these are required to slow down internal rotation and horizontal adduction of the humerus and to stabilize the humeral head in the glenoid cavity during the deceleration phase. Jobe and colleagues[43, 45] analyzed the throwing mechanism using electromyography and found that the muscles of the rotator cuff are extremely active during the deceleration phase. It has been reported that the posterior rotator cuff must resist as much as 300 pounds of force that is trying to pull the arm out of the glenohumeral joint.[10] Labrum tears at the attachment of the biceps long head, subluxation of the long head of the biceps by tearing of the transverse ligament, and various lesions of the rotator cuff can be incurred in this phase of throwing.[82]

Follow-Through

During the follow-through phase (see Fig. 11–5) the body moves forward with the arm, effectively reducing the distraction forces applied to the shoulder.[57] This results in tension being relieved on the rotator cuff muscles.

Because of the repetitive action of throwing, the baseball pitcher's shoulder undergoes adaptive changes that should be recognized and distinguished from pathologic lesions. The throwing shoulder has significantly increased external rotation and decreased internal rotation compared to those of the other side. In fact, a pitcher's shoulder not presenting with this increased external rotation and decreased internal rotation can be considered pathologic.

Injuries to the anterior aspect of the shoulder occur during the cocking phase of the throwing motion, whereas posterior shoulder injuries, particularly to the rotator cuff, are induced during the deceleration and follow-through phases. Injuries associated with the deceleration phase relate largely to the eccentric load placed on the shoulder's posterior structures.[41]

REHABILITATION PROGRAM OVERVIEW

The shoulder rehabilitation program presented in this chapter is designed to restore shoulder range of motion and strength in a functional progression. The exercises may be implemented with the contraindications kept in mind for certain motions, depending on the injury or surgical procedure. Often, emphasis is placed on the prime shoulder movers and not on the rotator cuff musculature. Rehabilitation exercises that concentrate on the cuff musculature are paramount following any shoulder injury, but are of particular importance to throwing athletes. All throwers should be placed on a preventative rotator cuff strengthening and flexibility program long before practice and the season begin and this should be maintained throughout the year. Shoulder rehabilitation should concentrate on increasing dynamic stability, particularly that of the rotator cuff, because the shoulder's static restraints are weak.

The entire kinematic chain should be considered when designing a shoulder rehabilitation program, remembering proximal stability for distal mobility. The synchronous interplay among the shoulder's joints is vital in contributing to joint stability and normal glenohumeral function. The scapula stabilizers (e.g., latissimus dorsi, rhomboids, serratus anterior) are often overlooked in addressing shoulder injuries. The scapula stabilizers play a large role during the deceleration phase of throwing to stabilize the scapular and glenohumeral relationship, and allow for normal kinematics during the pitching act.

Rotator cuff exercises have been evaluated by several investigators.[11, 42, 67] Jobe and Moynes[42] first examined the effect of specific exercises on the rotator cuff musculature. They reported that the supraspinatus can best be exercised apart from the other cuff muscles with the arm abducted to 90°, horizontally flexed 30°, and internally rotated (Fig. 11–6). The infraspinatus and teres minor can be exercised in the side-lying position with the arm held close to the side and the elbow flexed to 90° (Fig. 11–7). The subscapularis can be strengthened with the individual in the supine position, the affected arm held close to the side, and the elbow flexed to 90° (Fig. 11–8).

Since Jobe and Moynes's study,[42] Blackburn and associates[11] investigated rotator cuff activation using intramuscular electromyography (EMG) with particular rotator cuff exercises. During the deceleration phase of throwing the shoulder is most prone to injury, so intramuscular EMG was used to evaluate the muscle activity of the three posterior rotator cuff muscles (infraspinatus, supraspinatus, and teres minor) in various positions (supine, prone, standing). A 4-pound weight (resis-

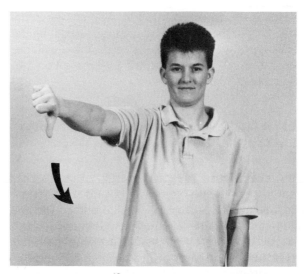

FIGURE 11–6   Jobe and Moynes[42] reported the supraspinatus muscle is best exercised with the arm abducted to 90°, horizontally flexed 30°, and internally rotated.

tance) was attached at the wrist. Although Jobe and Moynes[42] reported that the supraspinatus is best isolated and exercised with the arm abducted to 90°, horizontally flexed 30°, and fully rotated internally (see Fig. 11–6), Blackburn and co-workers[11] noted that the supraspinatus is involved whenever the arm is elevated, whether the subject is standing

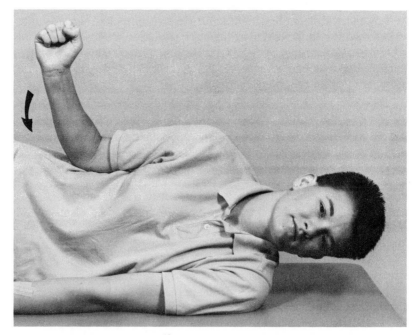

FIGURE 11–7   Jobe and Moynes[42] reported the infraspinatus and teres minor can be exercised in the side-lying position, with the arm held close to the side and the elbow flexed to 90°.

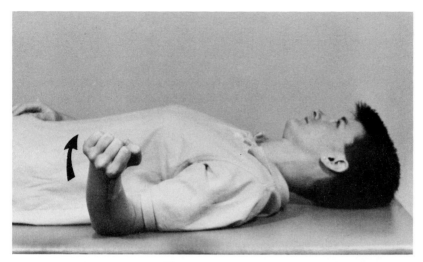

FIGURE 11–8   Jobe and Moynes[42] reported supine internal rotation with the arm held close to the side and elbow flexed to 90°. This exercises the subscapularis muscle.

or lying prone. Isolation of supraspinatus function appears to be demonstrated by pure abduction with neutral rotation of the arm while standing (Fig. 11–9). Also, a significant increase in supraspinatus function can be achieved in the prone position, maximum external rotation, and 100° of horizontal abduction (Fig. 11–10). It was concluded from

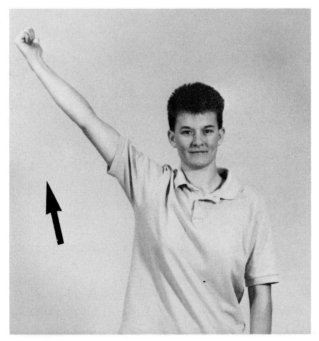

FIGURE 11–9   Blackburn and colleagues[11] reported the isolation of the supraspinatus muscle occurs in pure abduction with neutral rotation of the arm while standing.

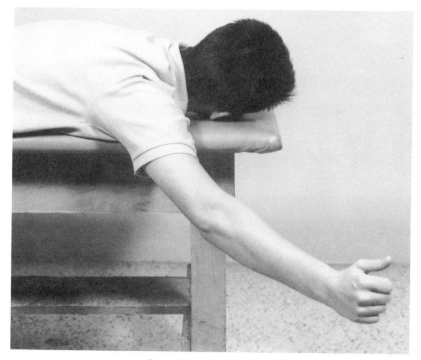

FIGURE 11–10　Prone horizontal abduction at 100°.

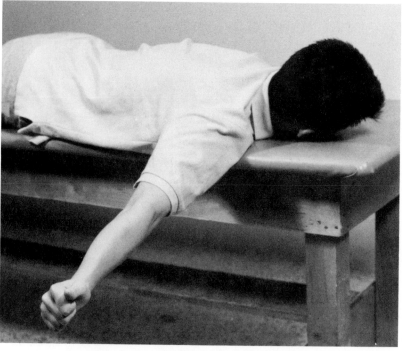

FIGURE 11–11　Prone horizontal abduction.

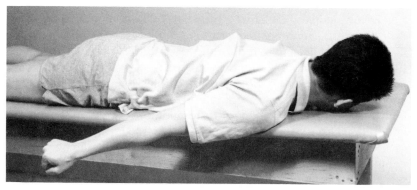

FIGURE 11–12   Prone extension with external rotation. This exercises the teres minor.

intramuscular EMG studies of the posterior rotator cuff muscles that (1) when using hand or wrist weights, the prone position allows for increased activity of the posterior rotator cuff muscles than when standing; (2) any exercise program using hand weights to strengthen the supraspinatus, infraspinatus, and teres minor muscles should include exercise positions similar to those shown in Figures 11–10 and 11–11; (3) teres minor isolation can be accomplished using a prone body position with extension of the arm in exernal rotation (Fig. 11–12); and (4) the infraspinatus acts in concert with the supraspinatus or teres minor in most of the exercises tested.[11] The exercises proposed by Blackburn and colleagues[11] are illustrated at the end of this chapter (see Figs. 11–48 to 11–54).

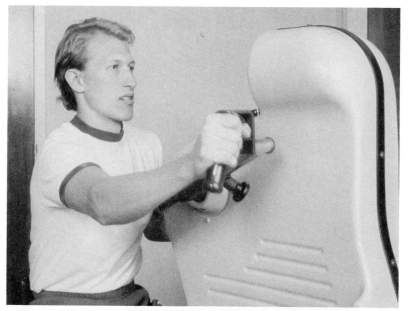

FIGURE 11–13   The upper body ergometer (UBE) can be used to restore upper extremity joint motion and muscular endurance. (Photo courtesy of Sports Medicine Update, Birmingham, AL. HealthSouth Rehabilitation.)

Following injury or surgery, modalities should be used as needed. Both preexercise and postexercise cryotherapy is recommended in the acute stages of healing to reduce the inflammatory process and should be used prophylactically after the acute phase has subsided. Moist heat and ultrasound may be indicated for chronic overuse injuries of the shoulder. The upper body ergometer (UBE) can be implemented in the early phases of rehabilitation for restoration of range of motion and in later phases for muscular endurance (Fig. 11–13). The Inertia machine (see Chap. 12) can be used to enhance coordination, timing, and eccentric strengthening, particularly for the decelerator shoulder muscles. Isokinetic equipment can be used at high speeds to help increase muscle contractile speed. With some isokinetic equipment, eccentric

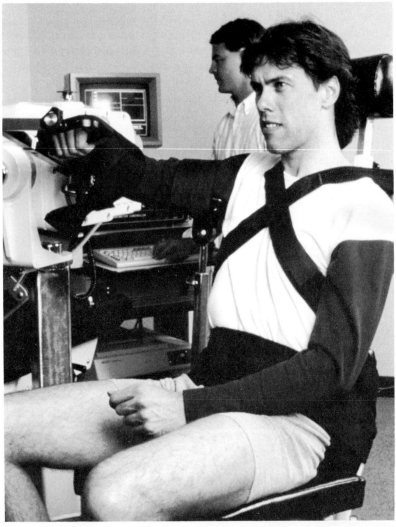

FIGURE 11–14 With some isokinetic equipment, eccentric contraction of the posterior cuff muscles and concentric contraction of the anterior muscles can be performed to increase exercise specificity. (Photo courtesy of Sports Medicine Update, Birmingham, AL. HealthSouth Rehabilitation.)

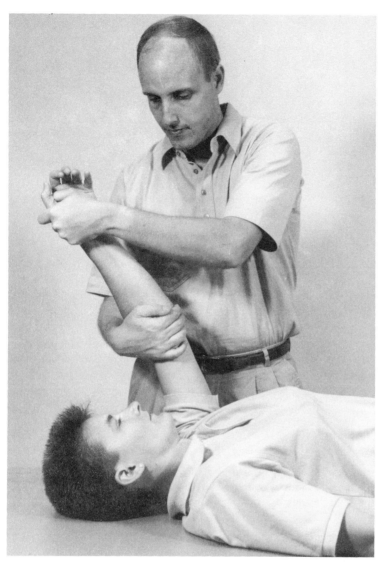

FIGURE 11–15   Proprioception neuromuscular facilitation (PNF) patterns can be used to simulate functional planes and enhance neuromuscular control of the shoulder girdle.

contraction of the posterior cuff muscles and concentric contraction of the anterior muscles can be performed to increase exercise specificity (Fig. 11–14). Most isokinetic equipment can be set up to simulate some functional planes; if not, proprioceptive neuromuscular facilitation (PNF) patterns can be used (Fig. 11–15). The use of upper extremity rhythmic stabilization cocontractions (Fig. 11–16) helps facilitate muscle synergistics. Surgical tubing can be used to simulate diagonal patterns of throwing and other functional activities (Figs. 11–17 and 11–18). This is a viable alternative for those clinicians who are inexperienced in PNF techniques. Later stages of rehabilitation should use surgical tubing in functional planes at a high rate of movement.

The use of glenohumeral mobilization techniques (see Chap. 6) is

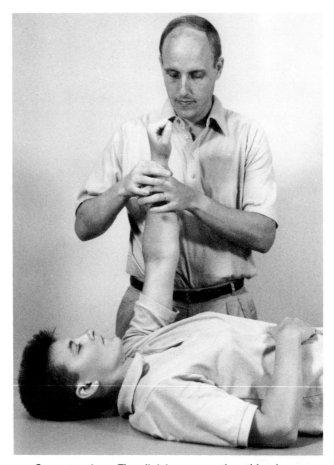

FIGURE 11–16   Cocontractions. The clinician moves the athlete's upper extremity in various directions with the athlete meeting that resistance by contracting his/her muscles helps facilitate muscle synergism of the shoulder girdle.

important in attaining accessory motion in the early stages of healing without subjecting the joint to the high forces of passive stretching. For instance, the use of grade I anterior-posterior, inferior-superior, and long arm distraction can be used early in the rehabilitation program, when an anterior capsule shift is performed, to prevent anterior dislocation or subluxation of the humeral head before aggressive passive external rotation stretching may begin.

Glenohumeral flexibility is paramount for the throwing athlete, particularly flexibility of the posterior shoulder structures that can contribute to poor joint mechanics if tight. This is particularly evident with inflexibility of the posterior capsule and musculature as seen with horizontal adduction and with internal rotation, creating increased stress to the posterior shoulder structures on follow-through during the pitching act. Tight posterior shoulder structures cause abnormal glenohumeral kinematics by forcing the humeral head superiorly into the acromion arch. The flexibility exercises illustrated at the end of this chapter should be undertaken not only following injury or surgery but also during the off-season to help prevent injury.

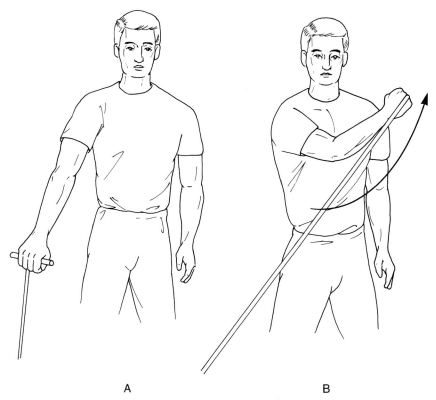

A   B

FIGURE 11–17   PNF diagonal pattern (D1) using surgical tubing. (Redrawn from Wilk, K.E., et al. (1990): Preventive and Rehabilitative Exercises for the Shoulder and Elbow, 3rd ed. Birmingham, AL, American Sports Medicine Institute, p. 23.)

Muscle strength and endurance in the scapula stabilizer musculature are important in maintaining correct joint arthrokinematics. The scapula musculature and the role of the scapulothoracic joint in maintaining a normal functioning shoulder are often overlooked. Spasm, weakness, and poor neuromuscular coordination of the stabilizing muscles directly affect glenohumeral motion. If the scapula cannot rotate on the thoracic cage, maintain the correct length–tension muscle relationship, and orient the glenoid fossa with the humeral head, asynchronous motion at the shoulder complex can result in injury. Scapula stabilizers can be strengthened by having the athlete perform reverse wall push-ups, prone horizontal abduction at 100°, shoulder shrugs, and scapula retraction exercises with tubing.

Because the rotator cuff muscles are mainly endurance-type muscles, the PRE (progressive resistance exercise) program is based on high weight and low repetition.[7] This not only increases muscular endurance but also decreases the potential of perpetuating the inflammatory process by performing the exercises with too much weight. The PRE program should be progressed by having the athlete work from 30 to 50 repetitions and not adding weight until 50 repetitions can be comfortably performed (see Chap. 7). The PRE program is begun with a

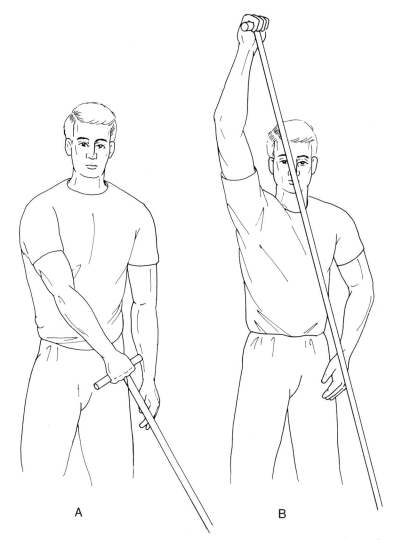

A   B

FIGURE 11–18   PNF diagonal pattern (D2) using surgical tubing. (Redrawn from Wilk, K.E., et al. (1990): Preventive and Rehabilitative Exercises for the Shoulder and Elbow, 3rd ed. Birmingham, AL, American Sports Medicine Institute, p. 23.)

gradual progression toward more dynamic exercises as healing occurs. The athlete should not use more than 5 pounds with the rotator cuff PRE program. This decreases the chance of cuff inflammation and trauma while still producing muscle strength and endurance of the rotator cuff.

The exercises at the end of this chapter are based on those of Blackburn and associates.[11] Added to this regimen are shoulder flexibility and concentric and eccentric tubing programs. Athletes should begin with the traditional PRE program and stretching exercises, with a gradual progression into eccentrics and isokinetics; this is followed by progression to a more dynamic program (Figs. 11–19 to 11–25) consisting of high-speed movements to muscle fatigue, proprioception, Inertia machine, and upper extremity plyometrics. Note that plyometrics should be performed only two or three times weekly

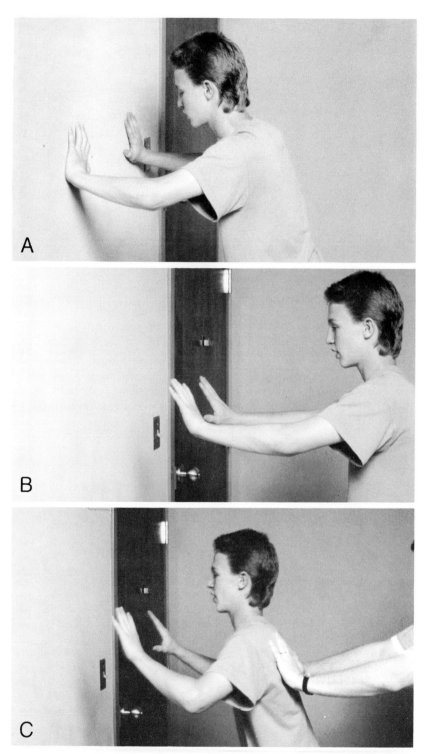

FIGURE 11–19 *A, B,* Progressive wall push-ups, as the athlete advances. *C,* Plyometric wall push-ups can be performed. (Photo courtesy of Sports Medicine Update, Birmingham, AL. HealthSouth Rehabilitation.)

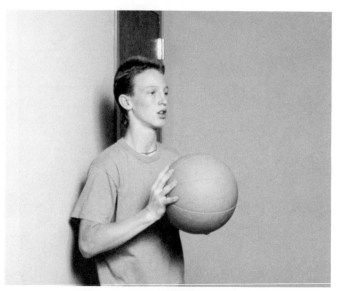

FIGURE 11–20   A 3-kg medicine ball can be used as rehabilitation progresses with various single- and double-arm overhead and double-arm chest passes. (Photo courtesy of Sports Medicine Update, Birmingham, AL. HealthSouth Rehabilitation.)

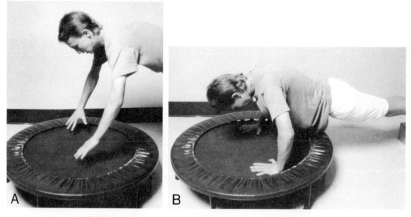

FIGURE 11–21   *A, B,* Plyometric push-ups bounding from minitramp. (Photo courtesy of Sports Medicine Update, Birmingham, AL. HealthSouth Rehabilitation.)

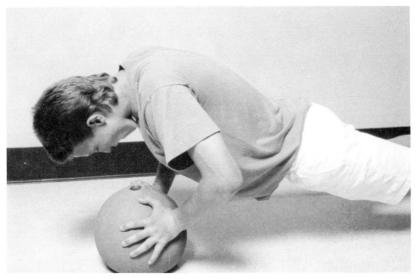

FIGURE 11–22   Medicine ball push-ups. (Photo courtesy of Sports Medicine Update, Birmingham, AL. HealthSouth Rehabilitation.)

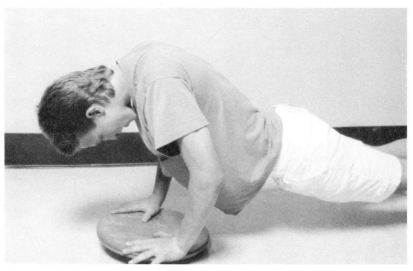

FIGURE 11–23   Balance board push-ups. (Photo courtesy of Sports Medicine Update, Birmingham, AL. HealthSouth Rehabilitation.)

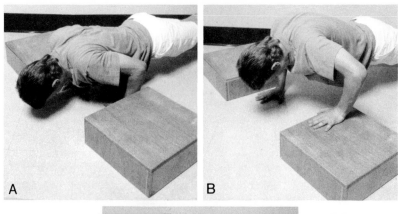

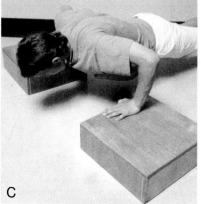

FIGURE 11–24 *A–C,* Modified push-ups using 6-inch boxes. (Photo courtesy of Sports Medicine Update, Birmingham, AL. HealthSouth Rehabilitation.)

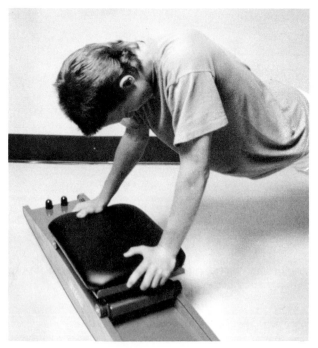

FIGURE 11–25 Upper extremity dynamic stabilization exercise using the Fitter. (Photo courtesy of Sports Medicine Update, Birmingham, AL. HealthSouth Rehabilitation.)

because of the microtrauma that occurs; everyday use of plyometrics can result in additional trauma. The athlete should return to throwing gradually by implementation of the Interval Throwing Program outlined in Appendix B.

COMMON POSTTRAUMATIC AND POSTSURGICAL COMPLAINTS

Following trauma or surgery to the shoulder joint the athlete may report several common complaints to the clinician, and these may affect the rehabilitation program.

Painful Arc

A painful arc or "catching point," particularly with shoulder abduction (but also in other planes), is characterized by specific points throughout a range of motion, where the pain intensifies, but once past that point it dissipates. There may be as many as three or four catching points through an arc of motion. The athlete should attempt to exercise through these points, and they should dissipate within 5 to 7 days after initiation of treatment.

Crepitus

Crepitus within the shoulder joint is a common occurrence and is usually asymptomatic. Generally, crepitus can be detected following shoulder surgery or rotator cuff tendinitis. If the crepitus remains asymptomatic, the athlete should attempt to exercise through it when performing the therapeutic exercise program. This should also dissipate within 7 to 10 days following initiation of the rotator cuff exercise program.

Middle Deltoid and Elbow Pain

Middle deltoid and elbow pain can be referred from the shoulder, most likely from a tight posterior capsule. It is usually exacerbated with external rotation in the 90–90° supine position and general glenohumeral tightness can also be detected (Fig. 11–26). This pain is usually seen in those with chronic shoulder problems or in individuals who have undergone prolonged immobilization. Often, the elbow pain at the end-range of shoulder external rotation may be greater than that of the actual shoulder pain. Such individuals usually respond well to moist heat and ultrasound to the posterior capsule and to glenohumeral joint mobilization. Glenohumeral joints in which external rotation is limited should not be aggressively stretched, because this exacerbates the elbow pain. Most patients can tolerate long arm distraction with imposed external rotation better than aggressive external

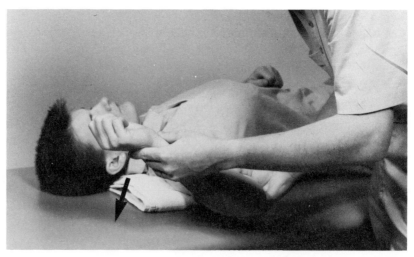

FIGURE 11–26 Increased deltoid and elbow pain can be experienced if the posterior shoulder capsule is tight. Note the towel under the arm and scapula, which facilitates exercise in the scapular plane.

rotation stretching in the 90–90° position (Fig. 11–27). As treatment proceeds and normal synchronous glenohumeral motion is restored, the athlete should report a decrease in elbow and middle deltoid pain.

Pain Above 90° of Flexion or Abduction

If impingement or rotator cuff tendinitis is present, pain above 90° in flexion or abduction is a common occurrence. Athletes with this complaint should begin active assisted rope-and-pulley exercises through a full range of motion, and use joint mobilization techniques as tolerated. The pain is often propagated by a decrease in muscular strength and usually improves with a gradual rotator cuff therapeutic exercise program. If symptoms are severe and the athlete has radiographic changes that could be classified as a grade III impingement, the therapeutic prognosis is poor.

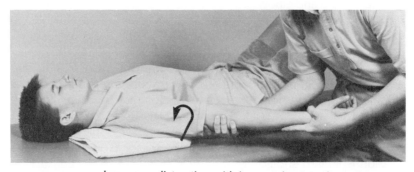

FIGURE 11–27 Long arm distraction with imposed external rotation.

SHOULDER INJURIES

Scapulothoracic Joint Lesions

The scapulothoracic joint is often overlooked in the initial evaluation following shoulder injury or surgery. This occurs particularly in chronic pain conditions, in which glenohumeral motion has gradually regressed and/or the glenohumeral joint has been immobilized for a long period. In most instances the scapulothoracic joint becomes involved as a secondary problem. Increased shoulder pain can result in muscle spasm in the supraspinatus, trapezius, rhomboids, latissimus dorsi, and subscapularis. As mentioned previously, for every 2° of glenohumeral abduction there must be an associated 1° of scapular motion to achieve 180° of abduction. If the scapulothoracic joint is not functioning properly, the athlete may be able to attain only 100 to 120° of passive abduction, and active abduction may be even more limited.

The scapulothoracic joint should be evaluated for spasm in the rhomboids, latissimus dorsi, upper and lower trapezius, subscapularis, teres minor, infraspinatus, and supraspinatus muscles. These areas should also be assessed for active trigger points, as discussed by Travell and Simons.[79] The activation of trigger points in these muscles may also cause referred pain to the middle deltoid and elbow and, in severe cases, down the arm. In addition, the clinician may find that the vertebral scapular border cannot be distracted off the thoracic cage; this results not only in increased pain for the athlete, but also in an increase in muscle spasm.

Before decreased glenohumeral motion can be treated, scapulothoracic motion must be restored. This is usually accomplished by reducing the muscle spasm with moist heat, ultrasound, electrical stimulation, and scapula mobilization (Figs. 11–28 and 11–29). In severe cases Travell and Simon's[79] spray-and-stretch technique using fluori-

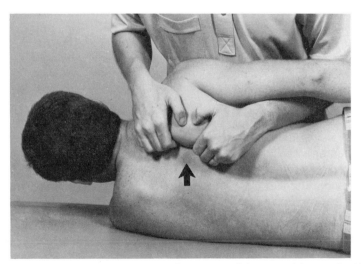

FIGURE 11–28 Scapula mobilization by distraction of the scapula's vertebral border and lateral glide.

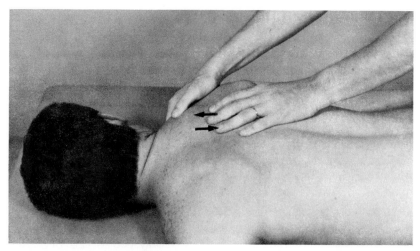

FIGURE 11–29   Scapula mobilization by superior and inferior scapula glides.

methane spray to desensitize the trigger points may be indicated; also, a home electrical muscle stimulation unit may be used over the trigger points to desensitize them and decrease muscle spasticity. In severe cases trigger point injection may be considered.[79] As trigger points are diminished the athlete should report a decrease in shoulder pain, neck stiffness, and referred pain, with an associated increase in glenohumeral abduction.

Impingement Syndrome

The term "impingement syndrome" was popularized by Neer in 1972.[62] He emphasized that the supraspinatus insertion to the greater tubercle and the bicipital groove lies anterior to the coracoacromial arch with the shoulder in the neutral position, and that with forward flexion of the shoulder these structures must pass beneath the coracoacromial arch, providing the opportunity for impingement.[56] He introduced the concept of a continuum in the impingement syndrome from chronic bursitis to partial or complete tears of the supraspinatus tendon, which may extend to involve ruptures to other parts of the rotator cuff.[56]

Impingement of the rotator cuff is commonly seen in baseball pitchers, quarterbacks, swimmers, and others whose activities involve repetitive use of the arm above the horizontal plane. Matsen and Arntz[56] have defined impingement as the encroachement of the acromion, coracoclavicular ligament, coracoid process, and/or acromioclavicular joint on the rotator cuff mechanism that passes beneath them as the glenohumeral joint is moved, particularly in flexion and rotation. Impingement usually involves the supraspinatus tendon. If the supraspinatus muscle depresses the head of the humerus sufficiently, the greater tubercle cannot butt against the coracoacromial arch (Fig. 11–30).[72] Whether impingement is the primary event causing rotator cuff tendinitis, or whether rotator cuff impingement occurs secondary to rotator cuff disease, is unproved.[72] In all likelihood both mechanisms of injury can occur.

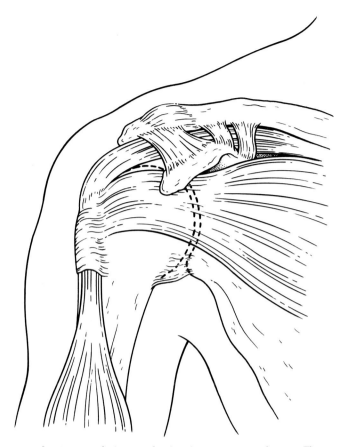

FIGURE 11–30 Anatomy relative to the impingement syndrome. The supraspinatus tendon is seen passing beneath the coracoacromial arch. (Redrawn from Matsen, F.A., III, and Arntz, C.T. (1990): Subacromial impingement. *In:* Rockwood, C.A., Jr., and Matsen, F.A., III (eds.): The Shoulder. Philadelphia, W.B. Saunders, p. 624.)

Usually there is approximately 1 cm of space between the humeral head and undersurface of the acromial arch. Thus, whenever the arm is elevated, some degree of rotator cuff impingement may occur.[72] The shoulder is most vulnerable to impingement when the arm is at 90° of abduction and the scapula has not rotated sufficiently to free the rotator cuff of the overhanging acromion and coracoacromial ligament. It is also vulnerable with horizontal adduction of the arm, which causes impingement against the coracoid process. Forward flexion or pronation of the arm also jams the greater tubercle under the acromion, coracoacromial ligament and, at times, the coracoid process.[72] If the arm is raised in supination, however, the greater tubercle is turned away from the acromial arch and the arm can be elevated without impingement.

Impingement syndrome is perpetuated by the cumulative effect of many passages of the rotator cuff beneath the coracoacromial arch. This results in irritation of the biceps (long head) and supraspinatus, and possibly the infraspinatus tendon, plus enlargement of the subacromial bursa, which can become fibrotic, thus further decreasing an already compromised space and resulting in a vicious cycle that severely limits the throwing motion. Furthermore, with time and progression of wearing and attrition, microtears and partial-thickness rotator cuff tears may result. If these continue, secondary bony changes (osteophytes) can occur under the acromion arch and produce full-thickness rotator cuff tears.

Etiology of the impingement syndrome is usually multifocal, and the supraspinatus tendon is the most likely to be involved. Several factors have been proposed that can contribute to the impingement syndrome. Tendon avascularity has long been thought to contribute to impingement. Lindblom,[51] in 1939, first reported avascularity of the rotator cuff at the supraspinatus attachment to the greater tubercle, describing this as the "critical zone"[19] where many lesions occur. Moseley and Goldie[61] concluded from their work, however, that the critical zone is no more avascular than the rest of the cuff. Finally, Iannotti and co-workers[38] have reported substantial blood flow in the critical zone of the rotator cuff using the laser Doppler.

Although it now appears that the rotator cuff is not a hypovascular structure, Rathbun and Macnab[71] and Sigholm and associates[77] have proposed two mechanisms that may compromise supraspinatus blood flow. Rathbun and Macnab[71] have noted that shoulder adduction places the supraspinatus under tension and "wrings out" its vessels, resulting in tissue necrosis. Sigholm and colleagues[77] demonstrated that active forward flexion increases subacromial pressure enough to reduce tendon microcirculation substantially.[56] Matsen and Arntz pointed out in interpreting these findings, however, that "since the shoulder is frequently moved, it is unclear whether either of these mechanisms could produce ischemia of sufficient duration to cause tendon damage."[56] The relationship among cuff vascularity, impingement, and rotator cuff lesions is still speculative, and more research is needed.

The shape of the acromion has been studied in individuals with impingement syndrome.[9, 62] It appears that rotator cuff lesions are more likely to occur if a hooked acromion is present,[9, 60] but it cannot be determined if the acromial shape is caused by or results from a cuff tear.[56]

Finally, a weakened cuff mechanism can predispose an athlete to rotator cuff impingement. The rotator cuff functions to stabilize the shoulder against the actions of the deltoid and pectoralis major muscles. In the presence of a weakened cuff mechanism, contraction of the deltoid causes upward displacement of the humeral head so that it squeezes the remaining cuff against the coracoacromial arch[56] (Fig. 11–31). Other factors that can result in rotator cuff impingement include the following:[56] degenerative spurs, chronic bursa thickening, rotator cuff thickening related to chronic calcium deposits, tightness of the posterior shoulder capsule (which forces the humeral head to rise up against the acromion during shoulder flexion), and capsular laxity.

Neer[62] has described four progressive stages of the impingement syndrome (Table 11–1). Stage I involves those individuals under 25

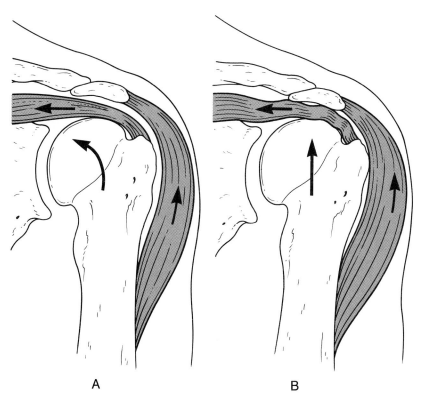

A　　　　　　　　　　　B

FIGURE 11–31 The supraspinatus helps to stabilize the head of the humerus against the upward pull of the deltoid. *A,* Subacromial impingement is prevented by normal cuff function. *B,* Deep surface tearing of the supraspinatus weakens the ability of the cuff to hold the humeral head down, resulting in impingement of the tendon against the acromion. (Redrawn from Matsen, F.A., III, and Arntz, C.T. (1990): Subacromial impingement. *In:* Rockwood, C.A., Jr., and Matsen, F.A., III (eds.): The Shoulder. Philadelphia, W.B. Saunders, p. 624.)

TABLE 11–1　NEER'S PROGRESSIVE STAGES OF IMPINGEMENT SYNDROME

Stage	Features
I	Edema and hemorrhage in the supraspinatus tendon resulting from excessive overhead use in sports or work; this tendinitis is localized and reversible
II	With repeated insults of inflammation the supraspinatus tendon, biceps tendon, and subacromial bursa become fibrotic and thickened
III	With further impingement wear, attritional changes occur in the supraspinatus and biceps tendons, which may even lead to partial tears
IV	Because of progressive changes in the supraspinatus tendon, a complete tear occurs

From Hill, J.A. (1988): Rotator cuff injuries. Sports Med. Update, 3(3):5. Reprinted with permission.

years of age, is a reversible lesion, and presents with a "tooth-like" discomfort in the shoulder. This stage usually only involves inflammation of the supraspinatus tendon and long head of the biceps brachii. Stage II is generally seen in individuals 24 to 40 years of age and involves fibrotic changes of the supraspinatus tendon, tendon of the long head of the biceps brachii, and subacromial bursa. Again, a "tooth-like" ache is present, pain may be increased at night, and there might be an inability to perform the movement that resulted in the impingement syndrome. This stage sometimes responds to conservative treatment but may require surgical intervention. Stage III seldom occurs in those under the age of 40; however, young baseball pitchers, 20 to 30 years of age, may present with this stage of the syndrome. In this stage the individual complains of a long history of shoulder pain, there is a frequent association with osteophytes and a partial and eventual full-thickness rotator cuff tear,[32] and there is obvious wasting of the supraspinatus and infraspinatus muscles. This stage usually does not respond well to conservative treatment. Stage IV is a complete rotator cuff tear.

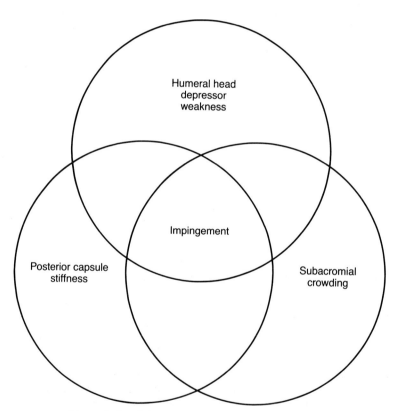

FIGURE 11-32   Normal shoulder tendon depends on normal function of the humeral head depressors, normal capsular laxity, and adequate subacromial space. Some effects of impingement (e.g., weakness of the humeral head depressors, stiffness of the posterior capsule, and crowding of the subacromial space with thickened bursa) may further intensify impingement, producing a self-perpetuating process. (Modified from Matsen, F.A., III, and Arntz, C.T. (1990): Subacromial impingement. *In:* Rockwood, C.A., Jr., and Matsen, F.A., III (eds.): The Shoulder. Philadelphia, W.B. Saunders, p. 624.)

Rotator cuff impingement is a self-perpetuating process. Matsen and Arntz[56] have noted the following (Fig. 11–32): (1) muscle or cuff tendon weakness causes impingement from loss of humeral head depressor function, leading to tendon damage, disuse atrophy, and additional cuff weakness (Fig. 11–33); (2) bursal thickening causes impingement from subacromial crowding, producing thickening of the bursa; and (3) posterior capsular stiffness can lead to impingement, disuse, and stiffness, because the tight capsule forces the humeral head to rise up against the acromion.

The goal in treating athletes with an impingement syndrome, whether conservatively or surgically, is reducing the compression and friction between the rotator cuff and subacromial space. This can be minimized by several factors:[56] (1) the shape of the coracoacromial arch, which allows passage of the subjacent cuff mechanism; (2) a normal undersurface of the acromioclavicular joint; (3) a normal bursa; (4) normal functioning of the humeral head depressors (rotator cuff); (5) normal capsular laxity; and (5) a smooth upper surface of the cuff mechanism. The primary complication of the impingement syndrome is a rotator cuff tear. If the impingement syndrome is diagnosed in its early stages, the prognosis is encouraging. In an acute impingement syndrome, time, rest from noxious stimuli, NSAIDs (nonsteroidal anti-inflammatory drugs), modalities such as cold, heat, and electrical stimulation, and a general shoulder rehabilitation program of flexibility and PRE (as outlined at the end of this chapter) are indicated.

On evaluation, active range of motion may be limited, with an open end-feel, as a result of pain. This may be caused by posterior capsule stiffness. In such cases moist heat, ultrasound, and deep friction massage to the posterior capsule, followed by joint mobilization and a general shoulder flexibility program, with emphasis on supine external rotation and horizontal adduction, are appropiate. Table 11–2 outlines the protocol for conservative treatment of the impingement syndrome.

Injection of the subacromial space with lidocaine in the presence of an impingement syndrome decreases the athlete's pain. Steroid injections in or near the cuff and biceps tendon may produce tendon atrophy, however, or reduce the ability of a damaged tendon to repair itself.[56] Kennedy and Willis[46] have found a substantial effect in the rabbit Achilles tendon following steroid injection. They concluded that physiologic doses of local steroids injected directly into a normal tendon weaken it significantly, up to 14 days postinjection. This weakness was attributed to cellular necrosis. The clinician must take this possibility into consideration when developing a rehabilitation program.

Surgical intervention for those with grade III impingement syndromes or those who do not respond to conservative care consists of subacromial decompression, referred to as an acromioplasty. The goal in performing a subacromial decompression is to relieve the mechanical impingement and prevent wear at the critical areas of the rotator cuff. Subacromial decompression consists of resection of the anteroinferior acromial undersurface to increase the space between it and the humeral head and rotator cuff; often, resection of the coracoacromial ligament to increase the rotator cuff space further is performed.

An acromioplasty may be performed in conjunction with a rotator

**TABLE 11–2   PROTOCOL: NONOPERATIVE ROTATOR
CUFF TENDINITIS, BURSITIS,
AND IMPINGEMENT**

I. Patient education
  A. Point out that such complaints as grinding, popping, and a "painful arc" are normal, and the crepitus should gradually decrease.
  B. The athlete should limit functional activities (e.g., throwing, tennis, golf, swimming, weight lifting) for 4 to 6 weeks with return to activity using an interval activity program (see Appendix B).
  C. A maintenance program during the off-season and in-season is important to help prevent symptoms from recurring.
  D. Do not exceed 5 pounds, 5 × 10 with the PRE program. Emphasis is on low weight, high repetition, and correct exercise technique.
II. Guidelines for program initiation
  A. Use modalities as indicated for pain (e.g., ice, electrical stimulation, phonophoresis). Use modalities in conjunction with home exercise program.
  B. Perform initial exercise program two or three times daily.
  C. It is important that athletes perform external rotation stretching in the three positions of 90°, 135°, and 180° of abduction.
  D. With PRE exercises, lifting technique and hand position are of the utmost importance. Stress this to the athlete.
III. Use preceding guidelines to initiate following exercises:
  A. Stretching
      1. Circumduction (if indicated)
      2. Overhead flexion with T-bar
      3. Supine abduction with T-bar
      4. External rotation with T-bar
      5. Internal rotation with T-bar
      6. Supine horizontal adduction
      7. Rope-and-pulley (active assisted)
          a. Flexion
          b. Abduction
  B. Progressive resistance
      1. Shoulder flexion
      2. Shoulder abduction
      3. Supraspinatus
      4. Prone extension
      5. Prone horizontal abduction
      6. Prone external rotation
      7. Shoulder shrugs
      8. Biceps curl
      9. Triceps curl
      10. Sitting dip
      11. Progressive push-up
  C. 4 to 6 weeks after program initiation
      1. Isokinetics at high speeds, PNF patterns, eccentric exercises, surgical tubing, and upper extremity plyometrics can begin as tolerated by the athlete.
      2. Begin Interval Throwing or Tennis Program when 5 × 10 with 3 to 5 pounds is reached (may begin sooner if asymptomatic and no deficiency can be detected with manual muscle testing). Interval Golf Program may begin sooner than 4 to 6 weeks if asymptomatic (see Appendix B).

cuff debridement or repair. Surgical correction of the impingement syndrome can be done using arthroscopy or arthrotomy techniques. Arthroscopy techniques consist of burring down the acromion undersurface. Similar techniques are undertaken with an arthrotomy. It is recommended that, in an open subacromial decompression, the "deltoid on" technique be employed, rather than taking down the deltoid. The deltoid on approach results in less morbidity and early postoperative motion, with almost no need for postoperative immobilization.[56] If the deltoid is taken down, rehabilitation should proceed more slowly to allow for deltoid healing restraints to gain strength.

Modalities can be used initially after surgery to help control pain and inflammation, with the concurrent initiation of early range-of-motion exercises. In the early stages the athlete may complain of joint crepitus and a painful arc or catching points; these should be worked through, as tolerable to the athlete, to regain the motion, with the crepitus and painful arc subsiding within 7 to 10 days after initiation of exercises. As active range of motion is restored, a PRE program can be initiated. The protocol outlined in Table 11−3 presents the general postoperative course for an arthroscopy or deltoid on type of acromioplasty. Coracoacromial ligament resection has no effect on the course of the rehabilitation. If a rotator cuff repair is performed in conjunction with the acromioplasty, a rotator cuff protocol should be followed.

Rotator Cuff Lesions

The act of throwing has been shown to be one of the movements that most consistently produces rotator cuff tears, with or without other pathology.[13] McLeod and Andrews[58] have reported that 122 of 178 baseball players in their study (68%) had rotator cuff tears. Again, the deceleration phase of throwing places greater stress on the posterior cuff musculature to contract eccentrically in an attempt to stabilize the glenohumeral joint and slow its forward motion. The rotator cuff's primary function is to provide dynamic stabilization and steer the humeral head. It appears that the cuff is well designed to bear tension and resist upward displacement of the humerus.[18, 19] The cuff balances the major forces applied by the prime mover muscles during motions such as flexion and abduction.[55]

The role of the rotator cuff in shoulder movements has long been and still is controversial. Poppen and Walker[68, 69] have reported that the pull of the supraspinatus is fairly constant throughout the range of motion, actually exceeding that of the deltoid until 60° of shoulder abduction has been reached. Norkin and Levangie[66] have found that EMG activity of the deltoid in abduction shows a gradual increase in activity, peaking at 90° of humeral abduction and not plateauing until 180°. Colachis and co-workers[20, 21] used selective nerve blocks and noted that the supraspinatus and infraspinatus provide 45% of abduction and 90% of external rotation strength. Additionally, Howell and colleagues[36] measured the torque produced by the supraspinatus and deltoid in the forward flexion and elevation planes. They found that the supraspinatus and deltoid muscles are equally responsible for pro-

TABLE 11–3 **PROTOCOL: ROTATOR CUFF DEBRIDEMENT, LABRUM TEAR, AND ACROMIOPLASTY**

I. Preoperative instructions
  A. Explain that the sling is used for the first day after surgery for comfort and that the athlete is then weaned out of it.
  B. Instruct in circumduction exercises, to be performed frequently.
  C. Explain about application of ice to shoulder at 20-minute intervals for pain and soreness.
II. Exercises*
  A. Initial phase: 2 to 7 days postoperatively
    1. Begin following exercises:
      a. Supine flexion
      b. Supine 90–90° external rotation
      c. Supine 90–90° internal rotation
      d. Supine abduction
      e. Horizontal adduction stretch
      f. Rope-and-pulley in abduction
      g. Rope-and-pulley in flexion
      h. Shoulder shrugs
    2. Goal: exercises above to be done 1 × 10, two times daily, progressing to 3 × 10. Expect soreness but do not discontinue. Reduce repetitions as needed.
    3. Use modalities as indicated for pain and inflammation.
  B. Intermediate phase: 7 to 10 days postoperatively
    1. Initiate the following active exercises after full active-assisted exercise is achieved:
      a. Shoulder flexion
      b. Shoulder abduction
      c. Supraspinatus
      d. Prone horizontal abduction
      e. Shoulder extension
      f. Prone external rotation
      g. Biceps curl
      h. Triceps or French curl
      i. Initiate PNF patterns for upper extremity, as tolerated
      j. Goal: begin with 3 × 10 as tolerated 2 or 3 times daily and progress to 5 × 10. When 5 × 10 is possible, begin adding weight 1 pound at a time, not to exceed 5 pounds. Always work from 3 × 10, progressing to 5 × 10 before increasing weight.
    2. Continue stretching exercises that began day 2 postoperatively
  C. Advanced phase: week 3 postoperatively
    1. Continue exercise program with additional exercises:
      a. Sitting dip
      b. Progressive push-up
  D. Weeks 4 to 6 postoperatively
    1. Begin medium- to high-speed isokinetic work in all planes.
    2. Begin eccentric shoulder program, if indicated.
  E. Weeks 8 to 10 postoperatively
    1. Begin Interval Golf Program, if indicated (see Appendix B).
    2. Begin PRE maintenance program.
  F. Weeks 12 to 16 postoperatively
    1. Begin Interval Tennis or Throwing Program, if indicated (see Appendix B).
    2. Begin upper extremity plyometrics.

* Continually monitor daily for residual pain and effusion. If this occurs reduce program in frequency and intensity.

ducing torque about the shoulder joint in functional planes of motions. Currently, it appears that both the deltoid and supraspinatus contribute to abduction throughout the full range of motion. Abduction is still possible with loss of the deltoid or supraspinatus, with a corresponding loss in power.[20, 21]

The etiology of cuff tears can be attributed to one or a combination of the following: trauma, overuse, and/or attrition. It has been postulated that rotator cuff tears result after the commonly diagnosed "cuff tendinitis," and may actually represent failure of rotator cuff fibers. This may explain why these individuals usually recover with time and conservative treatment.[55] Matsen and Arntz[55] have suggested the following as perpetuating rotator cuff failure:

> The traumatic and degenerative theories of cuff tendon failure can be synthesized into a unified view of pathogenesis. Let us assume that the normal cuff starts out well vascularized and with a full complement of fibers. Through its life it is subjected to various adverse factors such as traction, contusion, impingement, inflammation, injections, and age-related degeneration. Each of these factors places fibers of the cuff tendons at risk. Even though laboratory studies show that normal tendon does not fail before failure of the musculotendinous junction or the tendon bone junction, in the clinical situation the cuff tendon ruptures both at its insertion to bone and in its midsubstance. With the application of loads (whether repetitive or abrupt, compressive, or tensile), each fiber fails when the applied load exceeds its strength. Fibers may fail a few at a time or *en masse.* Because these fibers are under load even with the arm at rest, they retract after their rupture. Each instance of fiber failure has at least three adverse effects: (1) it increases the load on the neighboring fibers (fewer fibers to share the load); (2) it detaches muscle fibers from bone (diminishing the force that the cuff muscles can deliver); and (3) it risks the vascular elements in close proximity by distorting their anatomy (a particularly important factor owing to the fact that the cuff tendons contain the anastomoses between the osseous and muscular vessels). Thus, the initially well-vascularized cuff tendon becomes progressively avascular with succeeding injuries. Although some tendons, such as the Achilles tendon, have a remarkable propensity to heal after rupture, cuff ruptures communicate with joint and bursal fluid, which removes any hematoma that could contribute to cuff healing. Even if the tendon could heal with scar, scar tissue lacks the normal resilience of tendon and is, therefore, under increased risk for failure with subsequent loading (minor or major). These events weaken the substance of the cuff, impair its function, and render the cuff weaker, more prone to additional failure with less load, and less able to heal.

Whatever the etiologic factors involved in cuff damage, Figure 11–33 illustrates the vicious cycle of cuff degeneration that occurs if the problem is left untreated.

Arthroscopy has allowed investigators to examine cuff lesions and make the following observations:

1. Failure of the musculotendinous cuff is almost always peripheral, near the attachment of the cuff to the tubercles and nearly always begins in the supraspinatus part of the cuff near the biceps tendon.[56]

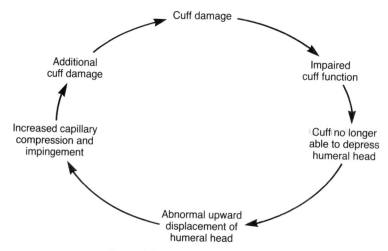

FIGURE 11-33   Potential pathogenesis of rotator cuff damage.

2. Partial-thickness tears appear to be twice as common as full-thickness lesions.[63, 84]
3. Most partial tears occur on the joint side and not on the bursal side.[29, 50]
4. Cuff tears begin deep and extend outward, therefore challenging the concept of subacromial impingement as the primary cause of defects.[26, 55, 83]

Full-thickness cuff tears appear to occur in tendons that are weakened by some combination of age, repeated small episodes of trauma, steroid injections, subacromial impingement, hypovascularity of the tendon, major injury, and previous partial tearing.[55]

Rehabilitation of rotator cuff lesions depends on the extent of the cuff lesion and the procedure used to carry out the repair. Athletes presenting with rotator cuff tendinitis generally respond well to therapeutic exercise (see Table 11-2). Their shoulders are usually stiff, especially in the posterior capsule, with detectable glenohumeral crepitus. The stiffness limits one or a combination of the following: forward flexion, internal and external rotation, and horizontal adduction. A tight posterior capsule can force the humeral head upward against the coracoacromial arch, further irritating the cuff tendon with resultant impingement. The athlete may also find it difficult to reach behind his or her back, because this elongates the musculotendinous unit and compresses it as it is pulled under the coracoacromial arch with internal rotation.[13] Modalities such as moist heat, ultrasound, mobilization, and stretching exercises for the posterior capsule are indicated. Rest from the noxious stimuli and NSAIDs are also appropriate. Initiation of a general shoulder flexibility program and a rotator cuff PRE program, as outlined at the end of this chapter, is necessary to prevent progressive cuff degradation. The PRE program should concentrate on the posterior rotator cuff muscles, because these muscles are responsible for humeral head depression and eccentric contraction to slow the arm down during the pitching act.

Return to throwing should not begin until 5 × 10 repetitions with 3 to 5 pounds is reached with the rotator cuff exercises outlined in this chapter, and restoration of full active range of motion (AROM) has been achieved. Return to throwing should be done using the Interval Throwing Program (Appendix B). The athlete should continue with a maintenance strength program of 5 × 10 repetitions with 5 pounds three times weekly, even after being released for unlimited participation and during the playing season.

Patients who do not respond to conservative care should undergo surgical correction. An acromioplasty is often performed in conjunction with the cuff repair. Rotator cuff tears seen and treated arthroscopically are incomplete tears that are noted on the undersurface of the muscle. Larger lesions may require an open procedure to repair. Many types of procedures can provide access to the rotator cuff for repair. The deltoid-on procedure is recommended to decrease morbidity and promote early range of motion. Tables 11−3 and 11−4 outline rehabilitation program protocols for arthroscopic debridement and open rotator cuff repair, using the deltoid-on surgical procedure. These protocols can easily be adapted to other rotator cuff procedures, if necessary. The use of an abduction pillow (Fig. 11−34) following rotator cuff repair can be used to alleviate stress placed on the cuff repair, because the adducted position causes undue early stress on the repair. Lesion size and extent of the repair determine how long the abduction pillow is used, usually for 2 to 5 weeks. As AROM is restored, the PRE program should focus on posterior cuff and scapular stabilizer muscle strengthening.

Rotator cuff injuries are induced by trauma, overuse, and/or attrition of the cuff. Because the pitching act is so violent and places an enormous amount of tension on the posterior rotator cuff muscles, most cuff lesions occur in pitchers. It has been postulated that chronic tendinitis results in microtrauma to the cuff through the tearing of the cuff fibers with each repeated episode. This gradually results in a weak-

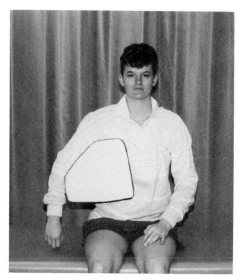

FIGURE 11−34   The use of an abduction pillow following rotator cuff repair can be used to help alleviate stress placed on the repair.

TABLE 11–4   ROTATOR CUFF REPAIR: DELTOID-ON PROCEDURE

I. Immediate postoperative phase
  A. Postoperative day 1: Hospital discharge
    1. Patient immobilization (abduction pillow)
       Sling with arm placed at side of body or 45° to 60° of abduction with neutral rotation (position varies with severity of tear)
    2. Range of motion
       a. Passive range of motion
       b. Rope and pulley
       c. T-bar exercises
       d. Pendulum exercises
       e. Gentle joint mobilization (grades I and II)
       f. Elbow, wrist, and hand range of motion
       g. Cervical range-of-motion exercises to deter neck stiffness
    3. Shoulder elevation, sagittal and scapular planes emphasized. Progress coronal elevation carefully.
       External rotation/internal rotation (ER/IR) (begin 0 to 20° abduction).
    4. Strengthening
       a. Shoulder isometrics as tolerated
       b. Hand putty
    5. Decrease pain/inflammation
       a. Ice 15 to 20 minutes every hour
       b. NSAIDs
       c. Other modalities as needed
II. Early motion phase (postoperative day 4 to week 6)
  A. Hospital discharge to 3 weeks post surgery
    1. Goals
       a. Increase range of motion
       b. Decrease pain/inflammation
       c. Minimize muscular atrophy
    2. Range of motion
       a. Passive range of motion (progress to active assisted range of motion)
       b. Rope and pulley
       c. Shoulder flexion/extension to 90°
       d. Shoulder abduction to 90°
          • Shoulder flexion/extension
          • ER to tolerance with arm abducted to 35°
       f. Pendulum exercises
       g. Joint mobilization (grades I and II) to scapulothoracic, sternoclavicular, and acromioclavicular joints
       h. Continue elbow, wrist, and hand range of motion
    3. Strengthening
       a. Isometrics (submaximal); may augment with electrical stimulation in flexion, abduction, external rotation, and internal rotation
       b. Hand putty
       c. Shoulder shrugs
    4. Decrease pain/inflammation
       a. Ice
       b. Other modalities as needed
  B. Week 3
    1. Goals
       a. Increase range of motion
       b. Promote healing
       c. Regain and improve muscle strength

Table continued on following page

    2. Range of motion
      a. Range-of-motion exercises continued (progress ER/IR range of motion from 40° abduction to 90° abduction)
      b. Continue joint mobilization
    3. Strengthening
      a. Isometrics (submaximal to maximal)
      b. Continue shoulder shrugs
      c. Initiate elbow flexion/extension isotonics
      d. Initiate surgical tubing for ER/IR at 30° abduction
    4. Promotion of healing
      a. Modalities as indicated
      b. Ice after treatment session

III. Intermediate phase (weeks 6 to 10)
    1. Goals
      a. Normalize range of motion
      b. Normalize arthrokinematics
      c. Increase strength/endurance
    2. Criteria to progress to next phase
      a. Normal range of motion
      b. Minimal pain/tenderness
      c. Manual muscle testing score of 4/5 in flexion, ER, IR
  A. Week 6
    1. Range of motion
      a. Continue shoulder range-of-motion exercises with T-bar
    2. Strength
      a. External/internal rotation with tubing
      b. Dumbbell isotonic exercises in shoulder flexion, abduction, extension, ER, and IR
      c. Initiate upper body ergometer (UBE)
      d. Diagonal PNF patterns, manually
      e. Initiate neuromuscular control exercises
      f. Continue joint mobilization (advance grades)
    3. Decrease pain/inflammation
      a. Modalities as needed
  B. Weeks 8 and 9
      a. Continue range-of-motion exercises
    1. Strength
      a. Continue isotonic/tubing exercises for rotator cuff/deltoid muscles
      b. Initiate empty-can exercise
      c. Begin dumbbell program for scapular muscles
      d. Initiate wall push-ups for serratus anterior
      e. Continue PNF patterns
      f. Continue upper extremity endurance exercises
      g. Continue neuromuscular control exercises
    2. Decrease pain/inflammation
      a. Modalities as needed
      b. Ice after treatment session as needed
  C. Week 10 to month 4
      a. Advance all exercises to tolerance

IV. Advanced strengthening phase (months 4 to 6)
  A. Dynamic strengthening phase
    1. Goals
      a. Normalization of muscle strength/power/endurance

Table continued on following page

TABLE 11–4   ROTATOR CUFF REPAIR: DELTOID-ON PROCEDURE (*Continued*)

        b. Improve neuromuscular control
        c. Prepare patient/athlete to return to preinjury activity level
  B. Criteria to progress to phase IV
        a. Full, pain-free range of motion
        b. No pain or tenderness
        c. Strength 70% to 80% vs contralateral side
    1. Range of motion
        a. Continue range-of-motion exercises as needed to maintain full range of motion
        b. Self capsular stretches
        c. T-bar (flexion, ER at 90°, IR at 90°)
    2. Strengthening
        a. Initiate tubing exercises
            (1) Diagonal patterns
            (2) Biceps
            (3) External/internal rotation
            (4) Scapulothoracic
        b. Initiate isokinetic exercises
        c. Continue isotonics
            (1) Deltoid
            (2) Supraspinatus
            (3) Triceps
        d. Continue PNF diagonals manually or with tubing
  C. Month 5
    1. Strengthening
        a. Continue isokinetic exercises
        b. Continue dumbbell program with emphasis on eccentrics and supraspinatus/deltoid muscles
        c. Initiate plyometrics for rotator cuff (slow/fast sets, ER/IR, 90/90)
        d. Continue PNF diagonals with tubing or isokinetics
        e. Medicine ball exercises (progress from below shoulder level to overhead)
        f. Isokinetic testing (shoulder strength should be 80% before sport-specific activities are started)
    2. Neuromuscular control
        a. Continue exercises for months 1 to 4
        b. Isokinetic examination fulfills criteria to throw
        c. Pass clinical examination
        d. No pain/tenderness
    4. Initiate interval program
    5. Upper extremity strengthening and stretching continued on a maintenance basis

ened cuff mechanism, allowing for abnormal upward diplacement of the humeral head, vascular compromise of the cuff tendon, poor ability of the cuff to heal itself, a subacromial inflammatory process propagating secondary bony and soft tissue changes caused by poor shoulder mechanics, and ultimately partial- and full-thickness rotator cuff lesions.

Anterior Instability

Shoulder instability is a common clinical problem, with anterior instability the most common. The arthrokinematics of the glenohumeral joint itself predisposes it to instability. The glenoid cavity is relatively small and shallow, the glenoid fossa faces laterally and forward, and the external rotators have an advantage over the subscapularis muscle. All these factors combine to make the shoulder susceptible to dislocations in the forward, medial, and inferior directions.[16, 40, 76] Anterior glenohumeral instability can be divided into acute traumatic dislocation and recurrent dislocation or subluxation. Most acute anterior dislocations occur with the arm abducted to 90° and externally rotated. This can occur when attempting an arm tackle in football, or an abnormal force to an arm that is executing a throw can produce a sequence of events that result in a shoulder dislocation or subluxation. The dislocated shoulder is characterized by a flattened deltoid contour, inability to move the arm, and severe pain. With this injury the head of the humerus is forced out of its articulation, past the glenoid labrum, and then upward to rest under the coracoid process.[2]

The dislocated shoulder is usually readily detectable, but the subluxing shoulder can be more subtle and may be overlooked. Anterior subluxation of the glenohumeral joint may develop without a history of trauma and is most common in throwers. The subluxing shoulder is often referred to as the "dead arm syndrome," because it is characterized by a loss in shoulder strength and power. Rowe and Zarins[74] have reported that, in 60 shoulders with dead arm syndrome, 26 patients were aware of shoulder subluxation and 32 patients were not aware of its occurrence. Clinically, the athlete presents with soreness over the anterior aspect of the shoulder and reports a reproduction of the signs and symptoms in the cocking and/or acceleration phase of the throwing act. Athletes may also report a loss in shoulder strength and power and a feeling of clicking or sliding within the shoulder.

Several mechanisms of injury exist to explain the insidious onset of anterior instability. One of the most prevalent views is that, in the cocking phase of throwing, external rotation places repeated stress on the anterior capsule and results in capsule attenuation and ultimately anterior instability.

Weakness of the scapula stabilizers is also believed to contribute to anterior instability.[44] The function of the scapula rotators (e.g., trapezius, rhomboids, serratus anterior) is to place the glenoid in the optimal position for the activities being performed, the rotator cuff seeks to stabilize the humeral head, and the glenohumeral ligament, particularly the inferior aspect, provides a static restraint at the margins of the joint.[44] Damage to the static restraints (gradual attenuation) results in instability, causing asynchronous firing of the scapula rotators and rotator cuff muscles. Greater stress is placed on the rotator cuff muscles in an attempt to stabilize the humeral head, producing rotator cuff damage and leading to rotator cuff impingement (described earlier). Thus, Jobe and associates[44] have reported that impingement problems are secondary to the primary lesion, glenohumeral instability. Support for this theory has been given by Glousman and colleagues,[31] who studied the throwing shoulder with glenohumeral instability using dynamic electromyographic analysis. They reported that a marked reduction in activity in the pectoralis major, subscapularis, and latissimus dorsi added to the anterior instability by decreasing the normal internal rotation force that is needed during the late cocking and acceleration phases. Diminished activity of the serratus anterior may decrease protraction of the scapula, causing the glenoid fossa to remain behind the forward flexing humerus during the late cocking phase. Diminished scapula protraction increases anterior laxity because of increased stress of the humeral head on the anterior part of the glenoid labrum and capsule.

Finally, it has been postulated[30, 44] that weakness of the posterior cuff muscles, attrition or attenuation of the anterior capsule, and/or hypertrophy of the internal rotators may result in excessive anterior displacement of the humeral head in the early acceleration phase of throwing. Because of the stresses placed on the posterior cuff to decelerate the arm, posterior shoulder pain is common with anterior subluxation as a result of the checkrein effect of the posterior structures, and can lead to a misdiagnosis.[70] Moreover, damage to the infraspinatus may aggravate the instability by inhibiting contraction of the infraspinatus.[17]

Shoulder instability can be associated with an anterior glenoid labrum tear as the humeral head slips past the anterior aspect of the labrum and then reduces itself. A small portion of the anterior labrum can be torn, resulting in joint crepitus and catching. Additionally, Hill–Sachs and Bankart lesions (Fig. 11–35) are common with anterior instability, and their presence can be used to confirm this injury. Bankart lesions result from an avulsion of the capsule and labrum from the glenoid rim. A Hill–Sachs lesion is a bony injury involving the humeral head as it strikes the rim of the glenoid at the time of dislocation.[73]

Whether the lesion is a subluxation or an outright dislocation with a reduction, conservative care should be attempted first. The success of conservative care is variable.[3, 4, 35] It should initially concentrate on decreasing the inflammation and pain, with gradual restoration of full shoulder motion. After normal motion is restored, an aggressive shoulder flexibility program is contraindicated because of the already present attenuated tissues. A PRE rotator cuff program should be implemented, concentrating on the posterior cuff muscles and scapula stabilizers.

If conservative treatment fails, several operative procedures can be used to restore function. These attempt to restore static restraints or to compensate for the insufficiency in static structures with a dynamic (muscle transfer) procedure. The most commonly used dynamic repair procedures are the Bristow, Magnuson–Stack, and Putti–Platt. The Bristow procedure involves transfer of the coracoid process with its

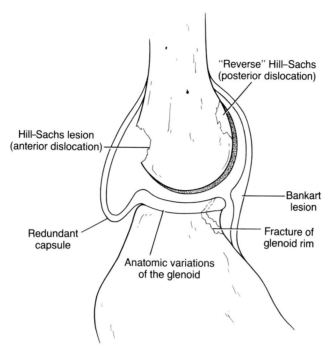

FIGURE 11–35 Anatomic lesions produced from shoulder instability. (From Rowe, C.R. (1988): The Shoulder. New York, Churchill Livingston, p. 177.)

tendon attachments through the subscapularis muscle to the neck of the glenoid. The coracoid process is held to the glenoid with a screw, producing a bony block to deter anterior subluxation of the humeral head. The Magnuson–Stack procedure involves detachment of the subscapularis muscle from the lesser tubercle and its lateral transfer across the bicipital groove to the shaft of the humerus. The Putti–Platt technique attempts to shorten the subscapularis muscle. There are many modifications of each of these techniques, but the basic principle remains the same. The major drawback to these dynamic procedures is the limitation imposed on external rotation. The Bristow and Magnuson–Stack procedures result in approximately a 10° loss in external rotation,[1, 14, 59] with as much as a 20° limitation on external rotation resulting from use of the Putti–Platt technique.[22]

The most common static reparative techniques include the Bankart and capsular shift (capsulorrhaphy) procedures, which address the glenohumeral ligament as the cause of instability. If a Bankart lesion is present the Bankart technique may be chosen, because it not only corrects the attenuated capsule but also the Bankart lesion. With this procedure the avulsed bone and capsule are reattached to the glenoid labrum and the redundancy of the capsule is taken up, resulting in a tighter anterior capsule. If no Bankart lesion is present the redundancy in the capsule may be taken up and attached at the capsule–labrum junction.

Because of the limitation on external rotation imposed by the use of dynamic repair procedures, static repairs are preferred for the throw-

TABLE 11–5   PROTOCOL: BRISTOW PROCEDURE

I. Preoperative instruction
   A. Explain that the sling is used for the first day after surgery for comfort, and then the athlete is weaned out of it.
   B. Instruct in circumduction and exercises (to be performed frequently).
   C. Explain about application of ice to shoulder at 20-minute intervals and as needed for pain and soreness.
   D. Explain rehabilitation progression.
II. Exercises
   A. Postoperative day 1
      1. Hand and elbow
         a. Putty
         b. Wrist ROM
         c. Elbow ROM
      2. Shoulder isometrics (with 0° shoulder adduction)
         a. Flexion
         b. Abduction
         c. Extension
         d. External rotation
         e. Internal rotation
      3. Shoulder ROM initiated as tolerated
         a. Circumduction ("saws, swings")
         b. Supine flexion
         c. Supine abduction
         d. Supine 0–90° external rotation
         e. Supine 0–90° internal rotation
         f. Supine horizontal adduction
         g. Rope-and-pulley in flexion and abduction
         h. Shoulder shrugs
      4. Gradually progress to 5 × 10, 2 or 3 times daily.
      5. Use ice pre- and postexercise for 20 minutes.
   B. Intermediate phase (weeks 2 to 8)
      1. Continue with above exercises twice daily.
      2. Add following exercises, as tolerated:
         a. External rotation stretch in 90–90° position, as tolerated
         b. UBE
         c. Shoulder flexion
         d. Shoulder abduction
         e. Supraspinatus
         f. Prone horizontal abduction
         g. Prone shoulder extension
         h. Prone external rotation
         i. Shoulder shrugs
         j. Biceps curl
         k. Triceps extension
         l. Rope-and-pulley in flexion and abduction, as tolerated.
      3. May progress PRE, as tolerated.
      4. Continue flexibility at 10 to 20 repetitions.
   C. Advanced phase (months 2 to 3)
      1. If progressing well, decrease program to maintenance 3 times weekly.
      2. Begin progressive return to functional weight lifting and activities.
      3. Begin eccentric shoulder program and isokinetics.
      4. Begin upper extremity plyometrics.
      5. Begin appropriate interval activity program if appropriate (Appendix B).

ing athlete, in whom restoration of full shoulder arthrokinematics is more likely. Some surgeons have experimented with arthroscopic stapling techniques to tighten the anterior capsule, but these procedures have met with only limited success.

Treatment following repair for anterior instability is similar whether a static or dynamic repair is performed. The main difference between these techniques is that, with dynamic repairs, external rotation can begin somewhat sooner than with a static procedure. Table 11–5 outlines a rehabilitation protocol for those athletes undergoing a Bristow repair, and Table 11–6 outlines a rehabilitation protocol following a capsular shift procedure.

Posterior Instability

Posterior dislocation or subluxation is not as common as its anterior counterpart, but it does occur. Usually, posterior subluxation results from overuse, which stretches out the posterior capsule; from one traumatic episode that results in subluxation with stretching of the posterior capsule, which recurs with repeated use of the shoulder (e.g., a pitcher stresses the posterior capsule repeatedly in the follow-through phase of throwing); or from a posteriorly directed force on the adducted, internally rotated arm, with the hand at a position below shoulder level. The diagnosis is frequently missed because physical

---

TABLE 11–6   PROTOCOL: ANTERIOR CAPSULAR SHIFT

I. Preoperative instructions
   A. Explain that athlete must wear immobilizer to sleep for 4 weeks, and then the athlete will be out of the immobilizer into a sling during the daytime as soon as possible. The sling should be used for 3 to 4 weeks.
   B. Stress *no* overhead activity for 6 weeks.
   C. Discuss rehabilitation program and progression.
II. Phase I (weeks 0 to 6)
   A. Weeks 0 to 2
      1. Use modalities (e.g., ice, electrical stimulation) for pain.
      2. Immediate postoperative hand and elbow exercises:
         a. Gripping with putty
         b. Wrist range of motion
         c. Elbow range of motion
         d. Goal: obtain full wrist and elbow range of motion on first postoperative day.
      3. Initiate following exercises:
         a. Pendulum
         b. Rope-and-pulley, active assisted
            (1) Shoulder flexion to 90°
            (2) Shoulder abduction to 60°
         c. T-bar exercises
            (1) External rotation to 45° with arm abducted at 40°
            (2) Shoulder flexion and extension
            (3) AROM—cervical spine
            (4) Isometrics
               (a) Flexion
               (b) Extension
               (c) Abduction

Table continued on following page

    (d) External rotation
    (e) Internal rotation
   d. Goal: 90° flexion, 45° abduction, 45° external rotation, active assisted
  B. Weeks 2 to 4
   1. All exercises performed to tolerance—take to point of pain and/or resistance and hold.
   2. Exercises:
    a. External rotation to 60° with 90° of shoulder abduction with T-bar
    b. Internal rotation to 65° with 90° of shoulder abduction with T-bar
    c. Shoulder flexion and extension to tolerance with T-bar
    d. Shoulder abduction to tolerance with T-bar
    e. Shoulder horizontal abduction and adduction with T-bar
    f. Rope-and-pulley in flexion and abduction, as tolerated
    g. Continue isometrics
    h. External and internal rotation with tubing at 0° shoulder abduction
   3. Begin PRE with elbow program.
   4. Begin joint mobilization techniques.
  C. Weeks 4 to 6
   1. Continue all exercises listed above to tolerance, except:
    a. External rotation to 75° at 90° of shoulder abduction with T-bar
    b. External rotation to 40° at 30° of shoulder abduction
    c. Internal rotation to 80° at 90° of shoulder abduction
III. Phase II (weeks 6 to 10)
 A. Weeks 6 to 8
  1. Range-of-motion exercises:
   a. Continue all T-bar exercises listed above.
   b. Gradually increase ROM to full ROM by week 8.
  2. Begin strengthening exercises (progress 0 to 5 pounds):
   a. Shoulder flexion
   b. Shoulder abduction
   c. Supraspinatus
   d. Prone extension
   e. Prone horizontal abduction
   f. Prone horizontal abduction at 100°
   g. Side-lying external rotation
   h. Biceps curls
   i. Triceps curls
   j. Shoulder shrugs
   k. Progressive push-ups
   l. Continue tubing at 0° of abduction for external and internal rotation
  3. Begin neuromuscular control exercises for scapular stabilizers.
 B. Weeks 8 to 10
  1. Continue all ROM and strengthening exercises listed above.
  2. Initiate tubing exercises for rhomboids, latissimus dorsi, biceps, and triceps.
IV. Phase III (weeks 11 to 16)
 A. Weeks 11 to 13
  1. Continue PRE program.
  2. Continue tubing program.
  3. Begin shoulder eccentric program.
  4. Begin tubing in diagonal patterns.
  5. Begin isokinetic exercise, as tolerated.
  6. Initiate high-speed tubing exercise, as tolerated.
 B. Weeks 14 to 16
  1. Continue all exercises above.
  2. Emphasize gradual return to recreational activities.
 Phase IV (weeks 18 to 26)
 A. Maintenance PRE, tubing, and ROM programs
 B. Isokinetic testing (18 to 20 weeks)
 C. Begin Interval Programs between weeks 20 and 24 (see Appendix B)

findings are not as dramatic as with an anterior dislocation. The inability to rotate the arm externally, the inability to supinate the forearm fully with the arm flexed forward and, possibly, glenohumeral subluxation with horizontal adduction are indicative of posterior instability.

Again, conservative treatment should be attempted first, with concentration on the posterior rotator cuff musculature. Strengthening of the posterior rotator cuff should be accomplished without placing the shoulder in the subluxed position.[65] An aggressive shoulder flexibility regimen is contraindicated because of the attenuated tissues. Engle and Canner[27] have reported success with a rehabilitation program that emphasizes proprioceptive neuromuscular facilitation (PNF) exercise techniques centered around development of the posterior cuff muscles.

Surgical management of those athletes who do not respond to conservative care is controversial. The results following surgical reconstruction for posterior instability have been disappointing.[33, 74] Surgical techniques include shifting of the posterior capsule (capsulorrhaphy) or a posterior osteotomy to help prevent dislocation.

Rehabilitation following posterior capsulorrhaphy is similar to the anterior capsulorrhaphy program except for the following: (1) no forward flexion or horizontal adduction for 4 to 6 weeks to avoid stress on the repaired capsule; (2) restoration of internal rotation should also proceed slowly—internal rotation in the 90–90° position should not begin until week 6 after surgery. Table 11–7 outlines a rehabilitation protocol following a posterior glenoid osteotomy. As rehabilitation progresses, emphasis is placed on the posterior cuff muscles and scapula stabilizers.

Multidirectional Instability

Athletes who are multidirectionally unstable pose a difficult problem, not only to the clinician but also to the surgeon. These individuals usually have a lax capsule in all directions and typically have generalized ligamentous laxity.[85] With evaluation under anesthesia, some surgeons elect to repair the most prominent instability and carry out other procedures at a later date.

Conservative care addresses the laxity in the muscles, ligaments, and capsule around the shoulder. PNF techniques could prove beneficial with this pathology, because neuromusucular control is vital in attempting to restore function. Flexibility exercises are definitely contraindicated, and exercises should focus on muscle strengthening.

Surgical intervention is controversial, with no satisfactory technique available at present. Bigliani[8] has addressed this problem with an inferior capsule shift that is believed to correct redundancy on all three sides: anterior, posterior, and inferior; however, there should be no hurry in regaining forward flexion, because the humerus must sublux posteriorly for forward flexion to be achieved and may damage the repair. Initial isometrics and hand–elbow exercises are recommended, with a gradual progression to range-of-motion (ROM) exercises by weeks 6 to 8. As ROM is restored and active motion becomes equal

**TABLE 11-7   PROTOCOL: POSTERIOR
GLENOID OSTEOTOMY**

I. Preoperative instructions
   A. Sling is to be used for 2 weeks after surgery.
   B. Circumduction exercises are performed frequently (1 minute/hour, as tolerated).
   C. Absolutely no straight forward flexion, internal rotation, or horizontal adduction
      should be carried out for 6 weeks.
   D. Perform exercise program two or three times daily.
   E. Explain about application of ice to shoulder at 20-minute intervals as needed for
      pain and soreness.
II. Exercises
   A. Initial phase (postoperative days 1 to 6)
      1. Hand and elbow:
         a. Putty
         b. Wrist ROM
         c. Elbow ROM
      2. Shoulder isometrics (with 0° shoulder abduction)—initiate as tolerated
         a. Flexion
         b. Abduction
         c. External rotation
      3. Shoulder range of motion—initiate as tolerated
         a. Circumduction
         b. Supine abduction to 90°
         c. Supine 0–90° external rotation
         d. Active assisted rope and pulley in abduction to 90° (*no* forward flexion)
      4. Shoulder isometrics—multiple planes from 0–90° abduction
      5. May progress light progressive resistive exercise with side-lying external rotation
         and biceps curls 1 to 5 pounds
      6. Gradual progression to 5 × 10, three times daily
   B. Intermediate phase (6 to 12 weeks)
      1. Shoulder ROM (may progress shoulder range of motion in all planes)
         a. Supine flexion
         b. Supine abduction
         c. Supine 90–90° external rotation
         d. Gradual supine internal rotation
         e. Gradual horizontal adduction
         f. Rope-and-pulley in flexion and abduction
      2. Initiate the following exercises after full active assisted exercise is achieved:
         a. Shoulder flexion
         b. Shoulder abduction
         c. Prone horizontal abduction
         d. Prone horizontal abduction at 100°
         e. Prone external rotation
         f. Prone extension
   C. Late phase (12 weeks)
      1. Begin PRE maintenance program. Continue with PRE program three times
         weekly.
      2. Begin progressive return to functional weight lifting and activities.

bilaterally, a PRE program may be initiated. Forward flexion may not be initiated for 6 to 12 weeks following surgery, depending on the amount of instability.

Glenoid Labrum Tears

Most glenoid labrum tears are the result of shoulder instability. The mechanism of tearing the rim of the glenoid is a forceful subluxation of the humeral head over the fibrocartilaginous labrum. If anterior instability is the primary cause of the labrum tear, simple resection of the torn labrum does not correct the ultimate problem, and additional labrum tears are probable as the humeral head is subluxed.

Isolated labrum tears can occur in the absence of anterior instability, such as in the pitcher because of the high-speed rotational velocities generated, which jeopardize the articulating surfaces.[58] If the rotator cuff is too weak to stabilize the humeral head, articulation may occur on the glenoid labrum rather than in the center of the glenoid fossa. Most isolated labrum tears occur during the acceleration and deceleration phases of throwing.

Labrum resections can be performed arthroscopically and result in minimal postoperative morbidity. Rehabilitation following arthroscopic resection of the glenoid labrum can proceed according to the rehabilitation program outlined in Table 11-3. The athlete can begin the interval throwing program at 4 to 6 weeks following arthroscopic glenoid labrum resections.

Acromioclavicular Separation

Injuries involving the acromioclavicular (AC) joint can occur insidiously, because of activities requiring repetitive overhead activity; acutely from direct trauma, in which the athlete falls on the tip of the shoulder and depresses the acromion process inferiorly; or from a fall on the outstretched arm, in which the forces are transmitted superiorly through the acromion process. The extent of AC separation depends on whether the acromioclavicular ligaments are traumatized or the main stabilizing coracoacromial ligaments are damaged. Neviaser[64] has classified AC joint injuries according to the amount of displacement. Grade I sprains are characterized by an incomplete injury to the supporting ligaments of the joint, without any degree of displacement. A grade II injury is identified by a rupture of the acromioclavicular ligaments with a sprain of the coracoclavicular ligaments. There is some displacement between the clavicular and acromial articular surfaces. A grade III injury results in no contact between the articular surfaces of the clavicle and acromion because of rupture of both the acromioclavicular and coracoclavicular ligaments. Grade III injuries may be further divided into subcategories.[64]

Treatment for grades I and II injuries is conservative, but grade III treatment is still controversial. Many physicians elect to treat grade III injuries nonoperatively, and believe that athletes do better than if they undergo a surgical procedure.[44, 64] A number of surgical measures are available, depending on the extent of damage. These include the following: (1) stabilizing the clavicle to the coracoid process with a screw; (2) transarticular fixation of the AC joint with pins following reduction; (3) resection of the outer end of the clavicle; and (4) transposing the coracoacromial ligament to the top of the AC joint. Biomechanical studies[28] have indicated that the superior acromioclavicular ligament is the most important for stabilizing the AC joint for normal daily activities. The conoid ligament is the most important for supporting the joint against significant injury.

Rehabilitation following first- and second-degree AC separations consists of progressing motion as tolerated and beginning a PRE program when active range of motion is equal bilaterally. Modalities may be used in the early stages of healing to help decrease inflammation and pain. Third-degree separations treated conservatively usually require 4 to 6 weeks of immobilization, with a gradual progression of motion and strengthening exercises following immobilization. Pendulum, elbow ROM exercises, isometrics in all planes, and rope-and-pulley exercises to 90° of flexion and abduction, as tolerated, can be initiated after immobilization. Precautions in rehabilitation following a surgical repair of the AC joint are similar to those following conservative care of grade III injuries, including limitation of abduction and flexion to 90° for approximately 3 to 4 weeks. Pendulum and isometric exercises in all planes are encouraged in the initial stages of rehabilitation. Range of motion is progressed to 90° in all planes, as tolerated after 4 weeks. Rehabilitation should concentrate on strengthening the rotator cuff and scapula stabilizers and on restoring neuromuscular control and arthrokinematics, not unlike rehabilitation following other shoulder injuries.

The shoulder joint's mobility comes at the expense of stability. Shoulder injuries can be induced acutely through traumatic injuries, or onset can be insidious as a result of repetitive stresses over time. Overuse injuries to the shoulder are common in athletes whose endeavors require repetitive overhead activities, particularly pitchers. Most shoulder injuries occur during the acceleration and deceleration phases of throwing. The most common shoulder injuries include rotator cuff tendinitis or tears, impingement syndrome, shoulder instability (most commonly anterior), and acromioclavicular joint injuries.

Rehabilitation of these injuries should concentrate on developing the posterior rotator cuff musculature. More importantly, those athletes who are susceptible to shoulder pathology should be on an off-season shoulder flexibility and rotator cuff strengthening program to help deter shoulder problems. They should continue this stretching and strengthening program two or three times weekly during the season. Preventative and postinjury exercises should also attempt to strengthen the scapular stabilizers that help orient the glenoid fossa with the humeral head to maintain stability. Weakness in the scapula stabilizers can predispose the athlete to anterior instability problems.

Following shoulder surgery or injury, emphasis should be placed on addressing the inflammation process and restoring motion. After initiation of a rotator cuff strengthening program, PNF techniques may be implemented to help restore neuromuscular control. In the late phases of rehabilitation, eccentric and isokinetic exercises may begin, followed by high-speed surgical tubing exercises in sports-specific planes.

The goals of shoulder rehabilitation are to prevent injuries through off-season and in-season flexibility and strengthening programs, strengthen scapular stabilizers, and develop neuromuscular control in the shoulder girdle. It is through proximal stability that distal mobility can be achieved and injuries prevented.

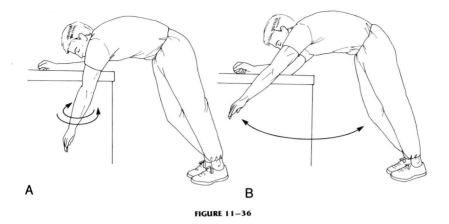

FIGURE 11–36

THERAPEUTIC SHOULDER EXERCISE PROGRAM

Range-of-Motion Exercises

Circumduction Pendulum Swings The athlete leans over the table, supporting the body with the uninvolved arm and allowing the involved arm to hang straight down in a relaxed position. The athlete gently swings the arm in circles clockwise and counterclockwise (Fig. 11–36A), in a pendulum motion forward and backward (Fig. 11–36B), and side to side, repeating 1 set of 10 repetitions each and progressing 5 sets of 10 repetitions each, as tolerated.

Supine Flexion The athlete lies on the back, grips the bar in both hands with the arms straight (Fig. 11–37A), raises both arms overhead as far as possible (Fig. 11–37B), and holds for 5 seconds before returning to the starting position. This is repeated 10 to 15 times. This may be performed with the thumb up as an alternate method, particularly if impingement syndrome is present.

Supine Abduction The athlete lies on the back with the involved arm at the side of the body, straightens the involved arm, and rotates the hand outward as far as possible. Then the athlete slides the arm along the table, bed, or floor, moving the arm away from the side as far as possible and using a T-bar to help pull (Fig. 11–38A and B). This is

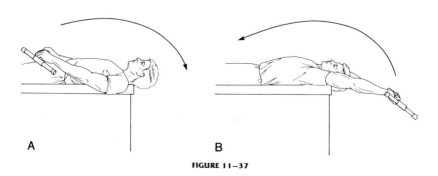

FIGURE 11–37

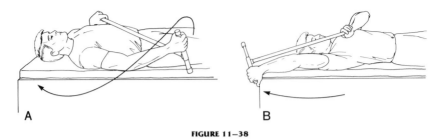

FIGURE 11–38

held for 5 seconds before returning to the starting position, and repeated 10 to 15 times.

Supine External Rotation

INITIAL EXERCISE   The athlete lies on the back with the involved arm out to the side of the body at 90° and the elbow bent at 90°. Gripping the T-bar in the hand of the involved arm and keeping the elbow in a fixed position (Fig. 11–39*A*), the athlete uses the opposite arm to push the involved arm into external rotation using the T-bar (Fig. 11–39*B*). This is held for 5 seconds before returning to the starting position and repeated 10 to 15 times. A towel can be placed under the arm to stretch in the scapular plane.

PROGRESSED EXERCISE   As shoulder abduction range of motion progresses, the athlete performs an external rotation stretch at 135° (Fig. 11–40) and full abduction (Fig. 11–41). This is repeated 10 to 15 times.

Supine Internal Rotation   The athlete lies on the back with the involved arm out to the side of the body at 90° and the elbow bent at 90°. Gripping the T-bar in the hand of the involved arm and keeping the elbow in a fixed position, the athlete uses the uninvolved arm to push the involved arm into internal rotation with a T-bar (Fig. 11–42). This is held for 5 seconds before returning to the starting position, and repeated 10 to 15 times.

Horizontal Adduction Stretch   The athlete grasps the elbow of the involved arm with the opposite hand and pulls the arm across the front of the chest (Fig. 11–43), holding for 5 seconds. The athlete then relaxes and repeats 10 to 15 times.

Inferior Capsular Stretch   The athlete holds the involved arm

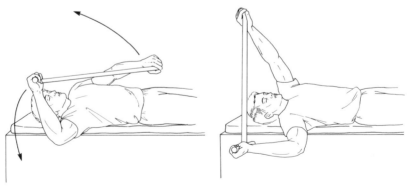

FIGURE 11–39

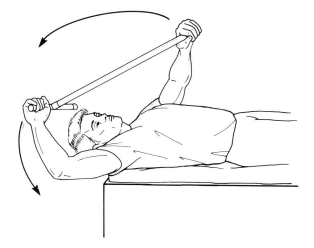

FIGURE 11—40

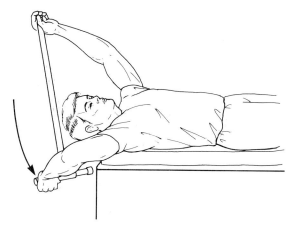

FIGURE 11—41

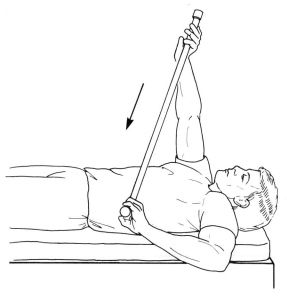

FIGURE 11—42

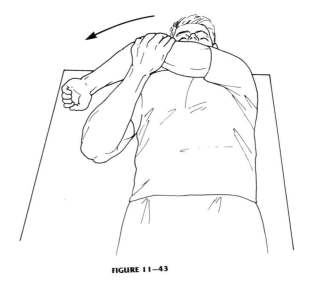

FIGURE 11–43

overhead with the elbow bent (Fig. 11–44*A*) and, using the uninvolved arm, stretches the arm further overhead (Fig. 11–44*B*) until a stretching sensation is felt. This is held for 5 seconds and repeated 10 to 15 times.

Anterior Capsular Stretch   The athlete stands in a doorway with the elbow straight and the shoulder abducted to 90° and externally rotated. With pressure on the arm, the arm is forced back to stretch the front of the shoulder (Fig. 11–45). This is held for 5 seconds and repeated 10 to 15 times.

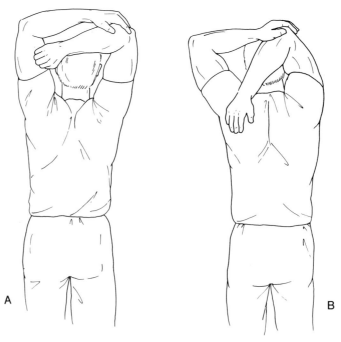

A

B

FIGURE 11–44

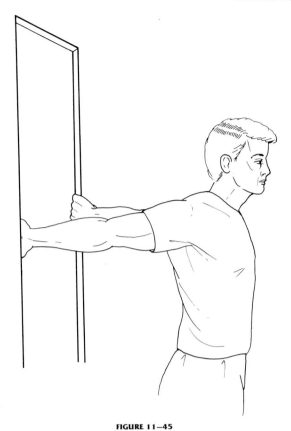

FIGURE 11–45

External Rotation (0° Abduction)   The athlete lies on the back with the involved arm against the body and the elbow bent at 90°. Gripping the T-bar handle and with the uninvolved arm, the involved shoulder is pushed into external rotation with the T-bar. This is held for 5 seconds before returning to the starting position and repeated. A towel should be placed under the arm to stretch in the scapular plane.

Rope and Pulley   The overhead rope and pulley should be positioned in a doorway. The athlete sits in a chair with the back against the door, directly underneath the pulley.

ACTIVE ASSISTED FLEXION   With the elbow straight and the back of the hand facing upward, the involved arm is raised out to the front of the body as high as possible (Fig. 11–46A), assisting as needed by pulling with the involved arm and holding for 5 seconds. The arm is lowered slowly, using the uninvolved arm to control lowering as needed. The athlete repeats 1 set of 10 repetitions, progressing to 5 sets of 10 repetitions as tolerated.

ACTIVE ASSISTED ABDUCTION   With the elbow straight and the hand rotated outward as far as possible, the involved arm is raised to the side of the body as high as possible (Fig. 11–46B), assisting as needed by pulling with the uninvolved arm and holding for 5 seconds. The arm is lowered slowly using the uninvolved arm to control lowering as needed. The athlete repeats 1 set of 10 repetitions, progressing to 5 sets of 10 repetitions as tolerated.

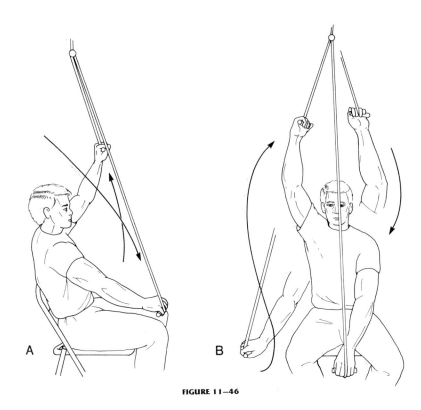

FIGURE 11—46

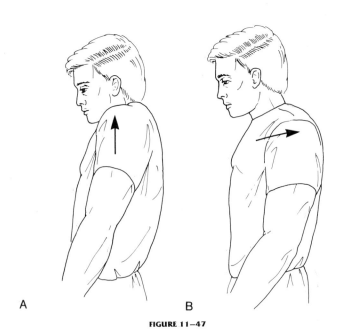

FIGURE 11—47

Progressive Resistance Program

Shoulder Shrugs   The athlete stands with the arms by the side, lifts the shoulders up to the ears, holds for 2 seconds (Fig. 11–47A), pulls the shoulders back, and pinches the shoulder blades together (Fig. 11–47B). This is held for 2 seconds and then the shoulders are relaxed and the exercise repeated.

Shoulder Flexion   The athlete stands with the elbow straight and the back of the hand facing upward, raising the involved arm out to the front of the body as high as possible (Fig. 11–48). This is held for 2 seconds and then the arm is slowly lowered. This may be performed with the thumb up as an alternate method, particularly if impingement syndrome is present.

Shoulder Abduction   The athlete stands with the elbow straight and the hand rotated outward as far as possible, raising the involved arm to the side of body as high as possible (Fig. 11–49). This is held for 2 seconds and then the arm is slowly lowered.

Supraspinatus ("Empty Can")   The athlete stands with the elbow straight and the hand rotated inward as far as possible, raising the arm to parallel to the floor at a 30° angle to the body (Fig. 11–50). This is held for 2 seconds and the arm is slowly lowered.

Prone Horizontal Abduction   The athlete lies on the table on the stomach with the involved arm hanging straight to the floor. With the hand rotated outward as far as possible, the arm is raised out to the side,

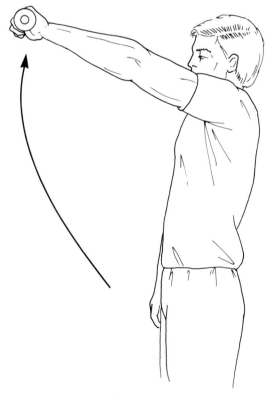

FIGURE 11–48

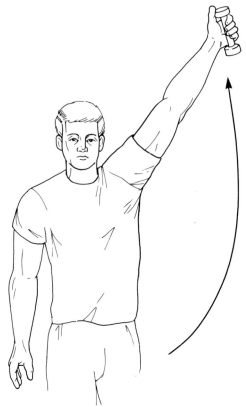

FIGURE 11–49

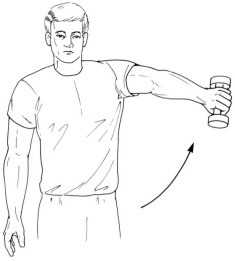

FIGURE 11–50

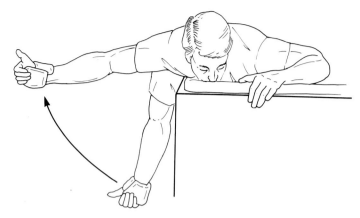

FIGURE 11-51

parallel to the floor (Fig. 11–51). This is held for 2 seconds and then the arm is slowly lowered.

Prone Horizontal Abduction (100°)   The athlete lies on the table on the stomach with the involved arm hanging straight to the floor. With the hand rotated outward as far as possible and the shoulder at approximately 100° of abduction, the arm is raised out to the side, parallel to the floor (Fig. 11–52). This is held for 2 seconds and then the arm is slowly lowered.

Shoulder Extension   The athlete lies on the table on the stomach with the involved arm hanging straight to the floor. With the hand rotated outward as far as possible, the arm is raised straight back into extension as far as possible (Fig. 11–53). When lifting the arm straight back the athlete continues to rotate the extremity externally as far as possible through the entire range of motion. This is held for 2 seconds and then the arm is slowly lowered.

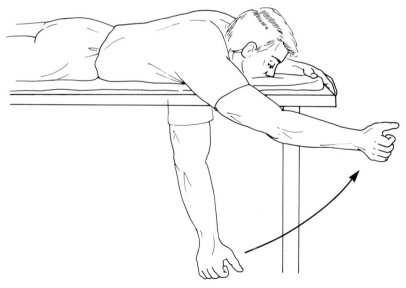

FIGURE 11-52

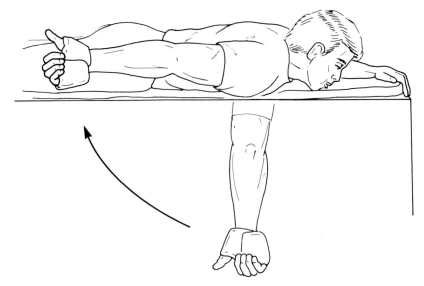

FIGURE 11–53

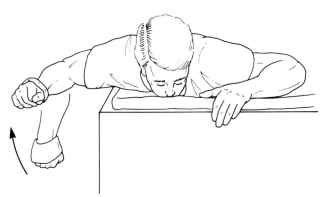

FIGURE 11–54

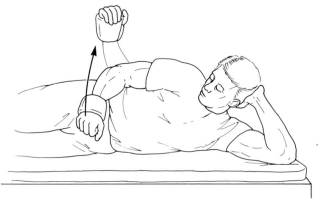

FIGURE 11–55

90–90° Degree External Rotation   The athlete lies on the table on the stomach with the shoulder abducted at 90° and the arm supported on the table with the elbow bent at 90°. Keeping shoulder and elbow fixed, the arm is rotated into external rotation (Fig. 11–54). This is held for 2 seconds and then the arm is slowly lowered.

Side-Lying External Rotation   The athlete lies on the uninvolved side with the involved arm at the side of the body and the elbow bent at 90°. Keeping the elbow of the involved arm fixed to the side, the arm is rotated into external rotation (Fig. 11–55). This is held for 2 seconds, and then the arm is slowly lowered.

Optional Progressive Resistance Exercise Program

Biceps Curl   The athlete supports the involved arm with the opposite hand and bends the elbow to full flexion. This is held for 2 seconds and then the arm is extended completely (Fig. 11–56).

French Curl (Triceps)   The athlete raises the involved arm overhead, providing support at the elbow with the opposite hand, and straightens the arm overhead (Fig. 11–57). This is held for 2 seconds and then the arm is slowly lowered.

Sitting Dip   The athlete sits on the edge of the chair, grips the sides of the chair with the hands, straightens the arms, and lifts the buttocks off the chair seat (Fig. 11–58). This is held in isometric contraction for 5 seconds and then the body is lowered, followed by relaxation.

Progressive Push-Up   The athlete starts with a push-up into the wall, gradually progressing to the tabletop (Fig. 11–59) and then to the floor, as tolerated.

External Rotation at 0° Abduction   Standing with the elbow fixed at the side, the elbow at 90° of flexion, and the involved arm across the front of the body, the athlete grips the tubing handle while the other end of the tubing is fixed (Fig. 11–60A), and pulls out with the arm

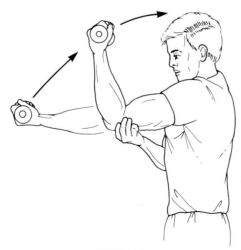

FIGURE 11–56

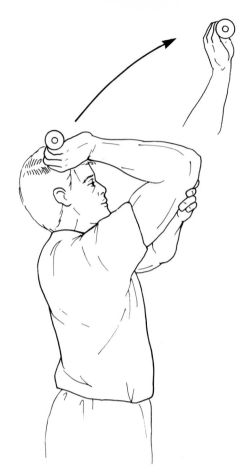

FIGURE 11–57

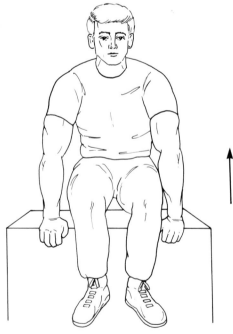

FIGURE 11–58

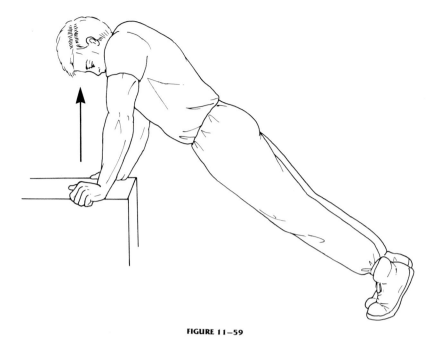

FIGURE 11–59

while keeping the elbow at the side (Fig. 11–60B). The tubing is returned slowly and with control.

Internal Rotation at 0° Abduction   Standing with the elbow at the side fixed at 90° and the shoulder rotated out, the athlete grips the tubing handle while the other end of the tubing is fixed (Fig. 11–61A) and pulls the arm across the body, keeping the elbow at the side (Fig. 11–61B). The tubing is returned slowly and with control.

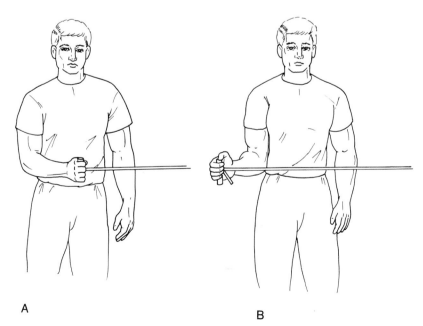

A   B

FIGURE 11–60

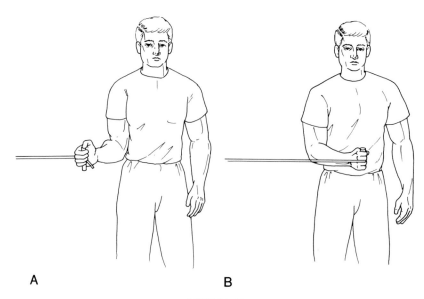

A   B

FIGURE 11–61

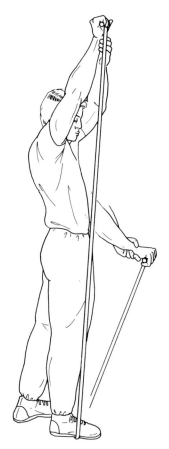

FIGURE 11–62

Eccentric Shoulder Program

Standing Flexion   The athlete stands with the tubing securely in the hand and the opposite end under the same foot of the involved side, controlling tension. Assisting with the opposite hand, the arm is lifted up and forward, in front of the body to the end point (Fig. 11–62), returning to starting position with a slow 5 count.

Standing Abduction   The athlete stands with the tubing securely in the hand and the opposite end under the same foot of the involved side, controlling tension. Assisting with the opposite hand, the arm is lifted outward away from the body to the end point (Fig. 11–63), returning to starting position with a slow 5 count.

Standing Empty Can (Supraspinatus)   The athlete stands with the tubing securely in the hand and the opposite end under the same foot of the involved side, controlling tension. Assisting with the opposite hand the arm is lifted horizontally at the 2 o'clock position parallel to the floor (Fig. 11–64). The athlete slowly returns to starting position with a 5 count.

Standing Internal Rotation   The athlete stands with the arm to

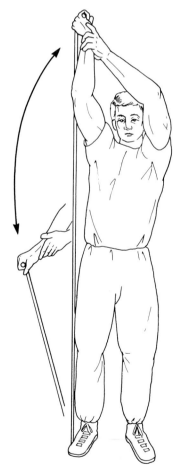

FIGURE 11–63

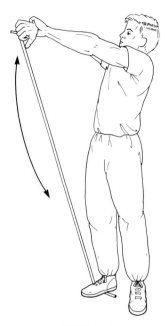

FIGURE 11–64

the side and the elbow bent at 90° and holds the tubing securely in the hand with the opposite end tied to a doorknob (Fig. 11–65A). Assisting with the opposite hand, the arm is internally rotated toward the chest (Fig. 11–65B), returning to starting position with a slow 5 count.

Standing External Rotation   The athlete stands with the arm to the side and the elbow bent at 90° and holds the tubing securely in the hand with the opposite end tied to a doorknob (Fig. 11–66A). Assist-

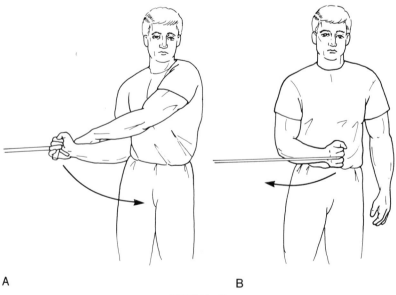

A   B

FIGURE 11–65

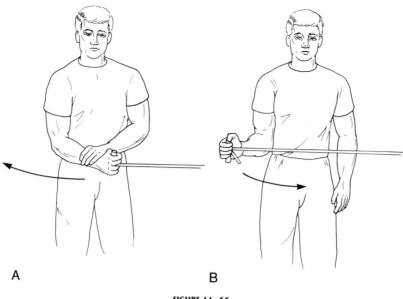

A   B

FIGURE 11–66

ing with the opposite hand, the arm is externally rotated away from the chest (Fig. 11–66B), returning to starting position with a slow 5 count.

Standing Elbow Flexion   The athlete stands with the tubing securely in the hand and the opposite end under the same foot of the involved side, controlling tension (Fig. 11–67A). Assisting with the opposite hand, the arm is flexed through a full range of motion (Fig. 11–67B), returning to starting position with a slow 5 count.

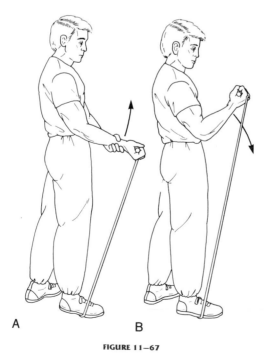

A   B

FIGURE 11–67

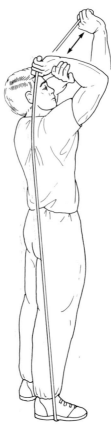

FIGURE 11–68

Standing Elbow Extension   The athlete stands with the tubing securely in the hand and the opposite end under the foot, controlling tension. The elbow is raised above the head with the tubing behind the shoulder. Assisting with the opposite hand, the arm is extended (Fig. 11–68), returning to starting position with a slow 5 count.

Prone Horizontal Abduction (100°)   The athlete lies face down

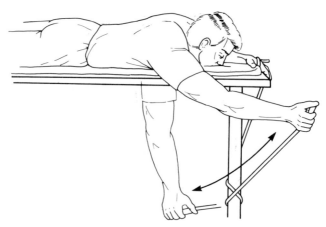

FIGURE 11–69

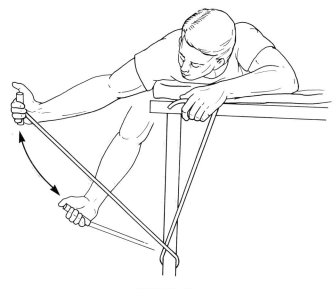

FIGURE 11–70

on the stomach with the tubing securely in the hand and the opposite end around the table leg and in the opposite hand to control tension. The arm is lifted straight up by the clinician to the end point (Fig. 11–69), returning to starting position with a slow 5 count.

Prone Horizontal Abduction   The athlete lies face down on the stomach with the tubing securely in the hand and around the table leg and in the opposite hand to control tension. The arm is lifted away from the body with the thumb up by the clinician to the end point (Fig. 11–70), returning to starting position with a slow 5 count.

Prone Extension   The athlete lies face down on the stomach with the tubing securely in the hand and the opposite end around the table leg and in the opposite hand to control tension. The arm is lifted straight back by the clinician to the end point (Fig. 11–71), returning to starting position with a slow 5 count.

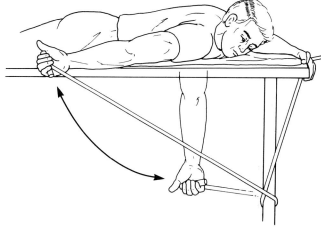

FIGURE 11–71

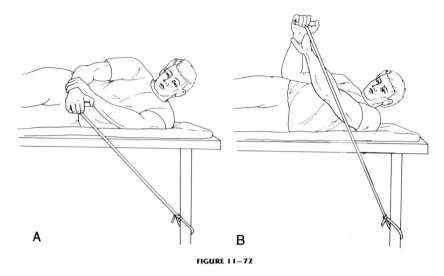

FIGURE 11–72

External Rotation on the Sides   The athlete lies on the side with the tubing securely in hand and the opposite end tied to the table leg (Fig. 11–72*A*) and rotates the arm away from the body to the end point (Fig. 11–72*B*), returning to starting position with a slow 5 count.

References

1. Ahmadain, A.M. (1987): The Magnuson–Stack operation for recurrent anterior dislocation of the shoulder. J. Bone Joint Surg. [Br.], 69:111–114.
2. Arnheim, D. (1985): Modern Principles of Athletic Training. St. Louis, C.V. Mosby.
3. Aronen, J.G. (1986): Anterior shoulder dislocation in sports. Sports Med., 3:224–234.
4. Aronen, J.G., and Regan, K. (1984): Decreasing the incidence of recurrence of first-time anterior shoulder dislocations with rehabilitation. Am. J. Sports Med. 12(4):283–291.
5. Basmajian, J.V. (1963): The surgical anatomy and function of the arm-trunk mechanism. Surg. Clin. North Am., 43:1475.
6. Bechtol, C. (1980): Biomechanics of the shoulder. Clin. Orthop. Rel. Res., 146:37.
7. Berger, R.A. (1982): Applied Exercise Physiology. Philadelphia, Lea & Febiger, p. 267.
8. Bigliani, L.U. (1990): Multidirectional instability. *In:* (ed.): 1990 Advances on the Knee and Shoulder. Cincinnati.
9. Bigliani, L.U., Morrison, D., and April, E.W. (1986): The morphology of the acromion and its relationship to rotator cuff tears. Orthop. Trans., 10:228.
10. Blackburn, T.A. (1987): Throwing injuries to the shoulder. *In:* Donatelli, R. (ed.): Physical Therapy of the Shoulder. New York, Churchill Livingstone.
11. Blackburn, T.A., McLeod, W. D., White, B. W., and Wofford, L. (1990): EMG analysis of posterior rotator cuff exercises. Athletic Training, 25(1):40–45.
12. Bland, J. (1977): The painful shoulder. Semin. Arthritis Rheumatol., 7(1):21.
13. Boissonnault, W.G., and Janos, S.C. (1989): Dysfunction, evaluation, and treatment of the shoulder. *In:* Donatelli, R., and Wooden, M.J. (eds.): Orthopaedic Physical Therapy. New York, Churchill Livingstone.
14. Braly, G., and Tullos, H.S. (1985): A modification of the Bristow procedure for recurrent anterior shoulder dislocation and subluxation. Am. J. Sports Med., 13(2):81–86.
15. Bratatz, J.H., and Gogia, P.P. (1987): The mechanics of pitching. Orthop. Sports Phys. Ther., 9(2):56–69.
16. Caillet, R. (1966): Shoulder Pain. Philadelphia, F.A. Davis.
17. Cain, P.R., Mutschler, T.A., Fu, F.A., et al. (1987): Anterior stability of the glenohumeral joint: A dynamic model. Am. J. Sports Med., 15:144–148.

18. Clark, J.C. (1988): Fibrous anatomy of the rotator cuff (abstr.). Presented at the 55th Annual Meeting of the American Academy of Orthopaedic Surgeons.

19. Codman, E.A. (1934): Rupture of the supraspinatus tendon and other lesions in or about the subacromial bursa. In The Shoulder. Boston, Thomas Todd.

20. Colachis, S.C., and Strohm, B.R. (1971): The effect of suprascapular and axillary nerve blocks and muscle force in the upper extremity. Arch. Phys. Med. Rehabil., 52:22–29.

21. Colachis, S.C., Strohm, B.R., and Brechner, V.L. (1969): Effects of axillary nerve block on muscle force in the upper extremity. Arch. Phys. Med. Rehabil., 50:647–654.

22. Collins, K.A., Capito, C., and Cross, M. (1986): The use of the Putti–Platt procedure in the treatment of recurrent anterior dislocation. Am. J. Sports Med., 14(5):380–382.

23. Davies, G.J., and Gould, J.A. (1985): Orthopaedic and Sports Physical Therapy. St. Louis, C.V. Mosby.

24. DeDuca, C.J., and Forrest, W.J. (1973): Force analysis of individual muscles acting simultaneously on the shoulder joint during isometric abduction. J. Biomech., 6:385–393.

25. Dempster, W.T. (1965): Mechanisms of shoulder movement. Arch. Phys. Med. Rehabil., 46A:49.

26. DePalma, A.F. (1973): Surgery of the Shoulder, 2nd ed. Philadelphia, J.B. Lippincott.

27. Engle, R.P., and Canner, G.C. (1989): Posterior shoulder instability approach to rehabilitation. J. Orthop. Sports Phys. Ther., 10(12): 488–494.

28. Fukuda, K., Craig, E.V., and An, K. (1986): Biomechanical study of the ligamentous system of the acromioclavicular joint. J. Bone Joint Surg. [Am.], 68:434–440.

29. Fukuda, H., Mikasa, M., Ogawa, K., et al. (1983): The partial-thickness tear of the rotator cuff. Orthop. Trans., 55:137.

30. Garth, W.P., Allman, F.L., and Armstrong, W.S. (1987): Occult anterior subluxations of the shoulder in noncontact sports. Am. J. Sports Med., 15(6):579–585.

31. Glousman, R., Jobe, F., Tibone, J., et al. (1988): Dynamic electromyographic analysis of the throwing shoulder with glenohumeral instability. J. Bone Joint Surg. [Am.], 70:220–226.

32. Hawkins, R., and Kennedy, J. (1980): Impingement syndrome in athletes. Am. J. Sports Med., 8(3):151–158.

33. Hawkins, R.J., Kippert, G., and Johnston, G. (1984): Recurrent posterior instability (subluxation) of the shoulder. J. Bone Joint Surg. [Am.], 66:169–174.

34. Hollingshead, W.H. (1958): Anatomy for Surgeons, Vol. 3. The Back and Limbs. New York, Hoeber & Harper.

35. Hovelius, L. (1987): Anterior dislocation of the shoulder in teenagers and young adults. J. Bone Joint Surg. [Am.], 69:393–399.

36. Howell, S.M., Imobersteg, A.M., Segar, D.H., and Marone, P.J. (1986): Clarification of the role of the supraspinatus muscle in shoulder function. J. Bone Joint Surg. [Am.], 68:398–404.

37. Hughston, J.C. (1985): Functional anatomy of the shoulder. In: Zarins, B., Andrews, J.R., and Carson, W.G. (eds.): Injuries to the Throwing Arm. Philadelphia, W.B. Saunders.

38. Iannotti, J.P., Swiontkowski, M., Esterhafi, J., and Boulas, H.F. (1989): Intraoperative assessment of rotator cuff vascularity using laser Doppler flowmetry (abstr.). Presented at the 1989 Meeting of the American Academy of Orthopaedic Surgeons, Las Vegas.

39. Inman, V., and Saunders, J.B. (1946): Observations of the function of the clavicle. Calif. Med., 65:158–166.

40. Inman, V., Saunders, M., and Abbott, L. (1944): Observations of the function of the shoulder joint. J. Bone Joint Surg. [Am.], 26:1–30.

41. Jobe, F.W., and Jobe, C.M. (1983): Painful athletic injuries of the shoulder. Clin. Orthop., 173:117–124.

42. Jobe, F.W., and Moynes, D.R. (1982): Delineation of diagnostic criteria and a rehabilitation program for rotator cuff injuries. Am. J. Sports Med., 10:336–339.

43. Jobe, F.W., Moynes, D.R., and Tibone, J.E. (1984): An EMG analysis of the shoulder in pitching: A second report. Am. J. Sports Med., 12:218–220.

44. Jobe, F.W., Tibone, J.E., Jobe, C.M., and Kvitne, R.S. Jr., (1990): The shoulder in sports. In: Rockwood, C.A., and Matsen, F.A., III (eds.): The Shoulder. Philadelphia, W.B. Saunders.

45. Jobe, F.W., Tibone, J.E., Perry, J., et al. (1983): An EMG analysis of the shoulder in throwing and pitching: A preliminary report. Am. J. Sports Med., 11:3–5.

46. Kennedy, J.C., and Willis, R.B. (1976): The effects of local steroid injections on tendons: A biomechanical and microscopic correlative study. Am. J. Sports Med., 4:11–21.

47. Kent, B. (1971): Functional anatomy of the shoulder complex: A review. Phys. Ther., 51:867–887.

48. Kessel, L., and Watson, M. (1977): The painful arc syndrome. J. Bone Joint Surg. [Br.], 59:166.

49. Kuland, D. (1982): The Injured Athlete. Philadelphia, J.B. Lippincott.

50. Lilleby, H. (1984): Shoulder arthroscopy. Acta Orthop. Scand., 55:561–566.

51. Lindblom, K. (1939): On pathogenesis of ruptures of the tendon aponeurosis of the shoulder joint. Acta Radiol., 20:563.

52. Lucas, D.B. (1973): Biomechanics of the shoulder joint. Arch. Surg., 107:425–432.

53. MacConnail, M., and Basmajian, J. (1969): Muscles and Movement: A Basis for Human Kinesiology. Baltimore, Williams & Wilkins.

54. Matsen, F.A., III (1980): Compartmental Syndromes. San Francisco, Grune & Stratton.

55. Matsen, F.A., III and Arntz, C.T. (1990): Rotator cuff tendon failure. In: Rockwood, C.A., Jr., and Matsen, F.A., III (eds.): The Shoulder, Vol. 2. Philadelphia, W.B. Saunders, pp. 647–677.

56. Matsen, F.A., III, and Arntz, C.T. (1990): Subacromial impingement. In: Rockwood, C.A., Jr., and Matsen, F.A. III (eds.): The Shoulder, Vol. 2. Philadelphia, W.B. Saunders, pp. 623–646.

57. McLeod, W.D. (1985): The pitching mechanism. In: Zarins, B., Andrews, J.R., and Carson, W.G. (eds.): Injuries to the Throwing Arm. Philadelphia, W.B. Saunders, pp. 22–29.

58. McLeod, W.D., and Andrews, J.R. (1986): Mechanisms of shoulder injuries. Phys. Ther., 66:1901–1904.

59. Miller, L.S., Donahue, J.R., Good, R.P., and Staerk, A.J. (1984): The Magnuson–Stack procedure for treatment of recurrent glenohumeral dislocations. Am. J. Sports Med., 12(2):133–137.

60. Morrison, D.S., and Bigliani, L.U. (1987): The clinical significance of variation in acromial morphology. Presented at the Third Open Meeting of the American Shoulder and Elbow Surgeons, San Francisco.

61. Moseley, H.F., and Goldie, I. (1963): The arterial pattern of rotator cuff of the shoulder. J. Bone Joint Surg. [Br.], 45:780.

62. Neer, C.S. (1972): Anterior acromioplasty for the chronic impingement syndrome in the shoulder: A preliminary report. J. Bone Joint Surg. [Am.], 54:41–50.

63. Neer, C.S. (1983): Impingement syndrome. Clin. Orthop. Rel. Res., 173:70–77.

64. Neviaser, R.J. (1987): Injuries to the clavicle and acromioclavicular joint. Orthop. Clin. North Am., 18:433–438.

65. Norwood, L.A. (1985): Posterior shoulder instability. In: Zarins, B., Andrews, J.R., and Carson, W.G. (eds.): Injuries to the Throwing Arm. Philadelphia, W.B. Saunders, pp. 153–159.

66. Norkin, C., and Levangie, P. (1983): Joint Structure and Function: A Comprehensive Analysis. Philadelphia, F.A. Davis.

67. Pappas, A.M., Zawacki, R.M., and Sullivan, T.J. (1985): Biomechanics of baseball pitching: A preliminary report. Am. J. Sports Med., 13(4):216–222.

68. Poppen, N.K., and Walker, P.S. (1976): Normal and abnormal motion of the shoulder. J. Bone Joint Surg. [Am.], 58:195.

69. Poppen, N., and Walker, P. (1978): Forces at the glenohumeral joint in adduction. Clin. Orthop., 135:165.

70. Protzman, R.R. (1980): Anterior instability of the shoulder. J. Bone Joint Surg. [Am.], 62:909–918.

71. Rathbun, J.B., and Macnab, I. (1970): The microvascular pattern of the rotator cuff. J. Bone Joint Surg. [Br.], 52:540.

72. Rowe, C.R. (1988): Tendinitis, bursitis, impingement, "snapping scapula" and calcific tendinitis. In: Rowe, C.R. (ed.): The Shoulder. New York, Churchill Livingstone, pp. 105–129.

73. Rowe, C.R. (1988): The Shoulder. New York, Churchill Livingstone.

74. Rowe, C., and Zarins, B. (1981): Recurrent transient subluxation of the shoulder. J. Bone Joint Surg. [Am.], 63:863–871.

75. Saha, A. (1961): Theory of Shoulder Mechanism: Descriptive and Applied. Springfield, IL, Charles C Thomas.

76. Sarrafian, S. (1983): Gross and functional anatomy of the shoulder. Clin. Orthop. Rel. Res., 173:11.

77. Sigholm, G., Styf, J., Korner, L., and Herberts, P. (1988): Pressure recording in the subacromial bursa. J. Orthop. Res., 6:123–128.

78. Steindler, A. (1955): Kinesiology of the human body. Springfield, IL, Charles C Thomas.

79. Travell, J.G., and Simons, D.G. (1983): Myofascial Pain and Dysfunction: The Trigger Point Manual. Baltimore, Williams & Wilkins.

80. Tullos, H.S., and King, J.W. (1973): Throwing mechanism in sports. Orthop. Clin. North Am., 4:709–721.

81. Turkel, S., Panio, M., Marshall, J., and Girgis, F. (1981): Stabilization mechanism preventing anterior dislocation of the glenohumeral joint. J. Bone Joint Surg. [Am.], 63:1208.

82. Walsh, D.A. (1989): Shoulder evaluation of the throwing athlete. Sports Med. Update, 4(2):24–27.

83. Wilson, C.F., and Duff, G.L. (1943): Pathologic study of degeneration and rupture of the supraspinatus tendon. Arch. Surg., 47:121–135.

84. Yamanaka, K., Fukuda, H., Hamada, K., and Mikasa, M. (1983): Incomplete thickness tears of the rotator cuff. Orthop. Traumatol. Surg. (Tokyo), 26:713.

85. Zarins, B., and Rowe, C.R. (1984): Current concepts in the diagnosis and treatment of shoulder instability in athletes. Med. Sci. Sports Exerc., 16(5):444–448.

CHAPTER 12

◆

Elbow Rehabilitation

Gary L. Harrelson, M.S., A.T.,C.

Elbow injuries are common in sports, whether induced by a direct blow (e.g., falling on an outstretched arm) or by overuse (e.g., as in baseball pitchers, quarterbacks, tennis players, and golfers). The incidence of elbow injuries in the throwing athlete has been well documented.[3, 11, 17, 23, 43, 55, 57] Schemmel and Andrews[48] have distinguished between throwing injuries of the elbow and injuries of the elbow in the throwing athlete. The term "throwing injuries of the elbow" refers to "overuse syndromes" that occur as a result of the repetitive stresses incurred by the structures about the elbow as a result of throwing over an extended period of time. Although the clinical manifestations may be acute at onset, the injuries are essentially the result of pathologic changes occurring at a subclinical level over varying periods of time. Injuries of the elbow in the throwing athlete are generally acute, traumatic injuries that occur as a result of a single injury or episode and are not specific to the throwing act itself.

Biomechanics of Throwing

The throwing act itself has been described by many authors.[24, 32, 51, 57, 58] Their analyses reveal that the elbow experiences distraction forces medially and compressive forces laterally. During the acceleration phase of throwing the valgus forces are maximum, causing the elbow to undergo medial tension and lateral compression. The acceleration phase places the elbow joint at the greatest jeopardy for injury. Medial tension produces such injuries as ulnar neuritis, medial epicondylitis, ulnar collateral ligament sprains, flexor muscle strains, and Little Leaguer's elbow in the adolescent. Laterally, compression can result in radial head and capitellum hypertrophy and osteochondritis dissecans in the young thrower.

The elbow is most vulnerable to injury during the acceleration and deceleration release phases of throwing. During the acceleration phase

443

an extension force is placed on the elbow. Elbow flexors resist this tendency to extend primarily by the brachialis and biceps muscles. Just before the end of the acceleration phase, the forearm is allowed to extend. The rate of extension can be high, causing high shear forces to be imposed on the articular cartilage.[32]

At the beginning of the deceleration release phase the humerus has a relatively high rate of internal rotation and the elbow is rapidly extending. After ball release this extension causes humeral internal rotation to present itself as forearm pronation. Large forces are applied to the biceps, brachialis, and brachioradialis to decelerate the rapidly moving forearm.[32] If the elbow extension velocity is not entirely decelerated, the overextension injuries common to the elbow can occur; conversely, if elbow extension is decelerated too rapidly, the extremely high flexion forces required can overstress the biceps tendon.[1] The curve ball has the highest rate of elbow extension and, theoretically, is the most destructive to the articular surfaces of the radial head and capitellum.[32]

As a result of the repetitive nature of throwing and the high shear forces produced, predictable osseous and muscular changes have been documented.[3, 17, 25, 28, 55] Medially, these changes are usually overuse injuries (e.g., tendinitis, muscle strains). The lateral side is prone to more serious damage (e.g., articular cartilage damage to the radial head and capitellum, with subsequent degeneration).[32] King and colleagues[29] have reported that 50% of all professional baseball pitchers have elbow flexion contractures and approximately 30% have cubitus valgus elbow deformities as a result of prolonged throwing.

Rehabilitation Program

Traumatic injuries to the elbow (e.g., elbow dislocation) usually require a period of immobilization or protected mobilization after injury. Range-of-motion and strengthening exercises should be started as quickly as possible, however, with wrist and hand exercises beginning during elbow immobilization. The opposite of an acute traumatic injury is an overuse syndrome (e.g., medial or lateral epicondylitis), which usually requires no immobilization. Here, the athlete's main complaint is that pain is exacerbated with a particular activity or motion. A therapeutic exercise program may immediately be initiated with chronic lesions. Overuse elbow injuries also respond well to such modalities as ice, heat, ultrasound, and iontophoresis in conjunction with a therapeutic exercise program.

Those athletes who engage in throwing types of activities should not neglect rehabilitation of the shoulder in conjunction with their elbow exercise program. Both joints are part of the total kinetic chain, and one would be remiss if one joint were addressed without a concurrent rehabilitation program for the other.

Postoperative elbow lesions, particularly those treated arthroscopically, can be treated aggressively with range-of-motion exercises beginning as early as the next postoperative day. Usually, the philosophy of instituting early range of motion can be followed whether an arthroscopy or arthrotomy is performed.

Exercise Program

The following therapeutic exercises can be used after arthroscopy or arthrotomy, as well as for conservative treatment of elbow lesions. In addition, they can be used for wrist injuries. The exercises include the following:

1. Therapeutic putty—for hand intrinsic muscle strength
2. Rice or sand bucket—for hand intrinsic muscle strength
3. Forearm flexor stretch
4. Forearm extensor stretch
5. Wrist curls
6. Reverse wrist curls
7. Ulnar deviation
8. Radial deviation
9. Pronation and supination
10. Broomstick curl-up with palms up and palms down
11. Biceps curls
12. French curls

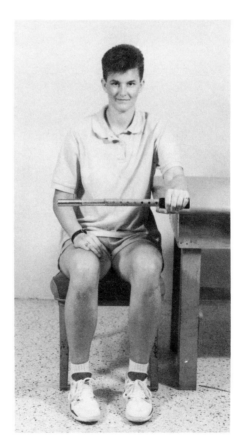

FIGURE 12–1 Use of an adjustable rod for elbow rehabilitation. As the lever arm is extended, the torque is increased.

These exercises emphasize all planes of elbow motion and flexibility. Guidelines for institution of this program are based on how quickly the athlete can advance and still allow the restraining structures time to heal. The use of an adjustable rod with a fixed weight on the end is excellent for concentric pronation–supination and radial-ulnar deviation exercises (Fig. 12–1). As strength increases and symptoms subside, the weight can be increased by lengthening the lever arm of the rod. If the rod proves to be too heavy in the early stages of rehabilitation a hammer can be substituted or the rod can be grasped in the middle, reducing the lever arm length and thus the weight.

As the athlete progresses with the exercises he or she can begin the following: (1) endurance training using the upper body ergometer—(UBE)* (it can also be used for range-of-motion restoration); (2) isokinetic exercises; (3) Inertia machine† for proprioception, eccentric muscle contraction, and high-speed functional planes (Fig. 12–2); and (4) eccentric elbow exercises (see Application, at the end of this chapter). Before returning to throwing, the athlete should participate in a high-speed surgical tubing program with emphasis on functional patterns. Emphasis should be on redevelopment of muscle concentric and eccentric synergistic contraction patterns. Exercise progression and restrictions for the most common injuries of the elbow and their rehabilitation are discussed below.

---

*Available from Cybex, Ronkonkoma, NY.

†Available from E.M.A., Newnan, GA.

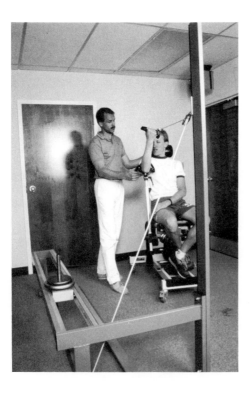

FIGURE 12–2 Inertia machine. This can be used in the later stages of elbow rehabilitation for proprioception, eccentric muscle contraction, and high-speed functional planes (From Courson, R. (1989): Rehabilitation of the thrower's elbow. Sports Med. Update, 4(2):7.)

COMMON ELBOW INJURIES IN ADULTS

Lateral and Medial Epicondylitis

Lateral epicondylitis was first described by Runge,[47] in 1873, who noted this condition in the general population. The prevalence of lateral epicondylitis surged with the increase in participation in tennis—thus, the generic name of "tennis elbow." Lateral epicondylitis is an overuse injury, with its pathology usually involving the origin of the extensor carpi radialis brevis (ECRB) and, to a lesser degree, the extensor carpi radialis longus and anterior portion of the extensor communis.[30, 53] Nirschl[36] has suggested that the pathology is primarily in the ECRB, with the development of fibroangiomatous hyperplasia as a result of chronic repetitive trauma. The ECRB is susceptible to increased stress when the wrist is flexed with ulnar deviation, the elbow extended, and the forearm pronated, because the ECRB muscle must lengthen by 1.1 cm to allow full wrist flexion and pronation.[6] This is the same biomechanical principle as that of the tennis backhand, thus predisposing the tennis player to lateral epicondylar pain. This pain is usually reproduced as the racket meets the ball. It is at the point of racket–ball contact that the extensor muscles must contract to stabilize the wrist and hold the racket. This results in repetitive muscle contraction, yielding chronic overload, and causing lateral epicondylar pain. If left untreated necrosis of the connective tissue in the lateral epicondylar area can occur.

Conversely, medial epicondylitis, which is less common, is generally seen in the throwing athlete as a result of valgus overload or overuse. Medial epicondylitis can be associated with the tennis forehand, serve, or overhead. Whatever the cause, medial epicondylitis is an overuse injury. The ratio of occurrence of lateral to medial epicondylitis is approximately 7:1.[30]

Individuals with epicondylitis usually complain of increased pain, either on the medial or lateral epicondyle. There is point tenderness over the involved epicondyle, and resisted wrist extension (lateral epicondylitis) or resisted wrist flexion (medial epicondylitis) exacerbates the symptoms, depending on the involved area. Grip strength can also decrease and refer pain to the symptomatic epicondyle.

Treatment of epicondylitis over the years has included the following: (1) nonsteroidal anti-inflammatory drugs (NSAIDs); (2) possible steroid injection; (3) rest; (4) ice; (5) counterforce bracing; (6) cock-up splint (lateral epicondylitis); (7) exercises to increase muscle strength and endurance; and (8) change in mechanics, if necessary. Treatment of medial and lateral epicondylitis is similar. A rehabilitation program should be initiated before the symptoms and pain escalate, because the longer medial or lateral epicondylitis is symptomatic, the more difficult and prolonged the treatment.[30]

Patients with acute epicondylitis obtain the best results with treatment.[30] The acute stage should be treated with a decrease in and/or avoidance of the noxious stimuli producing the symptoms. In severe lateral epicondylitis a cock-up splint may be used to decrease stress on the lateral epicondyle.[22] The athlete should remove the splint three or four times daily, however, to carry out elbow and wrist active range-of-motion exercises. In the initial stage, cryotherapy, electrical stimulation, and NSAIDs may be used to decrease the acute inflammatory reaction. As the acute phase subsides, the rehabilitation program can be progressed to include a more aggressive range-of-motion program and progressive resistance exercises.

Epicondylitis that is chronic or has passed the acute stage may respond well to thermotherapy techniques (e.g., moist heat, ultrasound), phonophoresis (using 10% hydrocortisone cream), or iontophoresis in conjunction with a stretching and therapeutic exercise program. The athlete with only mild pain or pain that does not increase may continue to play while undergoing treatment; however, if the activity exacerbates the symptoms, the athlete should stop the activity. Therapeutic exercises may worsen the symptoms for the first 7 to 10 days after initiation of the program, so the athlete should be instructed in the treatment of possible escalating symptoms. If the pain becomes severe, the exercises should be decreased or stopped. After 1 to 2 weeks with chronic lesions the increase in symptoms should dissipate and the athlete notices a decrease in pain. The interval tennis, golf, or throwing program (see Appendix B) can be used to return athletes back to their sport, if applicable.

Relatively few cases (5 to 10%) of lateral epicondylitis require surgery.[7] If performed, however, the postoperative course includes a posterior splint with the forearm in neutral position and the elbow at 90° of flexion for 7 to 10 days. The athlete may begin gentle active range of motion of the wrist and elbow on the first day postoperatively as pain allows. Active range of motion is progressed as tolerated, and the athlete may remove the posterior splint to exercise active elbow range of motion after 7 to 10 days postsurgery. Full, active, range of motion should return by the third postoperative week, and an elbow progressive resistance exercise (PRE) program may begin at this time. The athlete may gradually return to sports participation at about 2 months after surgery using the applicable interval program (see Appendix B). Nirschl[37] has reported that full power and flexibility in the extensor muscle mass returns in about 4 months.

Modalities should be used in the conservative treatment of epicondylitis to decrease pain, tenderness, and inflammation, thus allowing the athlete to exercise with less discomfort. Halle and associates[19] have compared the effectiveness of four treatment protocols (in association with a home program) on lateral epicondylitis: (1) ultrasound; (2) ultrasound with 10% hydrocortisone; (3) TENS (transcutaneous electrical nerve stimulation); and (4) subcutaneous steroid injection. It was determined that the four treatment protocols do not significantly differ in effectiveness. All are effective in decreasing pain and symptoms, but it should be noted that a home therapeutic exercise program is a common denominator in all four protocols.

Steroid injection has been recommended and been somewhat successful in treating epicondylitis symptoms, but this is only a palliative measure if not performed in conjunction with a therapeutic exercise program to increase muscular strength and endurance. Iontophoresis is a favorable alternative to hypodermic injection because of (1) decreased systemic side effects, and (2) short-term administration, and

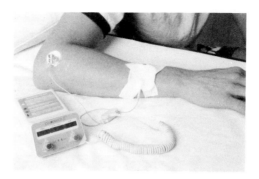

FIGURE 12–3 Administration of iontophoresis using the Phoresor. (From Courson, R. (1989): Rehabilitation of the thrower's elbow. Sports Med. Update, 4(2):4.)

because it (3) avoids associated discomfort of needle insertion at an already tender area and (4) avoids the use of a hypodermic needle, which prevents further tissue damage. The Phoresor* is an excellent device for administering iontophoresis (Fig. 12–3). For epicondylitis it is recommended that 2 ml of topical Xylocaine and 1 ml of dexamethasone be used with this device, treating every other day for five or six treatments (maximum).[15]

The use of counterforce bracing has long been advocated by many authors.[6, 7, 13, 22, 30, 36–38, 43] Froimson [13] and Ilfeld and Field[22] first reported the use of a counterforce brace for lateral epicondylitis. In 1966, Ilfeld and Field[22] described a tennis elbow brace designed to support the elbow between two lateral hinged metal stirrups that limited extension and rotation, somewhat different from the current proximal forearm band described by Froimson (Fig. 12–4).[13] The rationale behind the use of counterforce bracing for lateral epicondylitis is that the brace either decreases the amount of internally generated muscle contractile tension or it alters and directs potentially abusive force overloads to less sensitive tissues, and possibly to the brace itself.[18, 36] The counterforce brace is thought to exert its effect by gentle compression of musculotendinous areas, which partially decreases muscle expansion at the time of intrinsic muscle contraction or minimizes exaggerated tendon movement. A number of objective studies have supported the efficacy of counterforce bracing.[18, 52, 53, 60] In patients whose symptoms are severe, the counterforce brace can be used during the therapeutic excercise program.

Valgus Extension Overload

The repetitive nature of throwing results in muscular and osseous hypertrophy around the elbow.[28] This bony hypertrophy is usually located on the olecranon process, primarily posteromedially, and results in a bony block and loss of elbow extension. Valgus stress plus forced extension are the major pathologic mechanisms that produce scarring, fibrous tissue deposition in the olecranon fossa, and osteophyte formation on the tip or posteromedial aspect of the olecranon process.[1, 57] Traditionally, emphasis was placed on osteophyte formation on the

---

*Available from Iomed, Inc., Salt Lake City, UT.

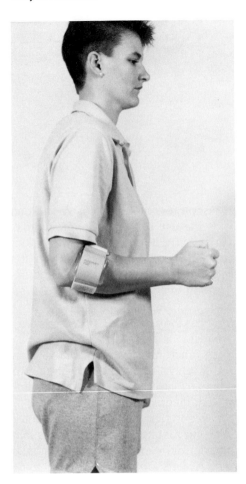

FIGURE   12–4 Counterforce brace for tennis elbow. These either decrease the quantity of internally generated muscle contraction tension or alter and direct potentially abusive force overloads to less sensitive tissues, and probably the brace itself.

posterior olecranon tip as a result of extension overload.[1, 29, 61] True symptomatic lesions, however, are caused by the posteromedial osteophyte as it abuts into the medial margin of the olecranon fossa.[2, 29, 61] This can result in osteochondrosis in this area.

Athletes suffering from valgus extension overload usually have already developed secondary soft tissue contractures as a result of fibrous tissue deposition in the olecranon fossa, olecranon osteophyte formation, loose bodies, or radial head hypertrophy. These athletes complain of elbow pain that is accentuated with throwing, as well as joint catching, locking, crepitus, and loss of elbow range of motion, particularly extension. The elbow end-feel is hard, painful, and unyielding when tested, clinical features that are generally associated with a mechanical block.

Conservative treatment is indicated for athletes with mild valgus extension overload. They usually respond favorably to rest from pitching and elbow range of motion, flexibility, and strengthening exercises. Therapeutic modalities include moist heat, ultrasound, and phonophoresis with 10% hydrocortisone cream.[1, 4] Although a flexion deformity is usually present, it does not appear to alter pitching performance.[1] Surgery is indicated for patients in whom pain persists and exercise increases symptoms.

Postoperative rehabilitation following arthroscopic or arthrotomy excision of loose bodies and osteophytes can begin the next day. The following outlines an early postoperative rehabilitation protocol following elbow arthroscopy for loose body removal and/or osteophyte excision:

1. Initial phase
   a. Day of Surgery—athlete begins gently moving elbow in bulky dressing.
   b. Postoperative days 1 and 2
      (1) Bulky dressing is removed and replaced with Band-Aids and elastic wrap or compressionette
      (2) Immediate postoperative hand and elbow exercises:
         (a) Putty
         (b) Wrist flexor stretch
         (c) Wrist extensor stretch
         (d) Wrist curls
         (e) Reverse wrist curls
         (f) Neutral wrist curls
         (g) Pronation
         (h) Supination
      (3) Goal: full wrist and elbow range of motion
   c. Postoperative days 3 to 7
      (1) Passive flexion and extension of elbow exercises
      (2) Progressive resistive exercises of elbow are begun with 1-lb. weight.
         (a) Wrist curls
         (b) Reverse wrist curls
         (c) Neutral wrist curls
         (d) Pronation
         (e) Supination
         (f) Broomstick curl-up
2. Intermediate phase—postoperative weeks 1 and 2
   a. Continue progressive resistive exercises three times daily
   b. Goal: Gradual advancement to 5 sets of 10 repetitions with 5- to 7-lb weight by increasing in 1-lb increments.
3. Advanced phase—postoperative weeks 4 to 6
   a. Gradual return to sport
      (1) Simulated activity in sport
      (2) Interval throwing program (see Appendix B)
   b. Eccentric and surgical tubing program
   c. Maintenance strength and flexibility program, once daily

If an arthrotomy is performed for removal of the osteophytes, a posterior splint should be used for 3 to 4 days, but the same exercises as those for an arthroscopy procedure are indicated. The athlete should exercise out of the splint during the early postoperative period. Initially, the use of ice pre- and postexercise is recommended. It is not unusual for the athlete to experience asymptomatic elbow crepitus. Depending on osteophyte or loose body size, and on the length of their presence within the elbow, a slight flexion contracture may be present from the lack of full extension for a prolonged period. The flexion contracture should be treated as soon as the athlete can tolerate passive stretching of the involved area. Proprioception neuromuscular facilitation (PNF) contract—relax techniques can be used in an attempt to facilitate the return to full extension. If pain has been relieved and the range of motion is equal bilaterally, then throwing for these athletes may begin as early as 4 to 6 weeks postoperatively using the interval throwing program (see Appendix B). If the athlete is a "thrower," the exercises should be performed a minimum of three times daily; for the non-throwing athlete, twice daily is sufficient.

Ulnar Nerve Lesions

The ulnar nerve is highly susceptible to the valgus forces encountered in throwing, which produce traction on the medial aspect of the elbow. The ulnar nerve can be injured by direct trauma, repetitive traction caused by ligament laxity, compression resulting from increased muscular hypertrophy, recurrent subluxation and/or dislocation of the nerve out of the ulnar groove, or fixation of the nerve in the cubital tunnel by adhesions. All these can be aggravated by repetitive throwing. Although protected proximally and distally by muscle mass within the cubital tunnel, the ulnar nerve is relatively unprotected and is vulnerable to compressive forces.[56] The ulnar collateral ligament (UCL) forms the floor of the tunnel and the roof is formed by the arcuate ligament. The arcuate ligament is taut at 90° of flexion and can compress the ulnar nerve as the degree of elbow flexion increases.[56, 59] Furthermore, any deficiency in the anterior oblique portion of the UCL that allows the elbow to open in valgus places undue stress on the ulnar nerve and sometimes may lead to "tardy ulnar nerve palsy."[13, 16]

Typically, once ulnar nerve lesions become symptomatic, they must be corrected surgically. Some athletes respond to conservative care, however, such as rest, cryotherapy, NSAIDs, and changes in pitching biomechanics. Surigical procedures usually transpose the ulnar nerve anteriorly. The nerve may be repositioned in the forearm musculature, but extensive scarring and compression of the nerve have been observed with this procedure.[5, 31] In addition, throwing athletes tend to have a hypertrophied forearm flexor mass and may compress the nerve during contraction.[5] Some surgeons elect to reflect the flexor mass and resect the medial epicondyle before anterior transposition.[14, 35] Subcutaneous transposition of the ulnar nerve has been advocated to avoid compression of the nerve by the forearm musculature.[12, 45, 46] Eaton and co-workers[12] have recommended the use of a fasciodermal sling to transpose the ulnar nerve anteriorly. Whatever surgical technique is used, the protocol outlined here for ulnar nerve transfer can be followed:

1. Posterior splint, 90° of flexion, used for 7 days
   a. Putty and grip exercises
   b. Wrist range of motion
2. At 7 days, splint taken off for exercises
   a. Last 15° of extension are avoided
   b. 30° initially, progressing to 15°

3. Splint is put back on except to bathe and exercise
4. Splint discarded 3 weeks after surgery
5. At 3 weeks following surgery, athlete
   a. Works for full extension
   b. Begins full elbow program
6. At 8 weeks, athlete begins interval throwing program (see Appendix B)

Loss of Range of Motion

Loss of elbow range of motion is a common complication, particularly in athletes who have suffered an elbow dislocation, radial head or olecranon fracture, osteochondritis, or osteochondritis dissecans. Because the elbow is susceptible to flexion contractures, initiation of early range of motion, even in a limited range, is an important deterrent. Immobilization for longer than 2 weeks after injury or surgery can affect the long-term outcome.[34]

High-intensity, short-duration stretching is contraindicated for any elbow with limited range of motion. This can stimulate ossification and result in traumatic myositis ossificans, additional loss of motion, and increased pain, ultimately worsening the patient's condition.[20, 39, 45] Flexion contractures are best treated in the subacute stage with modalities in conjunction with a therapeutic exercise program. The use of moist heat and ultrasound to stimulate vasodilation and increase collagen elasticity, in conjunction with range-of-motion exercises, may be helpful.

The athlete can perform range-of-motion exercises while immersing the elbow in a warm whirlpool, incorporating the heating effects with the buoyancy of the water. Also, the upper body ergometer (UBE) is an excellent range-of-motion tool. The seat and arm attachments can be adjusted to accommodate an athlete with a range-of-motion deficit, and it may be used for passive, active-assisted, or active range of motion. Exercise with the UBE increases local temperature and blood flow around the joint and stimulates synovial fluid disbursement. Heating of the joint by such methods prior to range-of-motion loading techniques increases collagen elasticity in the soft tissues, allowing greater elongation with less associated structural damage. When appropriate, soft tissue and joint mobilization techniques may be beneficial.

The tabletop terminal knee extension apparatus may be modified to assist in providing a low-load, prolonged elbow extension stretch (Fig. 12–5). This technique stabilizes the distal humerus adequately and allows a variable load to be placed on the distal forearm. Because the athlete does not have to hold a weight in the hand, the forearm flexor musculature may remain relaxed, enhancing the stretch. Therapeutic modalities such as moist heat, ultrasound, electrical muscle stimulation, or spray and stretch may easily be incorporated into this treatment regimen.

Application of a Dynasplint,* which applies a prolonged, low-

*Available from Dynasplint, Baltimore, MD.

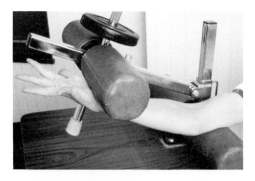

FIGURE 12–5 Use of Iso-Quad for regaining passive elbow extension. (From Courson, R. (1989). Rehabilitation of the thrower's elbow. Sports Med. Update, 4(2):5.

intensity force, has met with success in treating loss of elbow range of motion without the risk of traumatizing the joint by forceful and vigorous stretching (Fig. 12–6).[20] To obtain the best results, the Dynasplint is generally advocated for use at night while the athlete is sleeping, but it may be worn during the day. Usually, the athlete who can achieve from 0 to 10° extension is fully functional and does not notice the loss of extension.[1, 4, 29]

Some guidelines to be used when attempting to regain elbow range of motion include the following:

1. Avoid strong passive loading of the joint.
2. Once allowed by physiologic healing restraints, active range-of-motion exercises at the end ranges should be performed many times daily.
3. Exercises should be done only in the range of normal synergy.

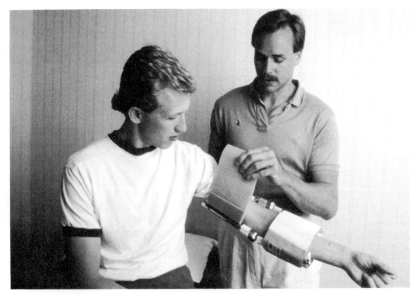

FIGURE 12–6 Elbow Dynasplint. This can provide a low-force long-duration stretch for an elbow with loss of range of motion. (From Courson, R. (1989): Rehabilitation of the thrower's elbow. Sports Med. Update, 4(2):6.)

4. The athlete should rest in a comfortable position to prolong the period of stretch stimulus.
5. Low-load, prolonged stretching should be done to minimize joint trauma.

Ulnar and Radial Collateral Ligament Sprains

Injuries involving the ulnar and radial collateral ligaments are induced by a direct blow, overuse, or elbow dislocation. The UCL suffers most of the ligamentous lesions around the elbow, particularly in throwers. Because of the distraction forces that occur medially, gradual attenuation of the UCL is not uncommon (Fig. 12–7). Furthermore, gradual laxity of the UCL results in increased compression laterally at the radiohumeral joint. This increased lateral compression can result in necrosis of the radial head articular cartilage, with the eventual formation of loose bodies.

The UCL is formed by three distinct bands—anterior oblique, posterior, and transverse portions (Fig. 12–8). The primary stabilizer to valgus stress is the anterior oblique part of the UCL.[49] This portion of the UCL is taut throughout its full range of motion, whereas the posterior aspect of the UCL is taut with flexion and lax with extension, and the transverse part of the UCL contributes little to medial stability.[49, 56] Sectioning of the posterior fibers of the UCL does not result in valgus instability, but resection of the anterior oblique UCL fibers alone results in valgus instability.[56] Also, resection of the radial head contributes to medial instability, even if the anterior oblique UCL fibers remain intact.[56]

In acute valgus instability direct repair of the UCL (usually the anterior portion), using the ligament itself is an appropriate option.[48] As

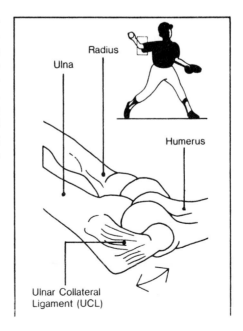

FIGURE 12–7 Because of the distractive forces that occur medially during the pitching act, the ulnar collateral ligament (UCL) can be injured from acute or subacute trauma. (From Schemmel, S.P., and Andrews, J.R. (1988): Acute and chronic ulnar collateral ligament injuries in the throwing athlete. Sports Med. Update, 3(3):10.)

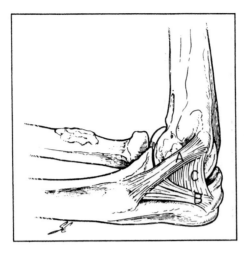

FIGURE 12–8 Medial aspect of the elbow, illustrating the three bundles of fibers that comprise the UCL. *A,* Anterior. *B,* Transverse. *C,* Posterior. (From Medich, G.F. (1989): Little League elbow. Sports Med. Update, 4(2):15.)

is usually the case at surgery, however, the ligaments are often found to be attenuated and are sacrificed; thus, primary repair is difficult, if not contraindicated. In such cases other connective tissues may be transferred to compensate for the insufficiency or a reconstruction may be attempted using a tendon graft, such as the palmaris longus, fascia lata, or long toe extensor. Jobe and colleagues[26] have described reconstruction of the UCL using autogenous tendon grafts to allow the athlete to return to the previous level of throwing. With this technique, 10 out of 16 throwing athletes successfully returned to their previous level of throwing ability.[26] Schwab and associates[49] have also described a procedure for osteotomy of the medial epicondyle with transfer to a proximal and anterior position on the humerus in the reconstruction of chronically lax UCL, with good results. Regardless of the surgical procedure performed for relief of UCL instability, the protocol outlined here can be followed:

1. Postoperative day 1
   a. Posterior splint at 90° of flexion
   b. Putty and grip exercises
   c. Wrist range-of-motion exercises
   d. Active wrist flexion and extension, PRE as tolerated
2. Postoperative day 10
   a. Hinged brace used, 30 to 60° of motion
3. Postoperative weeks 2 to 6
   a. Hinged Brace, 15 to 90° of motion
   b. Progress to full ROM in flexion and extension by 6 weeks
   c. Brace off for AAROM and AROM, with emphasis at end ranges of motion
   d. Full elbow program of active flexion–extension, pronation–supination, and forearm extension–flexion stretches;–progress PRE as tolerated
   e. Discontinue brace at 6 weeks
   f. Begin shoulder rehabilitation program, PRE as tolerated
4. Postoperative months 2 to 3

a. Isokinetic exercises with elbow flexion and extension at medium to high speeds
    b. Surgical tubing program at varying speeds
    c. Start functional activities at 3 months
5. Postoperative months 3 to 4
    a. Inertia machine in elbow flexion–extension
    b. Gradual decrease in isokinetic speed to 60°/sec
6. Postoperative months 4 to 6
    a. Begin interval throwing program (see Appendix B)
    b. Return to competitive activity

Conservative management of attenuated UCL lesions includes rest, avoidance of valgus stress, and initiation of a full elbow rehabilitation exercise program, with no limitations. Gradual return to throwing may be attempted at 6 to 8 weeks with initiation of the interval throwing program and monitoring of symptoms. This may be, however, only a palliative measure for those athletes who continue to throw and stress the elbow medially.

Athletes in contact sports, with acute first- or second-degree UCL sprains, should have the elbow taped or wear an orthosis that prevents the last 15 to 30° of extension and protects the elbow from valgus forces when the athletes return to participation (Fig. 12–9).

Contusions and Strains

Most elbow contusions occur to the bony projections, predominantly the medial and lateral epicondyles and the olecranon process. These injuries, depending on their severity, can result in a transitory loss of flexion, extension, or both. Initial treatment includes cryotherapy and electrical stimulation to decrease effusion and pain, and active or active-assisted range of motion. On the second or third postinjury day the athlete can progress with an elbow exercise program as tolerated and return to practice as early as the next day postinjury, with the area

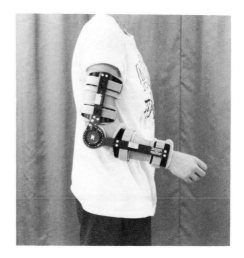

FIGURE 12–9 Hinged brace for limitation of range of motion with UCL repairs.

protected for contact sports. If the injury involves a "thrower," there should be a gradual return to throwing by accelerating the interval throwing program.

Dislocations

Most elbow dislocations result from a fall on an outstretched arm. Johansson,[27] however, has reported elbow dislocations caused by violent hyperextension and abduction forces, resulting in ruptures of the anterior oblique ligament and of the anterior portion of the joint capsule. Most elbow dislocations occur posteriorly or posterolaterally. Osborne and Cotterill[40] have maintained that the ligaments are the sole factors that prevent posterior dislocations while the elbow is in extension.

After reduction, the use of an arm sling and an elbow cast at approximately 90° of flexion for 6 weeks have traditionally been the accepted mode of treatment. Prolonged immobilization, however, is accompanied by detrimental effects (e.g., flexion contracture). The rationale for the use of prolonged immobilization is the prevention of a recurrent dislocation but this is rare even when early mobilization is initiated.[34, 49] Mehlhoff and co-workers[34] retrospectively examined the long-term effects of early mobilization on elbow dislocations. They found that prolonged immobilization after injury is strongly associated with an unsatisfactory result. The longer the immobilization, the larger the flexion contracture and the more severe the pain. From their data they recommended that immobilization not exceed 2 weeks following an elbow dislocation.[34] Their report is consistent with other findings that have promoted early elbow mobilization following dislocation; no recurrence of dislocation has been noted.[27, 44] Protzman[44] has noted no recurrence of dislocations in 27 patients treated with active range of motion less than 5 days postreduction. Even if some instability still exists, immobilizaiton should never exceed 3 to 4 weeks.[34] Outlined here is the protocol for rehabilitation following reduction of a dislocated elbow:

1. Immobilization in posterior splint for 3 to 4 days at 90° of flexion:
   a. Begin gripping exercises
   b. Wrist AROM in all planes
2. Splint removed for exercise after 3 to 4 days and gentle active motion begins several times daily, as tolerated by athlete; no passive range of motion:
   a. AROM in elbow flexion–extension, and pronation–supination
   b. Isometric flexion and extension at varying angles, as tolerated by athlete
3. Postinjury days 10 to 14, splint discarded with continuation of active exercises:
   a. Full elbow rehabilitation program
   b. PRE, as tolerated
   c. Hinged brace may be used 15 to 90° for 4 weeks postoperatively
4. Return to participation when muscular strength, power, and endur-

ance is 85 to 90% of the contralateral limb; should be braced and/or taped to prevent elbow hyperextension and protected against valgus forces when returning to play

ADOLESCENT INJURIES

Although adolescent pitchers subject their elbow to the same stresses as the adult pitcher, the manifestation of lesions is different because of the degree of maturation. In adolescent baseball players the elbow is the most frequent area of complaint. Most of the osseous changes seen in the adolescent as a result of the pitching act are manifested at the radiohumeral joint.[57] The two most common injuries in the adolescent pitcher are osteochondritis dissecans and Little Leaguer's elbow.

Osteochondritis Dissecans

Osetochondritis dissecans is considered the leading cause of permanent elbow disability in the young pitching athlete.[1, 23, 54] Andrews[1] has reported that this group usually has the most severe flexion contractures and obtain the least benefit from surgery. Osteochondritis dissecans is a lesion to the bone and articular cartilage that commonly occurs on the anterolateral surface of the capitellum (Fig. 12–10).[25] The condition results from repeated lateral compression of the radioca-

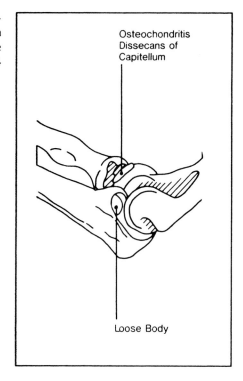

FIGURE 12–10 Osteochondritis dissecans of the capitellum. (From Medich, G.F. (1989): Little League elbow. Sports Med. Update, 4 (2):16.)

pitellar joint that can injure the articular cartilage, creating loose bodies.[38, 56] Unlike lesions occurring to the medial side of the elbow, lateral lesions can result in permanent elbow damage and often shorten or terminate a throwing athlete's career.[57]

The exact cause of osteochondritis dissecans is unknown, but it is believed that repeated traumatic impact of the radial head into the capitellum during the cocking and acceleration phases of throwing can result in a circulatory disturbance at the radiocapitellar joint. Primary changes occur to the bone and secondary changes to the cartilage.[41] Instead of presenting itself as loose body formation, as in mature throwers, aseptic necrosis of the radial head occurs in the adolescent. This can also result in a progression of loose bodies, overgrowth of the radial head, and early arthritic changes.

Osteochondritis dissecans represents a major threat to the elbow joint, and it is important that it be diagnosed early. The athlete complains of anterolateral elbow tenderness along with decreased pronation and supination, suggesting the diagnosis of radiocapitellum incongruity or radial head fracture.[56] The most common finding is a loss of full elbow extension. It is not unusual for the athlete to lack as much as 20° of full extension.[9, 54, 62]

Initial conservative treatment consists of avoidance of noxious stimuli and the use of modalities for the relief of pain and inflammation. The athlete may begin an elbow exercise program, as tolerated. An overly aggressive approach with osteochondritis dissecans, however, can result in progressive loss of motion. If avascular changes are noted on the lateral side of the elbow in the young thrower, abstinence from throwing should be maintained until revascularization of the affected area has occurred.

Most authors recommend surgical removal of symptomatic loose bodies and avoidance of other surgical procedures, unless there are changes that could compromise the architectural support of the capitellum.[42, 50, 62] Prognosis of osteochondritis dissecans after simple loose body removal is good if diagnosis is early and no degenerative changes are associated. There is slow recovery to normal function, however, and some limitation of full extension is likely to remain. Tivnon and colleagues[54] have reported an average elbow range of motion preoperatively of $-30°$ of extension with $-6°$ of full flexion, yielding an average arc of motion of 104°. Follow-up average range of motion was $-11°$ of extension and $-4°$ of full flexion, with an average arc of 125° of motion. Others have reported a similar response of range of motion following surgery.[9] Therefore, if range of motion is to be re-established or increased following loose body extraction in this condition, early mobilization is paramount.

Degenerative changes of the radiocapitellar joint have a poor prognosis for the athlete returning to pitching.[23] Although the osteophytes and loose bodies can be removed surgically, ankylosis may remain in the young athlete, who is then unable to throw.[21] Singer and Roy[50] reported that of five gymnasts treated for osteochondritis dissecans, four could not return to full workout without recurring symptoms in a 3-year follow-up period.

Little Leaguer's Elbow

Brogdon and Crow[8] initially coined the term "Little Leaguer's elbow" to describe an avulsion of the ossification center of the medial epicondyle caused by the pitching act in the adolescent athlete.[21] Since the initial description, several pathologic conditions have been included under this term, including strain of the flexor muscles, ulnar neuropathy, and osteochondritis dissecans.

The cause of this condition is the same as that for valgus extension overload except that the forces injure the epiphyseal plate because this is the weakest link in the adolescent kinetic chain. The injury occurs during the acceleration phase of throwing from traction forces medially as a result of repetitive throwing. Hypertrophy of the medial epicondyle may be present and usually represents a physiologic response to throwing. A widened growth line or displacement of the epicondyle is evidence of a fracture (Fig. 12–11).[33]

The adolescent athlete suffering from Little Leaguer's elbow most commonly presents with a history of progressive medial elbow pain over a few weeks, which worsens with pitching and is relieved by rest. Additional signs and symptoms include limitation of complete extension, tenderness over the medial epicondyle, and pain with passive extension of the wrist and fingers. Roentgenographic changes include accelerated growth and separation and fragmentation of the medial epicondylar epiphysis. Less commonly, the athlete may present with dramatic symptoms, including the report of a popping sensation followed by medial elbow pain, the inability to throw because of pain, and swelling accompanied by medial ecchymosis.

Prevention remains the best treatment for Little Leaguer's elbow. It is important that coaches and parents be educated about the proper warm-up, conditioning, and off-season pitching of the adolescent pitcher. Also, the throwing of curves and other breaking pitches by pitchers in the 9-to 14-year-old age group should be prohibited, because this stress considerably increases the force on wrist flexion and

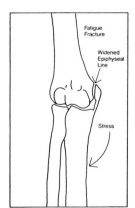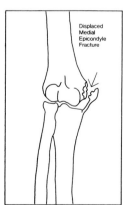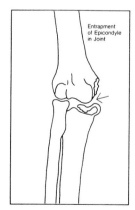

FIGURE 12–11 Little Leaguer's elbow characterized by a widening growth line and eventual epicondyle displacement. (From Medich, G.F. (1989): Little League elbow. Sports Med. Update, 4(2):17.)

pronation.[10, 42] Pitchers should be taught proper pitching mechanics and the establishment of a pitching maximum. Currently, Little League pitching rules advise six innings per week, with 3 days of rest between pitching turns, but no rules or recommendations govern the amount of practice pitching.

Treatment in the early stage of Little Leaguer's elbow includes rest from noxious stimuli, application of ice, and possibly immobilization. If roentgenographic findings reveal capitellum osteochondritis dissecans, it is recommended that the player stop pitching for the remainder of the baseball season.

After initial conservative treatment, if the athlete returns to throwing and there is any recurrence of symptoms, there should be complete abstinence from throwing until the next season. A medial epicondylar fracture that is displaced by more than 1 cm may occur in a small percentage of athletes. These injuries should be opened and fixed internally with a screw.[33] With open and internal fixation the athlete is immobilized for approximately 3 to 4 weeks and should not engage in any throwing activity until the following season. Also, sometimes in later stages, surgery may be indicated if loose bodies are present. Criteria for return to competition include no pain, normal elbow range of motion, and no muscle strength and endurance weakness in all planes of wrist and elbow ranges of motion. The return to throwing should be gradual and should follow the interval throwing program. Fortunately, most elbow injuries in the adolescent "thrower" are adequately treated by rest and cause no permanent disability.[33]

Elbow injuries, particularly in throwers, are a common complaint. Most elbow injuries are a result of subacute trauma over a period of time. The nature of the pitching act, which results in medial distraction and lateral compressive forces, causes predictable connective tissue and osseous changes. Some injuries seen in adult throwers, such as valgus extension overload, ulnar nerve irritation, and ulnar collateral ligament sprains, are usually a result of the volatile action of throwing, resulting in cumulative microtrauma to these structures. Most elbow lesions caused by overuse usually respond well to avoidance of noxious stimuli, the use of modalities, NSAIDs, and a low-weight, high-repetition rehabilitation regimen.

Although adolescent throwers subject themselves to the same mechanical elbow stresses as adult throwers, the injuries are different because of the maturation process and can be more debilitating. The two most common injuries reported in adolescents are osteochondritis dissecans, which involves the articular cartilage of the radiocapitellar joint, and Little Leaguer's elbow, which involves the epiphysis of the medial epicondyle. If these injuries are detected early they can be managed with no debilitating effects; but if left untreated, and the athlete continues to throw, permanent disability can ensue.

Initial treatment of elbow injuries after conservative management or surgery is concerned with decreasing the athlete's pain and inflammation and with restoring normal joint arthrokinematics. As pain decreases and healing restraints allow, range-of-motion exercises can be increased and a PRE regimen can be implemented. Later stages of rehabilitation should concentrate on the athlete performing exercises in functional planes at functional speeds to ready them for return to their sport. This return to competition should be preceded by an interval throwing program or by an interval program that is applicable for the individual athlete and allows for gradual return to participation.

APPLICATION*

Elbow Exercise Program

Deep Friction Massage.   Deep transverse friction massage is applied across the area of the elbow that is sore for 5 minutes, several times daily.

Grip.   The athlete uses a grip apparatus (e.g., putty, small rubber ball) frequently throughout the day.

Stretch Flexors.   The athlete straightens the elbow completely and, with the palm facing up, grasps the middle of the hand and thumb (Fig. 12–12). The wrist is pulled down as far as possible, holding for a 10 count, releasing and repeating 5 to 10 times before and after each exercise session.

Stretch Extensors.   The athlete straightens the elbow completely and, with the palm facing down, grasps the back of the hand and pulls the wrist down as far as possible (Fig. 12–13). This is held for a 10 count and released and repeated 5 to 10 times before and after each exercise session.

Progressive Resistance Exercises (PRE)

Each PRE session is begun with 3 sets of 10 repetitions (or 30 times) without weight, progressing to 5 sets of 10 repetitions (or 50 times) as

*All elbow exercises in this section (except ulnar and radial deviation) are from Middleton, K., Courson, R., Young, R., and Andrews, J.R. (1989): Preventative and Rehabilitative Exercises for the Shoulder and Elbow. Birmingham, AL, American Sports Medicine Institute.

FIGURE 12–12   (From Middleton, K., Courson, R., Young, R., and Andrews, J.R. (1989): Preventative and Rehabilitative Exercises for the Shoulder and Elbow, 2nd ed. Birmingham, AL, American Sports Medicine Institute.)

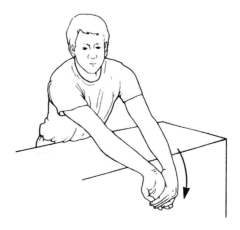

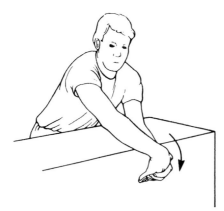

FIGURE 12–13 (From Middleton, K., Courson, R., Young, R., and Andrews, J.R. (1989): Preventative and Rehabilitative Exercises for the Shoulder and Elbow, 2nd ed. Birmingham, AL, American Sports Medicine Institute.)

tolerated. When the athlete can easily perform 5 sets of 10 repetitions, he or she may begin adding weight. Each PRE session begins with 3 sets of 10 repetitions with a 1-lb weight, progressing to 5 sets of 10, as tolerated over the next 2 to 3 days. When the athlete can easily perform 5 sets of 10 repetitions with a 1-lb weight, he or she may begin to progress the weight in the same manner.

Wrist Curls.   The forearm should be supported on a table with the hand off the edge; the palm should face upward. Using a weight, the athlete lowers the hand as far as possible and then curled up as high as possible (Fig. 12–14), holding for a 2 count.

Reverse Wrist Curls.   The forearm should be supported on a table with the hand off the edge; the palm should face downward. Using a weight, the athlete lowers the hand as far as possible and then curls the wrist up as high as possible (Fig. 12–15), holding for a 2 count.

Radial Deviation.   Standing with the arm by the side, the athlete holds an adjustable rod or hammer as depicted (Fig. 12–16), radially deviating the wrist, keeping the elbow straight, and holding for a 2 count.

Ulnar Deviation.   Standing with the arm by the side, the athlete

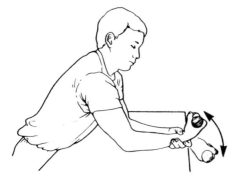

FIGURE 12–14 (From Middleton, K., Courson, R., Young, R., and Andrews, J.R. (1989): Preventative and Rehabilitative Exercises for the Shoulder and Elbow, 2nd ed. Birmingham, AL, American Sports Medicine Institute.)

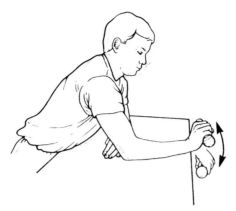

FIGURE 12–15   (From Middleton, K., Courson, R., Young, R., and Andrews, J.R. (1989): Preventative and Rehabilitative Exercises for the Shoulder and Elbow, 2nd ed. Birmingham, AL, American Sports Medicine Institute.)

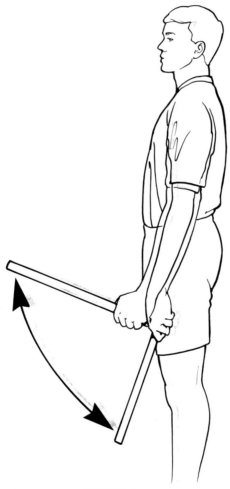

FIGURE 12–16

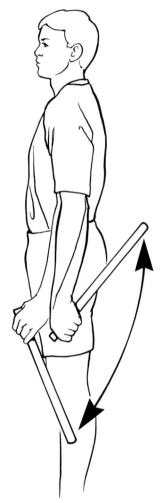

FIGURE 12–17

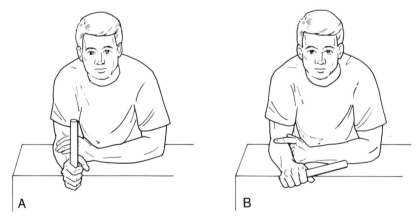

A   B

FIGURE 12–18   (Modified from Middleton, K., Courson, R., Young, R., and Andrews, J.R. (1989): Preventative and Rehabilitative Exercises for the Shoulder and Elbow, 2nd ed. Birmingham, AL, American Sports Medicine Institute.)

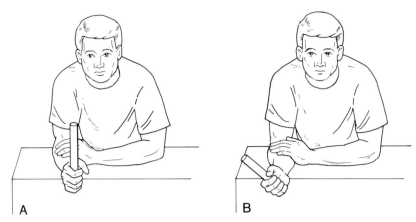

FIGURE 12–19 (Modified from Middleton, K., Courson, R., Young, R., and Andrews, J.R. (1989): Preventative and Rehabilitative Exercises for the Shoulder and Elbow, 2nd ed. Birmingham, AL, American Sports Medicine Institute.)

holds an adjustable rod or hammer as depicted (Fig. 12–17), ulnarly deviating the wrist, keeping the elbow straight, and holding for a 2 count.

Pronation. The forearm should be supported on a table with the wrist in the neutral position (Fig. 12–18A). Using a hammer or adjustable rod, the athlete rolls the wrist and brings the hammer or rod into pronation as far as possible (Fig. 12–18B), holding for a 2 count, and then raising back to starting position.

Supination. The forearm should be supported on the table with the wrist in the neutral position (Fig. 12–19A). Using a hammer or

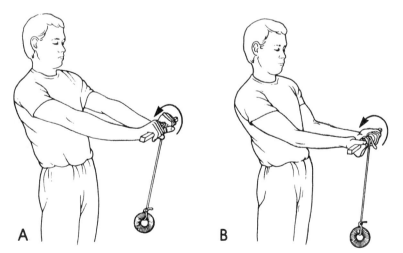

FIGURE 12–20A (From Middleton, K., Courson, R., Young, R., and Andrews, J.R. (1989): Preventative and Rehabilitative Exercises for the Shoulder and Elbow, 2nd ed. Birmingham, AL, American Sports Medicine Institute.)

FIGURE 12–20B (From Middleton, K., Courson, R., Young, R., and Andrews, J.R. (1989): Preventative and Rehabilitative Exercises for the Shoulder and Elbow, 2nd ed. Birmingham, AL, American Sports Medicine Institute.)

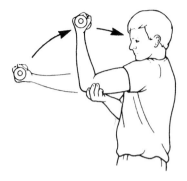

FIGURE 12–21 (From Middleton, K., Courson, R., Young, R., and Andrews, J.R. (1989): Preventative and Rehabilitative Exercises for the Shoulder and Elbow, 2nd ed. Birmingham, AL, American Sports Medicine Institute.)

adjustable rod, the athlete rolls the wrist and brings the hammer or rod into full supination (Fig. 12–19*B*), holding for a 2 count, and raising back to the starting position.

Broomstick Curl-Up.   A 1- to 2-foot broom handle with a 4- to 5-foot cord attached in the middle is used, with a 1-to-5-lb weight tied in the center.

EXTENSORS.   The athlete grips the stick on either side of the rope with the palms down (Fig. 12–20*A*). The cord is curled up by turning the stick toward the athlete (the cord is on the side of the stick away from the athlete). Once the weight is pulled to the top, the weight is lowered by unwinding the stick, rotating it away from the athlete. This is repeated 3 to 5 times.

FLEXORS.   This is the same as the exercise for the extensors, but the palms are facing upward (Fig. 12–20*B*).

Biceps Curl.   The athlete supports the arm on the opposite hand, bends the elbow to full flexion, and then straightens the arm completely (Fig. 12–21).

French Curl.   The athlete raises the arm overhead, using the opposite hand to support the elbow (Fig. 12–22). The elbow is straightened over the head, holding for a 2 count.

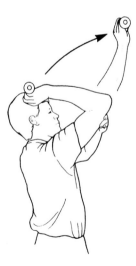

FIGURE 12–22 (From Middleton, K., Courson, R., Young, R., and Andrews, J.R. (1989): Preventative and Rehabilitative Exercises for the Shoulder and Elbow, 2nd ed. Birmingham, AL, American Sports Medicine Institute.)

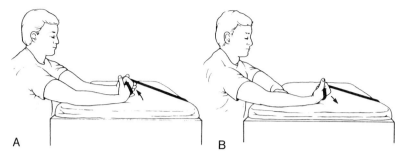

FIGURE 12–23   (From Middleton, K., Courson, R., Young, R., and Andrews, J.R. (1989): Preventative and Rehabilitative Exercises for the Shoulder and Elbow, 2nd ed. Birmingham, AL, American Sports Medicine Institute.)

Eccentric Elbow Program

Eccentric Flexion.   The athlete places the arm on the table, holding it straight with the hand facing up and off the table. Tubing is placed around the hand, with the opposite end tied tightly to the table leg (Fig. 12–23A). Assisting the hand with the palm up, the athlete works to starting position within a 5 count (Fig. 12–23B), repeating 3 to 5 sets of 10 repetitions.

Extension.   The athlete places the arm on the table, holding it straight with the hand facing down and off the table. The tubing is placed around the hand, with the opposite end tied tightly to the table leg (Fig. 12–24A). Assisting with the opposite hand to an extended position, the athlete works back to starting within a 5 count (Fig. 12–24B), repeating 3 to 5 sets of 10 repetitions.

Pronation.   The athlete places the arm straight on the table with the thumb up, holding the hammer with the tubing secure around the top of the hammer and the opposite end of the tubing tied to the table leg nearest the involved arm (Fig. 12–25A). The hammer is assisted with the opposite hand pushing the hammer and palm down, slowly returning to neutral within a 5 count (Fig. 12–25B). This is repeated for 3 to 5 sets of 10 repetitions.

Supination.   The athlete places the arm straight on the table with

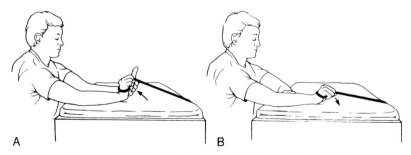

FIGURE 12–24   (From Middleton, K., Courson, R., Young, R., and Andrews, J.R. (1989): Preventative and Rehabilitative Exercises for the Shoulder and Elbow, 2nd ed. Birmingham, AL, American Sports Medicine Institute.)

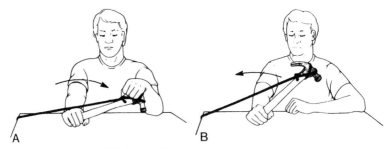

FIGURE 12–25   (From Middleton, K., Courson, R., Young, R., and Andrews, J.R. (1989): Preventative and Rehabilitative Exercises for the Shoulder and Elbow, 2nd ed. Birmingham, AL, American Sports Medicine Institute.)

the thumb up, holding the hammer with the tubing secure around the top of the hammer and the opposite end of the tubing tied to the table leg opposite the involved arm. The hammer is pushed down with the opposite hand, turning the involved hand palm up (Fig. 12–26A) and slowly returning to neutral position within a 5 count (Fig. 12–26 B). This is repeated for 3 to 5 repetitions.

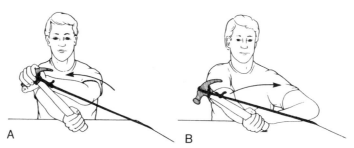

FIGURE 12–26   (From Middleton, K., Courson, R., Young, R., and Andrews, J.R. (1989): Preventative and Rehabilitative Exercises for the Shoulder and Elbow, 2nd ed. Birmingham, AL, American Sports Medicine Institute.)

References

1. Andrews, J.R. (1985): Bony injuries about the elbow in the throwing athlete. In Stauffer, E.S. (ed.): Instructional Course Lectures, Vol. 36. St. Louis, C.V. Mosby, pp. 323–331.
2. Andrews, J.R., and Wilson, F. (1985): Valgus extension overload in the pitching elbow In: Zarins, B., Andrews, J.R., and Carson, W.G. (eds.): Injuries to the Throwing Athlete. Philadelphia, W. B. Saunders, pp. 250–257.
3. Barnes, W.G., and Tullos, H.S. (1978): An analysis of 100 symptomatic baseball players. Am. J. Sports Med., 6(2):62–67.
4. Bennett, G.E. (1941): Shoulder and elbow lesions of the professional baseball pitcher. J.A.M.A., 117:510–514.
5. Berkely, M.E., Bennett, J.B., and Woods, G.W. (1985): Surgical management of acute and chronic elbow problems. In: Zarins, B., Andrews, J.R., and Carson, W.G. (eds.): Injuries to the Throwing Arm. Philadelphia, W.B. Saunders, pp. 235–249.
6. Bernhang, A.M., Dehner, W., and Fogerry, C. (1974): Tennis elbow: A biomechanical approach. J. Sports Med., 2:235–258.
7. Boyd, C.A., and McLeod, A.L. (1973): Tennis elbow. J. Bone Joint Surg. [Am.], 55: 1183–1187.

8. Brogdon, B.S., and Crow, M.D. (1960): Little Leaguer's elbow. Am. J. Roentgenol., 85:671.

9. Brown, R., Blazina, M.E., Kerlan, R.K., et al. (1974): Osteochondritis of the capitellum. J. Sports Med., 2(1):27–46.

10. DeHaven, K.E., and Evarts, C.M. (1973): Throwing injuries of the elbow in athletes. Orthop. Clin. North Am., 4:801–808.

11. Del Pizzo, W., Jobe, F.W., and Norwood, L. (1977): Ulnar nerve entrapment syndrome in baseball players. Am. J. Sports Med., 5(5):182–185.

12. Eaton, R.G., Crowe, J.F., and Parkes, J.C. (1980): Anterior transposition of the ulnar nerve using a non-compressing fasciodermal sling. J. Bone Joint Surg. [Am.], 62:820–825.

13. Froimson, A.I.(1971): Treatment of tennis elbow with forearm support. J. Bone Joint Surg. [Am.], 53:183–184.

14. Froimson, A.I., and Zahrawi, F. (1980): Treatment of compression neuropathy of the ulnar nerve at the elbow by epicondylectomy and neurolysis. J. Hand Surg., 5:391.

15. Garver, A.A. (1989): Iontophoresis Protocol: Tennis Elbow. Salt Lake City, Iomed.

16. Gay, J.R., and Love, J.G. (1947): Diagnosis and treatment of tardy paralysis of the ulnar nerve. J. Bone Joint Surg. [Am.], 29:1087.

17. Grana, W.A. (1980): Pitchers elbow in adolescents. Am. J. Sports Med., 8(5):333–336.

18. Groppel, J.L., and Nirschl, R.P. (1986): A mechanical and electromyographical analysis of the effects of various joint counterforce braces on the tennis player. Am. J. Sports Med., 14(3):195–200.

19. Halle, J.S., Franklin, R.J., and Karalfa, B.L. (1986): Comparison of four treatment approaches for lateral epicondylitis of the elbow. J. Orthop. Sports Phys. Ther., 8(2):62–68.

20. Hepburn, G.R., and Crivelli, R.J. (1984): Use of elbow Dynasplint for reduction of elbow flexion contractures: A case study. J. Orthop. Sports Phys. Ther., 5(5):269–274.

21. Hunter, S.C. (1985): Little Leaguer's elbow. In: Zarins, B., Andrews, J.R., and Carson, W.G. (eds.): Injuries to the Throwing Arm. Philadelphia, W.B. Saunders, pp. 228–234.

22. Ilfeld, F.W., and Field, S.M. (1966): Treatment of tennis elbow. J.A.M.A., 195:111–114.

23. Indelicato, P.A., Jobe, F.W., Kerlan, R.K., et al. (1979): Correctable elbow lesions in professional baseball players: A review of 25 cases. Am. J. Sports Med., 7(1):72–75.

24. Jobe, F.W., Moynes, D.R., Tibone, J.E., and Perry, J. (1984): An EMG analysis of the shoulder in pitching. A special report. Am. J. Sports Med., 12:218–220.

25. Jobe, F.W., and Nuber, G. (1986): Throwing injuries of the elbow. Clin. Sports Med., 5(4):621–636.

26. Jobe, F.W., Stark, H., and Lombardo, S.J. (1986): Reconstruction of the ulnar collateral ligament in athletes. J. Bone Joint Surg. [Am.], 68:1158–1163.

27. Johansson, O. (1962): Capsular and ligament injuries of the elbow joint: A clinical and arthrographic study. Acta Chir. Scand. [Suppl.], 287:5–71.

28. Jones, H.H., Priest, J.D., Hayes, W.C., et al. (1977): Humeral hypertrophy in response to exercise. J. Bone Joint Surg. [Am.], 59:204.

29. King, J.W., Brelsford, H.J., and Tullos, H.S. (1969): Analysis of the pitching arm of the professional baseball pitcher. Clin. Orthop., 67:116.

30. Leach, R.E., and Miller, J.K. (1987): Lateral and medial epicondylitis of the elbow. Clin. Sports Med., 6(2):259–272.

31. Levy, D.M., and Apfelberg, D.B. (1972): Results of anterior transposition for ulnar neuropathy at the elbow. Am. J. Surg., 123:304

32. McLeod, W.D. (1985): The pitching mechanism. In: Zarins, B., Andrews, J.R., and Carson, W.G. (eds.): Injuries to the Throwing Arm. Philadelphia, W.B. Saunders, pp. 22–29.

33. Medich, G.F. (1989): Little League elbow. Sports Med. Update, 4(2):15–17.

34. Melhoff, T.L., Noble, P. C., Bennett, J. B., and Tullos, H.S. (1988): Simple dislocation of the elbow in the adult. J. Bone Joint Surg. [Am.], 70:244–249.

35. Neblett, C., and Ehini, G. (1970): Medial epicondylectomy for ulnar palsy. J. Neurosurg., 32:55.

36. Nirschl, R.P. (1973): Tennis elbow. Orthop. Clin. North Am., 4:787–799.

37. Nirschl, R.P. (1975): The etioloby and treatment of tennis elbow. Am. J. Sports Med., 2:308–323.

38. Nirschl, R.P. (1986): Soft-tissue injuries about the elbow. Clin. Sports Med., 5(4):637–653.

39. O'Donoghue, D.F. (1970): Treatment of Injuries to Athletes, 2nd. ed. Philadelphia, W.B. Saunders, pp. 46–52, 239–240.

40. Osborne, G., and Cotterill, P. (1966): Recurrent dislocation of the elbow. J. Bone Joint Surg. [Br.], 48:340–346.

41. Pappas, A.M. (1981): Osteochondrosis dissecans. Clin. Orthop. Rel. Res., 158:59–69.

42. Pappas, A.M. (1982): Elbow problems associated with baseball during childhood and adolescence. Clin. Orthop. Rel. Res., 164:30–41.

43. Priest, J.D. (1976): Tennis elbow: The syndrome and a study of average players. Minn. Med., June:367–371.

44. Protzman, R.R. (1978): Dislocation of the elbow joint. J. Bone Joint Surg., [Am.], 60:539–541.

45. Raney, R.B., and Brasher, H.R. (1971): Shands' Handbook of Orthopaedic Surgery. St. Louis, C.V. Mosby, pp. 429–431.

46. Richmond, J.C., and Southmayd, W.W. (1982): Superficial anterior transposition of the ulnar nerve at the elbow for ulnar neuritis. Clin. Orthop., 164:42–44.

47. Runge, F. (1873): Žur Genese und Behandlung des Schreibekrampfes. Berl. Klin. Wochenschr., 21:245.

48. Schemmel, S.P., and Andrews, J.R. (1988): Acute and chronic ulnar collateral ligament injuries in the throwing athlete. Sports Med. Update, 3(3):10–11.

49. Schwab, G.H., Bennett, J.B., Woods, G.W., and Tullos, H.S. (1980): Biomechanics of elbow instability: The role of the medial collateral ligament. Clin. Orthop., 146:42–52.

50. Singer, K.M., and Roy, S.P. (1984): Osteochondrosis of the humeral capitellum. Am. J. Sports Med., 12(5):351–360.

51. Sisto, D.J., Jobe, F.W., Moynes, D.R., and Antonelli, D.J. (1987): An electromyographic analysis of the elbow in pitching. Am. J. Sports Med., 15(3):260–263.

52. Stonecipher, D.R., and Catlin, P.A. (1984): The effect of a forearm strap on wrist extensor strength. J. Orthop. Sports Phys. Ther., 6(3):184–189.

53. Snyder-Mackler, L., and Epler, M. (1989): Effect of standard and Aircast tennis elbow bands on integrated electromyography of forearm extensor musculature proximal to the bands. Am. J. Sports Med., 17(2):278–281.

54. Tivnon, M.C., Anzel, S.H., and Waugh, T.R. (1976): Surgical management of osteochondritis dissecans of the capitellum. Am. J. Sports Med., 4(3):121–128.

55. Torg, J.S., Pollack, H., and Sweterlitsch, P. (1972): The effect of competitive pitching on the shoulders and elbows in preadolescent baseball players. Pediatrics, 49:267–271.

56. Tullos, H.S., and Bryan, W.J. (1985): Examination of the throwing elbow. In: Zarins, B., Andrews, J. R., and Carson, W.G. (eds.): Injuries to the Throwing Athlete. Philadelphia, W.B. Saunders, pp. 201–210.

57. Tullos, H.S., and King, J.W. (1972): Lesion of the pitching arm in adolescents. J.A.M.A., 220:264–271.

58. Tullos, H.S., and King, J. W. (1973): Throwing mechanism in sports. Orthop. Clin. North Am., 4:709–721.

59. Vanderpool, D.W., Chalmers, J., Lamb, D.W., and Winston, T.B. (1968): Peripheral compression lesion of the ulnar nerve. J. Bone Joint Surg. [Br.], 50:792–803.

60. Wadsworth, C.T., Nielson, D.H., Burns, L. T., et al. (1989): Effect of the counterforce armband on wrist extension and grip strength and pain in subjects with tennis elbow. J. Orthop. Sports Phys. Ther., 11(5):192–197.

61. Wilson, F.D., Andrews, J.R., and McClusky, G. (1983): Valgus extension overload in the pitching elbow. Am. J. Sports Med., 11(2):83–87.

62. Woodward, A.H., and Bianco, A.J. (1975): Osteochondritis dissecans of the elbow. Clin. Orthop. Rel. Res., 110:35–41.

CHAPTER 13

◆

Aquatic Rehabilitation*

Glenn McWaters, B.S.

There are three primary objectives in rehabilitating the injured athlete: (1) returning the athlete to play as soon as possible, (2) with the injury at or near 100% of preinjury strength levels, and (3) the athlete's conditioning level equal to the preinjury level. Only a decade ago, few people understood the advantages of water and still fewer were using aquatic exercises to return athletes to competition. Although research is still limited, evidence has suggested a 40 to 50% reduction in the duration of rehabilitation time.

The use of water to treat injuries is not a new concept. Physical therapists and athletic trainers have long used water, primarily in the form of a whirlpool. The whirlpool provides a soothing, massage-like effect to the muscles, increasing the amount of blood and oxygen to the traumatized area while reducing effusion. The use of water as a treatment for various maladies, however, precedes the use of the whirlpool by centuries. Ancient Rome was noted for its public bathing pools, and the Greeks immersed themselves in thermal springs to treat various ailments.

Currently, it is not the whirlpool but the (re)discovery of the swimming pool that is making aquatic rehabilitation an exciting area to explore. Extensive use of the pool is helping clinicians return injured athletes to participation sooner than with the use of conventional rehabilitation techniques. When the athlete is ready to return to participation, the aquatically rehabilitated athlete is usually near 100% of preinjury strength levels, and the overall conditioning level is equal to or greater than that of the preinjury state. It appears that almost all sports-related injuries (e.g., of the knee, ankle, hip, back, shoulder) can be rehabilitated in a shorter period of time using "water therapy" or "aquatic therapy" than with previously used methods of "dry land" rehabilitation.

---

* Figures 13-2 to 13-32 are © copyrighted by Glenn McWaters.

HISTORY OF AQUATIC THERAPY

My first encounter with water as something other than for drinking, bathing, cleaning, or playing occurred in 1970. As a Marine Corps helicopter pilot in Vietnam, my tour of duty was cut short by a gunshot wound to the left thigh. Following the initial operation, a second surgery was performed after I returned to the United States.

I had been a competitive middle distance runner in college and in the Marine Corps and had planned to renew my competitive career. My first thought after being wounded was to get my leg healed so my training could resume. The Navy surgeon who repaired my damaged left thigh said there was little hope of my ever running again. He suggested taking up his former sport, swimming. He indicated that swimming was nonweight-bearing and could be done even with an imperfect leg. A couple of weeks following the second surgery, after the wound had healed sufficiently to immerse my leg in water, I submerged myself into a new athletic world. After three or four laps of swimming, however, I lay back on the side of the pool, gasping for breath—I had discovered that I was not a swimmer. Swimming is a skilled sport, and, although I had spent many hours in the pool while growing up, little time was devoted to swimming. In the 1960s, only competitive swimmers swam laps. Now, several years later, I found myself unable to swim more than a few lengths. Instead, I braced myself in the corner of the deep end of the pool and began kicking my legs. The only limiting factor was fatigue to my arms and shoulders. After about 15 minutes, I had to stop and rest my arms. I began going to the pool twice a day and exercising for 30 to 45 minutes each session. Within a week the swimming was dropped altogether, but the kicking exercises were expanded to whatever could be imagined. Within 5 months of entering the pool I was on dry land, running again. Two months later, I ran my first race. The doctors were not only amazed at how quickly I recovered, but also at how completely. Today my leg wound remains asymptomatic.

From that unlikely beginning in 1970, water has become a close ally. Throughout the early 1970s I used water strictly for rehabilitation. I found deep water to be more beneficial for the rehabilitation of most running injuries than shallow water. Consequently, most of my work has revolved around exercise in the deep end of the pool.

I discovered that athletes not only recovered rapidly, but maintained or improved their conditioning while recovering from their injury. This led me to experiment with using deep water as a supplement to a training program. Initially, life jackets and ski belts were used to provide buoyancy, and the injured athletes used them because there was no other alternative, but once healed they quickly left the pool. Out of frustration, I designed a lightweight, snug-fitting, buoyant vest that provided total freedom of movement in deep water. This became known as the Wet Vest* and it has received widespread acclaim. Research has confirmed that it is the only training aid that allows specificity

---

* Available from Bioenergetics, Pelham, AL.

of movement in deep water, which is essential to training and rehabilitation.[4, 8, 10, 13, 14, 16, 20]

With the advent of this aquatic training aid, the field of aquatic rehabilitation and supplementary training has exploded. For example, over 50% of all runners in the 1988 Olympic Games used deep water running as part of their training routine. This supplementary water training not only promotes faster rehabilitation but can also increase speed, endurance, and flexibility. Although supplementary training is another beneficial aspect of the use of aquatic therapy, this chapter will concentrate on the rehabilitation phase.

Dr. Igor Burdenko has done much for the advancement of aquatic rehabilitation. For more than a decade, Dr. Burdenko worked with elite Soviet athletes at the Comprehensive Sports Rehabilitation Training Center in Moscow. He had cross-country skiers, speed skaters, gymnasts, hockey players, and runners attending this unique facility, and they all used the swimming pool as an adjunctive training tool. He devised sophisticated training programs of walking, running, and other activities, all performed in varying depths of water. Dr. Burdenko not only relied on the pool for rehabilitation, but also used it to increase balance, coordination, flexibility, speed, strength, and endurance.

Dr. Burdenko left Russia for the United States in 1981. Dr. Lyle Micheli, Director of Sports Medicine at the Children's Hospital in Boston, who was familiar with Dr. Burdenko's popular Soviet exercise books, assisted Dr. Burdenko in establishing his practice. Soon Dr. Burdenko was extolling the "magical" powers of water as he developed a loyal following among those in the athletic community of Boston. Burdenko[2] has stated that "With no gravity to impede movements, individuals can rehabilitate much faster in the pool than on land."

CASE HISTORY 1

◆

One of Dr. Burdenko's most well-known success stories is that of the Boston Celtics' forward, Kevin McHale.[2] Dr. Burdenko began aquatic rehabilitation exercises with McHale only 4 days after foot surgery. McHale returned to basketball, in top condition, 5 months earlier than expected.

Dr. Burdenko felt it extremely important to begin aquatic therapy immediately, even though McHale's foot was casted. The cast was enclosed in a waterproof covering and the program was started. McHale's initial rehabilitation was performed in deep water. Warm-up exercises consisted of running in deep water followed by a series of deep water activities to increase balance, flexibility, strength, and speed. Dr. Burdenko has also been a proponent of specificity of training: the athlete should do in the pool what he or she normally does on dry land. Although McHale was unable to dribble in the water, Dr. Burdenko used a basketball to throw high, arching lobs; McHale would leap as high as possible in the deep water, catch the ball, and immediately throw it back to Dr. Burdenko. This simulated rebounding and the beginning of a fast break, and McHale made thousands of catches and tosses in this manner.

Dr. Burdenko directs injured tennis players to swing rackets, injured baseball players to swing bats, and injured golfers to swing golf clubs while in the water.[2]

◆

CASE HISTORY 2

◆
―――

Back patients have also benefitted from Dr. Burdenko's water therapy program. One female patient, a former competitive figure skater, had been plagued by a mysterious back ailment for 10 years.[2] She was often bedridden for weeks and wore a neck-to-navel brace for more than a year. Many physicians and physical therapists had been unable to reduce the pain or locate its cause. She sought Dr. Burdenko's assistance. During her 40-minute pool sessions, Dr. Burdenko had her move and bend in every conceivable manner. The recovery was remarkable. For the first time in a decade, she is now pain-free. She believes herself to be in better shape at age 50 than she was at age 30.

―――
◆

"Active rest" is the key to Dr. Burdenko's success. He hates passive recovery and has stated that "Nothing can come from nothing. Even an injury can benefit from the right activity, the right orderly regimen."[2]

Dr. Burdenko does not limit rehabilitation to the pool. He uses other dry land activities such as surgical tubing, extending arms and legs throughout increasing ranges of motion, walking and running in unusual manners in the gym, and running uphill in sand. However, the basis for his rehabilitation program revolves around and in the water. Without the water to improve mobility and eliminate pain, other dry land activities would not be feasible.

Dr. Burdenko breaks up a workout session into the following:[2]

Warm-up: 15 to 20% of the total session
Main workout: 70 to 80% of the total session
Cool down: 5 to 10% of the total session

Both the warm up and cool down are vital parts of each workout. A muscle has a "brain" that remembers if it is stretched or not. If the athlete forgets to stretch at the end of a workout session, the muscle remains tense longer than normal.

Dr. Burdenko has recommended that, if the water temperature is warm (above about 29° C, or 84° F), a shorter warm up is needed, and, if the water temperature is cool, a longer warm-up is preferable. In all cases, however, the patient should use a Wet Vest prior to exercising in deep water. Burdenko has noted that a little more buoyancy relaxes the muscles and improves circulation.[2] If a muscle is tight it constricts the circulation, and a person needs to be relaxed and at ease in the water.

BENEFITS OF AQUATIC THERAPY

Buoyancy

The buoyancy factor is the most obvious reason why water is a beneficial rehabilitative medium. It eliminates approximately 90% of the gravitational pull and the Wet Vest eliminates the remainder, so the body has neutral buoyancy in the water. Movements that may be painful on dry land can be undertaken in water with little or no pain. Deep water allows the athlete to exercise all muscle groups and move all joints through a complete range of motion while benefitting from the cushioning effect of water's buoyancy.[16] Water therapy is implemented in postsurgical rehabilitation programs to lessen pain, increase mobility, and accelerate the healing process.[16] For example, a runner recovering from knee surgery can run suspended in the water without ever placing any pressure on the injured extremity. By exercising in this manner, the athlete maintains cardiovascular fitness and increases strength and mobility in the recovering knee.[16] Currently, aquatic therapy is used to achieve faster rehabilitation than dry land activities, because it reduces gravity and pain.[13]

Increased Resistance

The increased resistance of water is another factor. Even though the gravitational pull is almost eliminated, the resistance to movement is increased. Water resistance is directly proportional to the speed of movement. If the athlete walks easily in the water, the fluid resistance may be only five to six times greater than that of air. If the athlete attempts to run fast in the water, however, the fluid resistance increases to more than 40 times that of air (Table 13–1).[14]

In Table 13–1 the vertical column on the right lists times achieved running 12.5 yards in the water at various speeds, from slowest to fastest (reading top to bottom). The top time (188 seconds) means it

TABLE 13–1   **RATIOS OF THE RESISTANCE ENCOUNTERED RUNNING IN DEEP WATER VERSUS RUNNING IN AIR AT VARIOUS SPEEDS***

	Resistance, Water Versus Air (Ratio)							12.5-Yard Pace Time in Water (sec)
	16.0	12.6	10.2	8.5	7.1	6.1	5.2‡	188
	19.0	15.0	12.2	10.1	8.5	7.2	6.2	94
	22.3	17.6	14.3	11.8	9.9	8.5	7.3	63
	25.9	20.4	16.6	13.7	11.5	9.8	8.5	47
	29.7	23.5	19.0	15.7	13.2	11.3	9.7	38
	33.8	26.7	21.6	17.9	15.0	12.8	11.0	31
	38.1	30.1	24.4	20.2	17.0	14.4	12.5	27
	42.7†	33.8	27.4	22.6	19.0	16.2	14.0	23
440-Yard Pace Time on the Track (sec)	122.1	104.6	91.6	81.4	73.3	66.6	61.0	

* Several factors were used in computing these ratios, including the absolute viscosity and density of air and water, the velocity of the extremities relative to body movement, the average diameter of the extremities, body roughness, and the Reynolds factor (a method allowing mathematical comparisons of one substance to another).

† Resistance when running in water at the fastest pace and running a quarter mile on the track at the slowest pace.

‡ Resistance when running in water at the slowest pace and running a quarter mile on the track at the fastest pace.

took 3 minutes, 8 seconds to run forward 12.5 yards. The bottom time (23 seconds) corresponds to a very fast pace—running 12.5 yards forward in the water in 23 seconds. The last row of numbers along the bottom represents times achieved running 440 yards (a quarter mile) on a track at various speeds. The slowest times are on the left, and the fastest are on the right. The left-most time (122 seconds equals $\frac{1}{4}$ mile) corresponds to running a mile in 8 minutes and 8 seconds. The right-most time (61 seconds equals $\frac{1}{4}$ mile) corresponds to running a mile in 4 minutes and 4 seconds.

Let us first consider the resistance encountered when running 12.5 yards in water at the fastest pace (23 seconds), compared to the resistance encountered when running a quarter mile on the track at the slowest pace (122 seconds). The resistance of the water is 42.7 times greater than that of air (see dotted arrows, Table 13–1).

The other extreme occurs if the resistance encountered when running 12.5 yards in water at the slowest pace (188 seconds) is compared to the resistance encountered when running a quarter mile at the fastest pace (61 seconds). The resistance of the water is still 5.2 times greater than air (see dashed arrows, Table 13–1).

When running at the same exertion level in water as on land, the resistance of the water is 12 to 14 times greater than air. Every muscle submerged below the water is subjected to an increased resistance. Consequently, a better overall workout can be achieved in water.

Isodynamic Exercise

Exercise can be classified into four categories—isometric, isotonic, variable resistance, and isokinetic. Isometric muscle contractions occur when the muscle is subjected to tension without changing length. Isotonic exercises involve both concentric and eccentric muscle contractions. Isotonic actually means same tension, but this is a misnomer. There are large fluctuations in the tension applied to the muscles throughout a range of motion, even though the resistant force (or weight) does not change. Even with variable resistance machines, the tension does not remain constant on the muscles throughout a full range of motion. A more proper definition of isotonic is same weight. The fourth type of activity is isokinetic, meaning same speed, but this is also an incomplete definition. An individual can actually vary the speed of movement on most isokinetic machines. A more complete definition of isokinetic is a positive contraction that occurs when a muscle is subjected to an even amount of tension at a constant speed over the full range of motion.

Of the four exercise categories, water therapy is considered isokinetic. Aquatic activity performed in deep water is almost totally isokinetic. Even though an individual can change the speed of movement in the water, the amount of tension on the muscles throughout the range of motion remains constant. The most appropriate term for deep water exercise is probably "isodynamic"—an equal or uniform force applied to the muscles throughout a full range of motion.

Because only four categories are normally used to classify exercise, and for the purpose of relating the benefits of aquatic rehabilitation, it is included here under the heading of isokinetic exercise. Isokinetic activities have provided the best results in regard to both training and rehabilitation.[2, 5, 7, 10, 13, 14, 16, 17] Fox stated that "From a theoretical viewpoint isokinetic contractions, and thus isokinetic training programs, appear to be best suited for improving athletic performance."[7] This was based on studies that showed more enhanced performance following isokinetic activities than after other activities. This is also proving to be true for rehabilitation. A 5-year study of over 5000 postsurgical knee rehabilitation patients showed that isokinetic rehabilitation exercises are more efficient and effective than any other type of activity for long-term success.[17] At the end of the first year following surgery, all patients who had undergone rehabilitation with a home program or who had no rehabilitation returned to their physician for additional treatment of the affected knee. Those in the isotonic rehabilitation program fared much better, but still only 7% remained pain-free at the end of the 5-year period. Patients who underwent an isokinetic rehabilitation program had superb results, with 61% showing no recurring knee problems after 5 years.

From empirical studies, it can be surmised that isodynamic aquatic activities provide equal or greater benefits than isokinetic, dry land activities.[1–4, 6, 8, 9–11, 13–16, 18–21] These include enhanced performance as a result of optimizing neuromuscular responses, improved motor unit contraction synchrony, and facilitation of maximal muscle contraction at each point in an available joint's range of motion. Water activities also appear to provide increased muscle fiber and motor unit recruitment, and both slow- and fast-twitch muscle fibers are stimulated.[2, 4, 6, 7, 10, 11, 14, 17, 19]

Whereas isotonic exercise is submaximal because of concentric and eccentric muscle loading occurring only at the extremes of movement, isokinetic (and isodynamic) exercise concentrically loads the muscle equally throughout the full range of motion. Some individuals have suggested that aquatic activity is not as beneficial as isotonic movements because there is almost no eccentric contraction. A study has shown that concentric isokinetic training not only improves concentric strength levels, but also increases eccentric strength levels in tennis players.[5] Another group, which underwent only eccentric isokinetic exercises, showed no gain in eccentric strength levels. The same study also determined that concentric isokinetic training produces a significant increase in serving speed among the tennis players tested, whereas those in the eccentric isokinetic training group actually showed a decrease in serving speed.[5]

Psychologic Effects

The worst thing an athlete can hear is that "You will have to remain inactive for . . ." Inactivity represents a death knell to an active person. The injured athlete fluctuates among depression, anger, and acceptance. By keeping the active person involved in some activity, even if not the chosen sport, the individual is not subjected to the roller coaster of emotional feelings experienced by the inactive person. Burdenko has stated that "Doctors tell you to take it easy, but how can you have healing circulation if you take it easy? Movement is life!"[2] Kuland[11] has advocated water therapy for injuries for several years and has noticed that rehabilitation seems to be accelerated if an individual can maintain an exercise program without interruption. Perhaps the body interprets an individual's ability to continue to train without discomfort as a sign that the injury has healed, a response that may in itself speed healing.[11]

Shortened Rehabilitation Time

The ultimate objective of injured athletes is to participate in their chosen sport again, and as soon as possible. Empirical studies have shown that water therapy accelerates the healing process faster than any other method.[2, 4, 10, 11, 13, 14, 16, 18–20] Tony Kennon,[10] who oversees the University of Alabama's aquatic rehabilitation program for the football team, has noted that, since the university implemented aquatic therapy, rehabilitation time has been reduced by 40 to 50%.

Bill McDonald, head athletic trainer at the University of Alabama and a proponent of water rehabilitation, has stated that "Rehab often means pain and discomfort, but this discomfort is not experienced in the water. The frequency, duration, and intensity can be increased with no adverse affects. This cannot be done with conventional rehab, thus enabling players to return to competition sooner."[13]

CASE HISTORY 3

On September 13, 1988, David Smith, University of Alabama's starting quarterback, injured his right knee during a practice session.[10] The following day, Smith underwent a lateral meniscectomy and debridement of the anterior cruciate ligament. The news media reported that the senior quarterback's career was over—he would not return. The next day Smith began quad setting, range-of-motion exercises, and electrical muscle stimulation.[10, 13] Smith began deep water exercise 1 week following surgery. This allowed the exterior wound to heal and prevented infection.

Smith's aquatic rehabilitation regimen began in deep water. Warm-up consisted of slow running followed by a series of exercises designed to move his injured knee through as full a range of motion as possible. As range of motion improved, additional activities such as overstriding drills and sprinting were added. Following 1 week in deep water his range of motion was almost completely restored and he could bear full weight on the injured leg. During week 2, Smith carried out deep water drills followed by shallow water activities consisting of standing in chest-deep water and performing kicks and paddling exercises. There was a ledge inside the pool, and Smith submerged himself about halfway down the wall, where he would stand on his good leg and use his injured leg as a paddle, pulling and pushing against the water. He performed knee and hip extension and flexion exercises under the trainer's supervision.

Smith returned as the starting quarterback in the seventh game of the year, only 4 weeks following injury. The trainers speculate that the water exercises strengthened Smith and brought him back faster than anyone thought possible.[10] Even after he was healthy, Smith continued to use the pool to gain strength. He practiced hundreds of drop backs and lateral movements in shallow water, just as if he were taking the snap from center.[10] By season's end he was not only stronger but also quicker.[13]

Kennon and McDonald[10, 13] are such strong proponents of water therapy that, at one time or another, almost every one of their players has used the pool. Kennon[10] has reported that hamstring strains were a problem for years, especially for wide receivers. In particular, one wide receiver had hamstring problems throughout his first 2 years at the University of Alabama. After being subjected to water therapy during his third year, the player played out his remaining 2 years with no hamstring problems.

Bill McDonald[13] has suggested that water rehabilitation is especially beneficial for those individuals or institutions who cannot afford the enormous array of rehabilitation equipment presently on the market. He believes that an athlete can perform almost all the necessary movements and activities in the water.

CASE HISTORY 4

Priscilla Welch won the 1987 New York City Marathon at the age of 42. She was the oldest competitor ever to win a major marathon. She used the pool to intensify training and to maintain conditioning while recovering from injuries. She incorporated deep water running into her training program on a regular basis and also found that relaxing runs in the pool readily reduced her postrace soreness.[20]

In early 1988 a bone scan confirmed a stress fracture in her foot, and she was told not to run for 8 weeks. She continued her training by running in deep water. Four weeks later, the foot pain had totally dissipated. A second bone scan confirmed that her foot had totally healed. It was believed that the water exercise had reduced the normal rehabilitation time by half. Additionally, she found she was in better condition after resuming her road running than she was prior to injury. She ran an impressive time of 2:30.48 at the Boston Marathon only 4 weeks after resuming dry land running.

Brody[1] has confirmed the benefits of water running in a study in which five volunteer runners, two of whom were suffering from stress fractures, were placed on a supervised water training regimen. For 3 months, the only exercise these volunteers performed was long slow distance and interval training runs in the pool. At the end of 3 months both stress fractures had healed, and all five runners reported improved performance. It was concluded that even marathon runners can maintain cardiovascular fitness levels without dry land running.[1] Burdenko[2] has postulated that aquatic therapy hastens fracture healing because the exercise expedites bone remodeling.

CASE HISTORY 5

---◆---

Tim Krumrie suffered a fracture of the left tibia during the 1989 Super Bowl.[12] The tibia was fractured in two places and the fibula in one. Krumrie underwent closed reduction of the fibula fracture and internal fixation of the fractured tibia.

Krumrie's rehabilitation began 3 weeks following surgery. The initial pool therapy consisted of deep water running three times per week, as well as massages and manual therapy of the lower leg. After 3 months of water therapy, strength training was added to his program.[12] Although the initial prognosis for Krumrie's return was poor, the next year he returned to the starting line-up, playing the nose tackle position with the same intensity as that prior to injury.

---◆---

Watkins[19] has noted that, a decade ago, physicians told injured athletes to rest for a few weeks until the injury healed. Now it is recognized that rest and inactivity may be the worst treatment for an injury—muscles atrophy and weaken, and the athlete loses physical conditioning and often becomes depressed and anxious. Unfortunately, for most injuries, normal exercise is not possible, and aquatic therapy is a viable alternative.[18, 19]

The aquatic rehabilitation exercises described at the end of this chapter were developed over a period of years. They benefit almost everyone, athlete or nonathlete. Baseball players can regain the use of injured shoulders and elbows, football and basketball players can rehabilitate and strengthen lower body muscles, soccer players can improve their kicking ability, tennis and golf players can enhance their swings, and runners can improve speed and endurance. Aquatic therapy is one way to recover from an injury while maintaining or improving performance.[6, 14]

Brody[1] has devised a plan whereby individuals can know when they are ready to return to dry land activities. The athlete should rate the pain on a scale of 0 to 10 (0 represents no pain, and 10 represents severe pain). When individuals can honestly rate the pain level at 0, they can return to dry land training. The athlete should consider encompassing deep water exercises into the regular training routine, however, even when healthy.

CONTRAINDICATIONS AND GUIDELINES

Water is a forgiving medium. Most injuries benefit from aquatic therapy by responding faster and healing sooner. As with any rehabilitation program, however, there are a few guidelines and contraindications.

Open Wounds.   Wounds should be healed sufficiently before submerging in the water. Some physicians allow a patient to enter the water immediately after removal of sutures, whereas others prefer to wait a little longer. Generally, 7 to 10 days following surgery is ample time for the wound to heal before immersing in water.

Contagious Infections.   Anyone with a contagious infection should not risk passing the illness to others who share the pool. The athlete should wait until the contagious stage has passed before undergoing aquatic activities.

Chronic Ear Infections.   Most aquatic activities can be performed with the head maintained comfortably above water. As a safety precaution, however, individuals susceptible to ear infections should wear an ear protection device while in the water.

Excessive Fear of Water.   It has been postulated that at least half of the United States population cannot swim. Many nonswimmers are terrified of the water, and special concerns should be given to these athletes. Many of the exercises can be performed in shallow water but, for athletes with lower extremity injuries, deep water is preferred. The regular Wet Vest provides enough buoyancy for everyone but about 3% of the population who are considered "sinkers." These are normally athletes with dense bones, heavy musculature, and very low body fat. Such individuals may require a double flotation Wet Vest, which assures them enough buoyancy to maintain the head well above the water line. Even then, exercises should be started slowly, allowing the athlete to gain confidence in the water. The rehabilitation phase may take a little longer, but the athlete emerges with greater confidence and improved self-esteem.

Severe Pain.   If the athlete experiences any pain, he or she should stop that activity because progress cannot be made in rehabilitation if pain is present.[2] If the athlete is not experiencing pain when in a nonweight-bearing position on dry land, it is all right to begin aquatic therapy. Movements that cause pain should be stopped and tried again in a few days. If the athlete is overseeing his or her own rehabilitation program, pain should be the guide.

Buddy System.   *Never, never* allow individuals to exercise alone, even if they are excellent swimmers. Another person should always be present in the pool area, such as the clinician, lifeguard, or a buddy.

Aquatic therapy is often overlooked as a rehabilitation modality but recently has been advocated in many medical circles for various ailments. In the orthopedic community aquatic rehabilitation is used to promote early range of motion and exercise, attempting to negate the deleterious effects of inactivity. Water's greatest asset is its buoyancy effect, allowing for early weight-bearing and even running that may not be possible on dry land following injury or surgery. Water also provides an isokinetic-like exercise, and sports-specific patterns can be implemented.

Although the Wet Vest is the aquatic device of choice for this chapter because it allows freedom of movement, many other water appliances are available and can be used (e.g., kick boards, fins, hand paddles). Most athletes can begin aquatic therapy 5 to 7 days postsurgery with early implementation of a cardiovascular component through deep water running, modified as needed to protect the healing restraints. Although certainly not a panacea, aquatic therapy can be advantageous in the overall recovery of the injured athlete.

AQUATIC REHABILITATION EXERCISES

Aquatic exercises may not be applicable in the early stages of rehabilitation for those with certain injuries. Some movements may need to be avoided initially or limited to a specific range of motion.

Warm-Up Phase

The first phase involves the warm-up, and deep water running is often preferred (Fig. 13—1). Depending on the location and extent of injury, this may vary from an easy walking to an easy running motion. The warm-up should last from 8 to 10 minutes, with the athlete attempting to maintain a proper running motion (Fig. 13—2).

Running Motion.   The athlete leans slightly forward in the water, as if running outdoors (Fig. 13—2A), but should not reach out and pull with the arms as if swimming. The athlete's arms are kept next to the body and the elbows bent at a 90° angle. The athlete will move forward in the pool. If attempting to stay in one place, the athlete should do more of a bicycling motion (Fig. 13—2B). To increase upper body resistance, the hands are cupped. If less resistance on the upper torso is desired, the hands are left open. Runner A receives maximum benefits. Leaning too far forward reduces resistance on the lower body, thus decreasing workout effectiveness (Fig. 13—2C). Dry land running form should be duplicated as closely as possible in the water.

Cross-Country Skiing Motion.   An alternative to the running motion is the cross-country skiing motion (Fig. 13—3). Running is done with the legs stiff and knees locked. Athletes with upper body injuries should keep their arms stiff. This activity may be less painful for athletes with a serious knee injury.

Horizontal Jumping Jack.   This is an excellent warm-up activity. The athlete begins by floating on the back with the arms by the sides and the feet together (Fig. 13—4A). Simultaneously, the athlete spreads

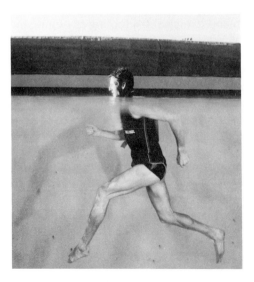

FIGURE 13—1   Deep water running. (Courtesy of Bioenergetics, Inc., Pelham, AL.)

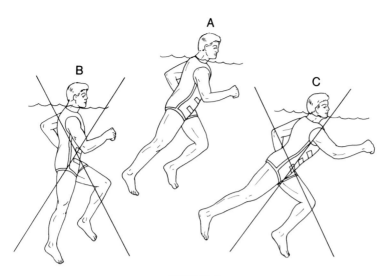

FIGURE 13—2

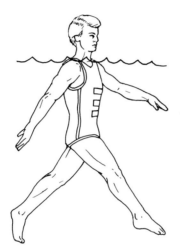

FIGURE 13—3

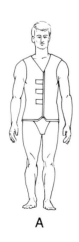
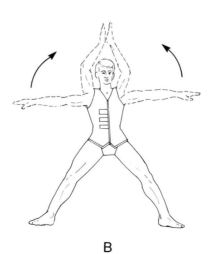

A   B

FIGURE 13—4

the legs as far to the sides as possible (Fig. 13–4B), bringing the arms above the head as far as possible while keeping the arms in the water (on the same plane as the body), and returning to the starting position. This is 1 repetition (same movement as for jumping jacks).

Sidestroke.   The sidestroke may also be used for a warm-up activity for those who do not have an upper body injury. The athlete lies on the left side (Fig. 13–5A), reaching and pulling primarily with the left arm (Fig. 13–5B). The legs should bend at the knee, bringing the left leg upward toward the chest as far as possible while swinging the right leg backward, and with the heel coming upward toward the buttocks. After 10 strokes on the left side, the athlete rolls over and repeats the activity on the right side. This exercise involves the muscles of the side that an individual does not often use.

Following the warm-up, the athlete is ready to move to specific exercises oriented toward rehabilitation of the injured area. Initially, the muscles around the injured area are exercised, not the injured area itself. As strength is recovered and pain eliminated, the injured area can be exercised. The athlete should not perform any activities that cause joint pain, especially at the injury site.

Lower Body Injuries

Ankle

Rotations.   The athlete stands in chest-deep water or holds onto the pool side, rotating each ankle clockwise and counterclockwise.

Ankle Plantar Flexion and Dorsiflexion.   The athlete stands in chest-deep water or holds onto the pool side, plantar flexing and dorsiflexing each ankle.

Alphabet.   The athlete stands in chest-deep water or holds onto the pool side and spells the alphabet using the big toe of the injured foot, beginning with the letter A.

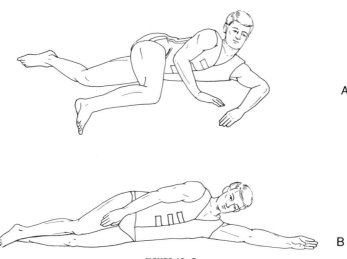

A

B

FIGURE 13–5

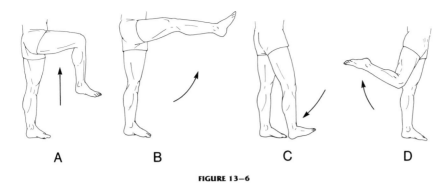

A   B   C   D

FIGURE 13–6

Knee

Hip Flexion, Knee Extension, Hip Extension.   The athlete stands on the uninjured extremity in shallow water or on a ledge in deep water. The injured leg is raised until it is parallel to the pool bottom (Fig.13–6A). The knee is then extended as far as possible (Fig. 13–6B). On reaching full knee extension, the athlete immediately pulls the entire leg into hip extension as far as possible (Fig. 13–6C), while simultaneously flexing the knee as far as possible (Fig. 13–6D). This is 1 repetition.

These exercises can be broken down into three separate components. The athlete may do one or two of these components separately instead of the complete activity.

Hip Flexion.   The athlete stands on the uninjured leg in shallow water or on a ledge in deep water, flexing the hip until the injured leg is parallel to the pool bottom (Fig. 13–7A). The leg is then lowered (hip extension) back to the starting position (Fig. 13–7B). This is 1 repetition.

Hip Flexion with Knee Extensions.   The athlete stands on the uninjured leg in shallow water or on a ledge in deep water, flexing the hip until the injured leg is parallel to the pool bottom (Fig. 13–8A). The knee is then extended as far as possible (Fig. 13–8B), flexing the knee and returning the extremity back to a perpendicular position (Fig. 13–8C). This is 1 repetition.

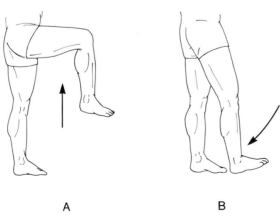

A   B

FIGURE 13–7

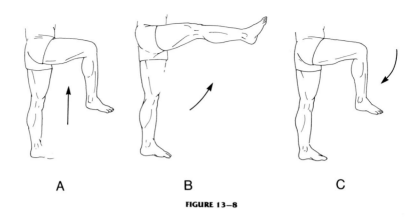

A   B   C

FIGURE 13–8

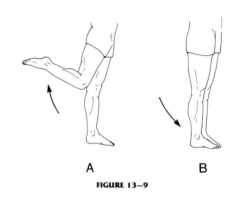

A   B

FIGURE 13–9

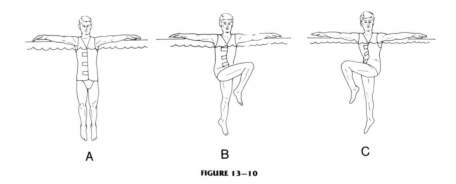

A   B   C

FIGURE 13–10

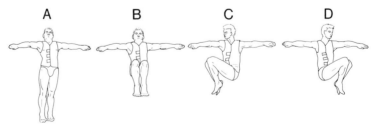

A   B   C   D

FIGURE 13–11

Hamstring Curls.   The athlete stands on the uninjured leg in shallow water or on a ledge in deep water, flexing the knee of the injured leg as far as possible (Fig. 13–9A). The leg is then returned to the starting position (Fig. 13–9B). This is 1 repetition.

Bent Knee Lifts.   The athlete begins with the back against the side of the pool and the hands and arms holding onto the pool gutter or edge (Fig. 13–10A). The right hip and knee are flexed, bringing the right knee upward toward the left shoulder (Fig. 13–10B). The leg is lowered completely and the exercise repeated with the opposite leg (Fig. 13–10C). This is 1 repetition.

Bent Knee Trunk Twists.   The athlete begins in open water, floating on the back with the arms out to the side (Fig. 13–11A), and drawing the knees as close to the chest as possible (Fig. 13–11B). The athlete twists at the waist, turning the knees to the right and pushing down in the water with the left hand, to ensure remaining stationary (Fig. 13–11C). Then, twisting the knees to the left, the athlete pushes down in the water with the right hand (Fig. 13–11D). This is 1 repetition.

Soccer kicks.   This exercise can be performed in deep water or while holding onto the pool side in shallow water. With an injury that requires no weight-bearing, it is best to perform this activity in deep water. In a vertical position (Fig. 13–12A), the athlete swings the right leg upward and to the left, through as full a range of motion as possible (Fig. 13–12B), using the arms to balance as if on land. The athlete then returns to the vertical starting position (Fig. 13–12A). This is 1 repetition. After completing the prescribed number of repetitions with one leg, the athlete repeats the exercise with the opposite leg.

Back

Deep Water Sit-Ups.   The athlete begins in deep water with the body leaning back at a 45° incline and the arms out to the side (Fig.

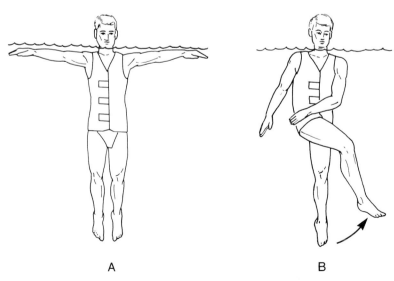

A   B

FIGURE 13–12

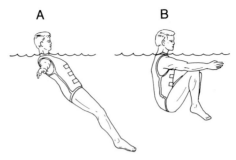

FIGURE 13—13

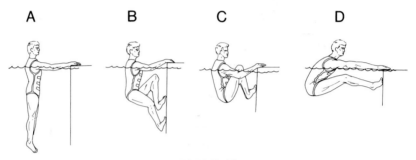

FIGURE 13—14

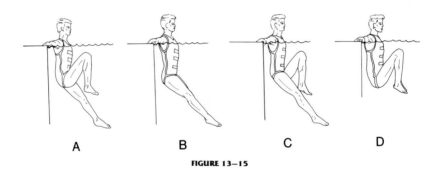

FIGURE 13—15

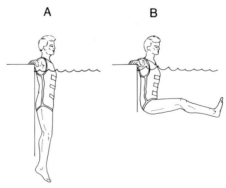

FIGURE 13—16

13–13*A*). The athlete brings the knees to the chest and the arms forward in a clapping motion with the palms facing forward (supinated) (Fig. 13–13*B*). The athlete returns to the starting position (Fig. 13–13*A*) by extending the legs to a straight position and pushing the arms out to the side with the palms facing backward (pronation). Keeping the palms facing backward as the athlete swings the arms toward the rear prevents bobbing up and down and maintains the athlete in a stationary position in the pool. This is 1 repetition.

Crab Crawl. The athlete begins by facing the side of the pool with the hands on the pool gutter or edge and the feet together (Fig. 13–14*A*). Pretending there is a ladder directly in front, the athlete slowly climbs the pool wall, keeping the knees flexed (Fig. 13–14*B*). When the toes near the surface of the water, the athlete slowly pulls the buttocks into a tuck position with the knees between the hands (Fig. 13–14*C*). Slowly pushing away from the wall, the athlete extends the knees as far as possible (Fig. 13–14*D*), holding for about 10 seconds and returning to the tuck position (Fig. 13–14*C*) with the knees flexed. This is held for about 10 seconds. This is 1 repetition.

Back Stretcher. The athlete begins with the back against the pool side, legs angling away from the pool side at about 45° and the hands and the arms holding onto the pool gutter or edge. The athlete slowly flexes the right knee (Fig. 13–15*A*) and draws it as close as possible to the chest, lowering the leg to the starting position (Fig. 13–15*B*). Slowly flexing the left knee and drawing it as close as possible to the chest (Fig. 13–15*C*), the athlete lowers the leg to the starting position, slowly flexing both knees and drawing them as close as possible to the chest (Fig. 13–15*D*). Both legs are then lowered to the starting position. This is 1 repetition.

Straight Leg Lifts. This is an advanced back exercise and should not be performed by an athlete who is experiencing back pain. It should be used to strengthen the back and abdomen after pain has been eliminated. The athlete begins with the back against the pool side and the hands and arms holding onto the pool gutter or edge (Fig. 13–16*A*). The athlete bends at the waist and draws the toes toward the water surface, keeping the knees locked (Fig. 13–16*B*), and lowers the legs to the starting position. This is 1 repetition.

Hips

Vertical Trunk Twist. The athlete begins in deep water in a vertical position with the feet directly below and the arms out to the side (Fig. 13–17*A*). Keeping the right leg straight, the athlete crosses it over the left leg and extends it as far as possible (Fig. 13–17*B*). Simultaneously, the athlete twists the upper body in the opposite direction (to the right), crossing the left arm over the torso and extending it to the right as far as possible. This is repeated to the opposite side (Fig. 13–17*C*). This is 1 repetition.

Abduction and Adduction. This can be done in deep water or by holding onto the pool edge. In deep water, the athlete begins in a vertical position with the feet directly below and the arms out to the side (Fig. 13–18*A*). Keeping the legs straight and the knees locked, the

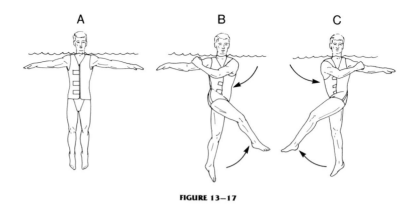

FIGURE 13–17

athlete spreads the legs out to the sides as far as possible (Fig. 13–18*B*). At the same time, the arms are lowered slightly in a paddling motion to help deter bobbing up and down. The athlete brings the legs back together and raises the arms to horizontal (Fig. 13–18*A*). This is 1 repetition. If the side of the pool is used, the leg motions are the same.

Scissors.   This activity can be performed in deep water or by holding onto the pool side. In deep water, the athlete holds the arms out to the side and the legs extended downward (Fig. 13–19*A*). The athlete begins crisscrossing the lower legs, alternately bringing the right leg in front of the left (Fig. 13–19*B*) and then the left leg in front of the right (Fig. 13–19*C*).

If the athlete is holding onto the pool wall the exercise may be done in a vertical position, as indicated above, or a straight leg lift may be performed first (Fig. 13–20*A*), then commencing the scissors activity (Fig. 13–20 *B, C*).

Leg Rotations.   The athlete stands in shallow water or holds onto the pool side (Fig. 13–21*A*), raising one leg about 45° and then rotating it in circles (Fig. 13–21*B*). Small circles are made at first, slowly increasing to large circles. After completing all rotations with one leg, the athlete repeats with the opposite leg.

Upper Body Injuries

Shoulder

Breast Stroke.   The breast stroke is a good beginning activity for shoulder problems. It can be adjusted from small strokes for those just beginning rehabilitation to full range-of-motion strokes for those more advanced. Additionally, the breast stroke can be performed in the traditional horizontal method or in the vertical position.

TRADITIONAL HORIZONTAL.   The athlete lies forward in the water, bringing the hands together, with the elbows flexed. At the same time the knees are flexed, abducting the thighs to the side as far as possible (Fig. 13–22*A*). The athlete reaches forward with the hands in sweeping circles and makes a frog-kicking motion with the legs (Fig. 13–22*B*).

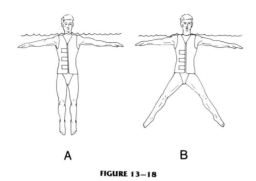

A   B

FIGURE 13–18

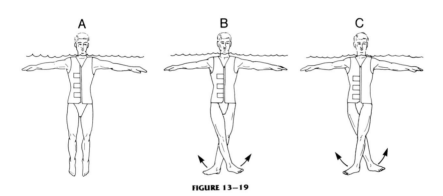

A   B   C

FIGURE 13–19

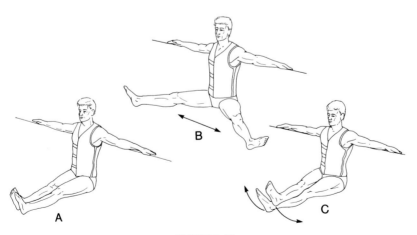

B

A   C

FIGURE 13–20

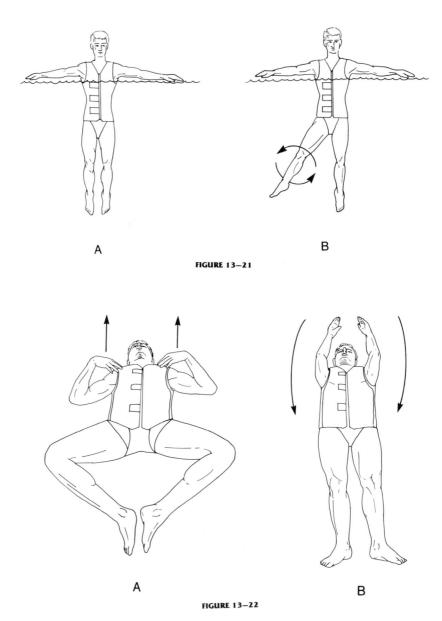

A   B

FIGURE 13–21

A   B

FIGURE 13–22

A   B

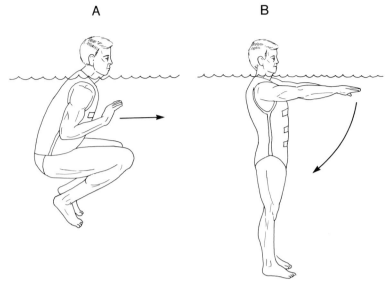

FIGURE 13-23

VERTICAL. This position is more suited for individuals who have a fear of getting their face in the water. The athlete remains upright in the water, bringing the hands together in front of the body in the same manner as the horizontal breast stroke. However, the knees come up in the front and the thighs are abducted to the side as far as possible (Fig. 13–23A). The athlete reaches forward with the hands in sweeping circles and makes a downward frog-kicking motion with the legs (Fig. 13–23B).

Front and Back Clapping. The athlete begins in deep water in a vertical position with the feet directly below and the arms out to the sides (Fig. 13–24A). The athlete claps the hands straight out in front (Fig. 13–24B), reversing the palms (pronation) and moving the arms to

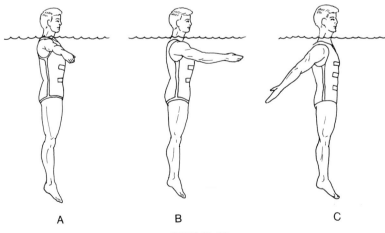

A   B   C

FIGURE 13-24

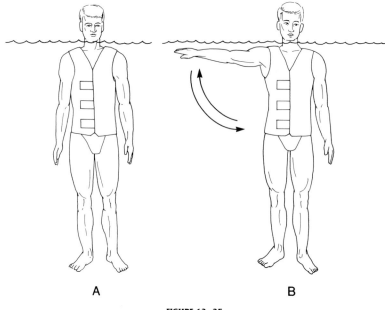

A   B

FIGURE 13–25

the rear in an effort to clap the hands behind the back (Fig. 13–24C). The palms are kept facing forward as the hands move toward the rear to prevent bobbing up and down and to keep the athlete stationary in the pool.

Abduction and Adduction.   The athlete stands in chest-deep water (Fig. 13–25A), flexing the knees so the water comes to chin level. The athlete raises one arm directly out to the side to the 90° position (Fig. 13–25B) (or as close as possible without pain), keeping the palm open and returning to the starting position (Fig. 13–25A). This is 1 repetition. As pain subsides, range of motion should be increased.

Front Shoulder Raise and Circle.   The athlete stands in chest-

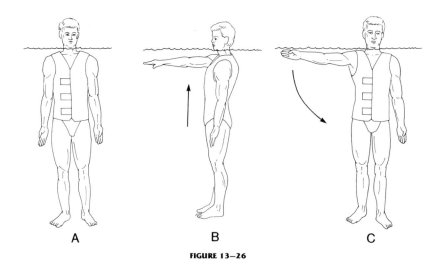

A   B   C

FIGURE 13–26

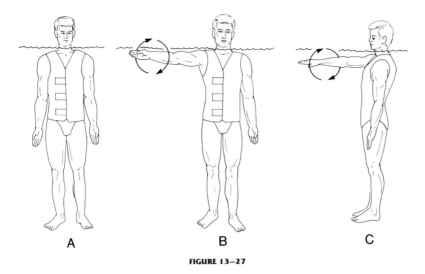

FIGURE 13–27

deep water (Fig. 13–26A), flexing the knees so the water comes to chin level. One arm is raised directly in front of the body to the 90° position (Fig. 13–26B)(or as close as possible without pain), keeping the palm open. The arm is then rotated out to the side of the body (Fig. 13–26C) and down to the starting position (Fig. 13–26A). This is 1 repetition.

As range of motion improves, the athlete continues to expand the arc of the circle further toward the rear of the body before returning the arm to the starting position.

Arm Rotations.   The athlete stands in chest-deep water (Fig. 13–27A), flexing the knees so the water comes to chin level. With the elbow

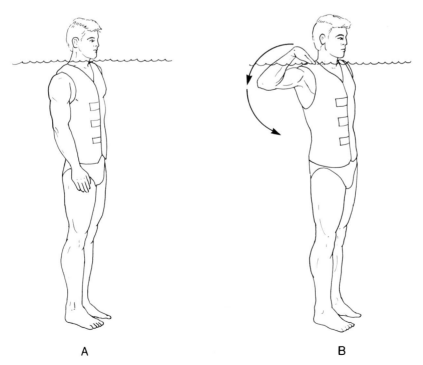

FIGURE 13–28

locked in extension, the arm is rotated in circles, beginning with small circles and slowly increasing to large circles (Fig. 13–27B). All rotations are completed with one arm prior to beginning the rotations with the opposite arm. Additionally, the athlete may perform a set of arm rotations out to the side and a set with the arm in front of the body (Fig. 13–27C).

Bent Arm Rotations.   The athlete stands in chest-deep water (Fig. 13–28A), flexing the knees so the water comes to chin level. The athlete flexes the elbow and places the hand on the shoulder (Fig. 13–28B), rotating the arm in small circles and slowly increasing to large circles. The arm is rotated toward the back as far as possible.

Bent Elbow Swing.   The athlete stands in chest-deep water (Fig. 13–29A), flexing the knees so the water comes to chin level. The elbow is flexed to 90° (Fig. 13–29B), keeping the palm open and externally rotating the arm as far as possible (Fig. 13–29C).

Elbow

Flexion and Extension.   The athlete stands in chest-deep water (Fig. 13–30A), flexing the knees so the water comes to chin level and keeping the palm open and using it as a paddle. The elbow is flexed and the palm brought toward the shoulder as far as possible without pain (Fig. 13–30B). The elbow is extended back to the starting position (Fig. 13–30A). This is 1 repetition.

Bent Elbow and Shoulder Abduction and Adduction.   The athlete stands in chest-deep water (Fig. 13–31A), flexing the knees so the water comes to chin level. The elbow is flexed to 90° with the palm open (Fig. 13–31B). The arm is abducted to the 90° position (or as

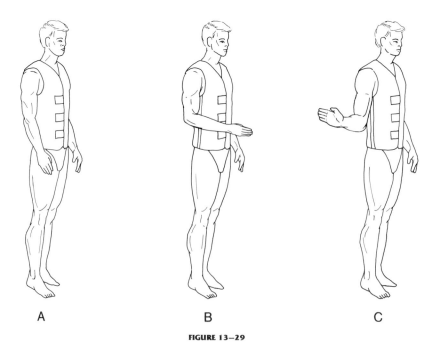

A   B   C

FIGURE 13–29

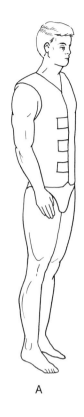

A

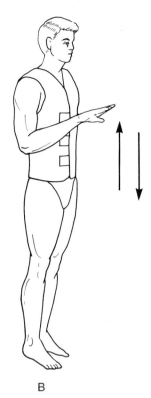

B

FIGURE 13—30

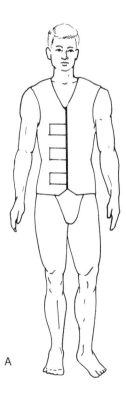

A

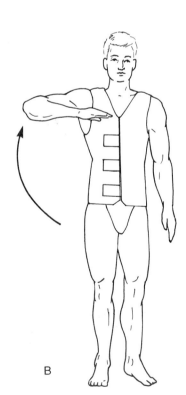

B

FIGURE 13—31

close as possible without pain). The athlete returns the arm to the side, maintaining the 90° elbow flexion. This is 1 repetition.

Wrist

Circle Eights.   The athlete stands in chest-deep water, flexes the elbow to 90° and makes a figure eight with the hand. The athlete begins with small figure eights and increases to larger figure eights as range of motion improves.

Wrist Rotations.   The athlete stands in chest-deep water, flexes the elbow to 90°, and rotates the wrist clockwise and counterclockwise.

Radial and Ulnar Deviations.   The athlete stands in chest-deep water, flexes the elbow to 90°, keeps the palm open, and radial and ulnar deviates the wrist.

Flexion and Extension.   The athlete stands in chest-deep water, flexes the elbow to 90°, keeps the palm open, and flexes and extends the wrist.

Supination and Pronation.   The athlete stands in chest-deep water, flexes the elbow to 90°, keeps the palm open, and supinates and pronates the wrist.

Alphabet.   The athlete stands in chest-deep water, flexes the elbow to 90°, keeps the palm open, and spells the upper-case letters of the alphabet with the injured hand, using the index finger as a guide.

Other Exercises

After completing the activities for a specific area, the athlete may perform other exercises for an overall conditioning program or can return to deep water running to increase speed and endurance. Speed can be increased by performing overstriding drills and sprints in deep water. The overstriding drill increases strength levels in the hip flexors and extensors, buttocks, shoulders, and back. It is effective for increasing stride length and speed. This activity is performed at a controlled pace and for short periods, usually 1 to 2 minutes. Sprints help increase leg speed and strength. They can be performed at an all-out effort for very short periods, usually 15-30 seconds.

Overstriding Drill.   The athlete assumes a natural running position in deep water. The body is kept almost erect, without leaning too far forward or bending at the waist (Fig. 13–32A). The athlete lifts the lead knee high (Fig. 13–32B), then reaches out with the lower leg as far as possible, getting full knee extension (Fig. 13–32C). Simultaneously, the other leg is extended as far to the rear as possible. The triceps touches the top of the water on one arm while the fist touches the top of the water on the opposing arm (Fig. 13–32D). In smooth, fluid movements, the athlete continues to alternate the legs, just as if running on dry land, (Fig. 13–32E,F), except the legs are stretched as far forward and backward as possible.

Endurance.   Endurance can be enhanced by continuous running

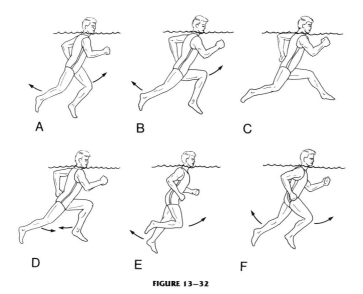

FIGURE 13–32

at a steady speed or by alternating fast runs with easy runs, all while buoyed at neck level in the deep end of the pool.

The amount of time spent running and the number of repetitions of each exercise vary, depending on the athlete's overall condition and extent of injury. If doubts exist about how much the athlete can do, 10 repetitions of each exercise should be attempted. If this is too much, decrease the amount. If it appears insufficient, increase the workload. The harder the athlete pushes against the water, the more resistance is encountered. If little force is applied, the resistance is minimal. If a greater force is exerted, the resistance is stronger.

If one of the exercises elicits pain, discontinue that particular exercise; it may be attempted again in a few days. If it still causes pain, wait several more days. As the injured body part increases in strength, the athlete should be able to perform all exercises without pain.

Sample Program

The regimen below is an example of a weekly program of deep water exercises. After full recovery, the athlete may want to incorporate deep water exercise into a regular exercise routine; this can be advantageous in reducing the risk of future injuries while maintaining a top level of conditioning.

Monday—8 to 10 minutes of easy deep water running and other warm-up exercises, followed by concentrated exercises for the lower or upper body and then by 20 minutes of steady running for endurance. Conclude with stretching exercises, either in water or at poolside.

Tuesday—8 to 10 minutes of easy deep water running and other warm-up exercises, followed by concentrated exercises for the lower or upper body and then by speed running: 2×2 minutes of overstriding with a 2-minute rest between, then, 5 $\times$ 30 seconds of hard running with 30 to 45 seconds of rest between. As the injury heals, the athlete may rest for 5 minutes and repeat this drill. Conclude with stretching exercises, either in water or at poolside.

Wednesday—8 to 10 minutes of easy deep water running and other warm-up exercises, followed by concentrated exercises for the lower or upper body and then by 20 minutes of steady running for endurance. Conclude with stretching exercises, either in water or at poolside.

Thursday—8 to 10 minutes of easy deep water running and other warm-up exercises, followed by concentrated exercises for the lower or upper body and then by speed running: 2×2 minutes of overstriding with a 2-minute rest between, then, 10 $\times$ 15 seconds of sprinting with 30 to 45 seconds of rest between. As the injury heals, the athlete may rest for 5 minutes and repeat this drill. Conclude with stretching exercises, either in water or at poolside.

Friday—8 to 10 minutes of easy deep water running and other warm-up exercises, followed by concentrated exercises for the lower or upper body, and then by 20 minutes of steady running for endurance. Conclude with stretching exercises, either in water or at poolside.

Saturday—8 to 10 minutes of easy deep water running and other warm-up exercises, followed by concentrated exercises for the lower or upper body, and then by 20 minutes of steady running or a speed workout, whichever is preferred. Conclude with stretching exercises, either in water or at poolside.

Sunday—off.

References

1. Brody, D.M. (1980): Clinical symposia: Running injuries. Ciba. Found. Symp., 32: 1–37.
2. Burdenko, I. (1990): Personal communication. Boston, MA.
3. Crane, C., Tacia, S., and Thompson, J. (1987): A comparison of land and water exercise programs for older individuals. Master's thesis. Rochester, MI, Oakland University.
4. Edlich, R. (1989): Personal communication. Charlottesville, VA.
5. Ellenbecker, T.S., Davies, G.T., and Rowinski, M.J. (1988): Concentric versus eccentric isokinetic strengthening of the rotator cuff. Am. J. Sports Med., 16(1):64–69.
6. Evans, B.W., Cureton, K.J., and Purvis, J.W. (1978): Metabolic and circulatory responses to walking and jogging in water. Res. Q. 49(4):442–449.
7. Fox, E.L. (1984): Sports Physiology. New York, CBS College Publishing.
8. Glass, B. (1986): Personal communication. Auburn, AL.
9. Katz, J. (1985): The W.E.T. Workout. New York, Facts on File Publications.
10. Kennon, T. (1990): Personal communication. Tuscaloosa, AL.
11. Kuland, D.N. (1986): Poolex for the Injured Runner. Charlottesville, VA, Sports Medicine and Rehabilitation Center.
12. Lieber, J. (1989): Broken but unbowed. Sports Ill., 70(12):104–107.
13. McDonald, B. (1990): Personal communication. Tuscaloosa, AL.

14. McWaters, G. (1988): Deep Water Exercise for Health and Fitness. Laguna Beach, CA, Publitec Editions.
15. Navia, A.M. (1986): Comparison of energy expenditure between treadmill running and water running. Master's thesis. Birmingham, AL, University of Alabama.
16. Silver, D. (1989): Personal communication. Los Angeles, CA.
17. Timm, K.E. (1988): Postsurgical knee rehabilitation. Am. J. Sports Med., 16(5):463–468.
18. Watkins, R.G., Buhler, B., and Lovelock, P. (1988): The Water Workout Recovery Program. Chicago, Contemporary Books.
19. Watkins, R.G. (1988): Personal communication. Inglewood, CA.
20. Welch, P., and Welch, D. (1989): Personal communication. Boulder, CO.
21. Welsh, D.G., and Rhodes, E.C. (1988): Cardiovascular and respiratory parameters during immersion and treadmill training. Master's thesis. Vancouver, B.C., University of British Columbia.

APPENDIX A

---◆---

Knee and Leg
Rehabilitation Exercises

Patella Mobilization. With the leg straight and the thigh musculature relaxed, the athlete or clinician places the fingers of each hand on either side of the patella and gently mobilizes the patella side to side for 1 to 2 minutes. This is repeated, mobilizing the patella up and down for 1 to 2 minutes.

Heel Slide. The athlete pulls the heel toward the buttocks, flexing the knee; holds for 5 seconds; straightens the leg by sliding the heel downward; and holds for 5 seconds. In later stages of rehabilitation the athlete may grasp the lower leg with both hands and pull the heel toward the buttocks. When straightening the leg, pressure may be put on the leg above the patella to aid in regaining extension.

Quad Set. With the leg as straight as possible, the athlete tightens the front thigh muscles (quadriceps), trying to pull the patella superiorly; holds for 5 seconds, contracting the muscles as tightly as possible; completely relaxes the thigh; and rests for 2 seconds. This exercise may be performed standing, sitting, or lying down.

6-Inch Straight Leg Raise. The athlete tightens the quadriceps as in a quad set, keeps the leg straight; lifts the heel off the table approximately 6 inches (Fig. A–1); pauses; slowly lowers the leg down; and then completely relaxes the thigh and rests for 2 seconds.

Static Weight Loading. Sitting on the edge of a chair, the athlete straightens the

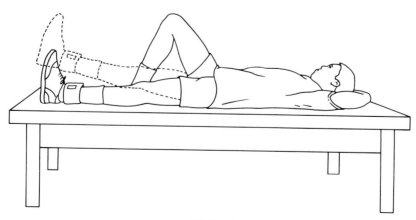

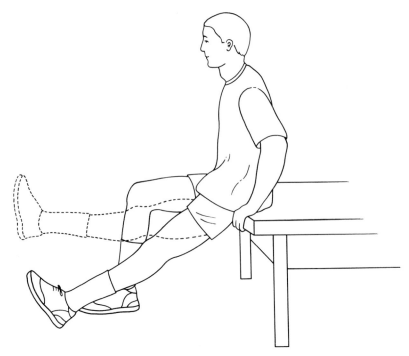

FIGURE A–2

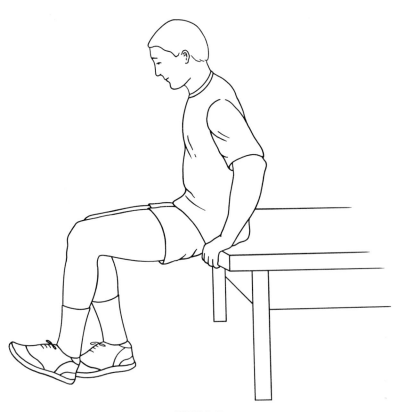

FIGURE A–3

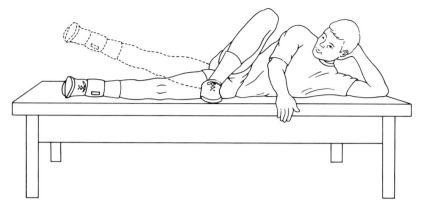

FIGURE A—4

leg with the foot resting on the floor; tightens the quadriceps as in a quad set; keeps the leg straight; raises the leg until parallel with the floor (Fig. A—2); and holds for 10 seconds. The athlete then lowers the leg to the floor, rests, and repeats the exercise, performing 10 repetitions. This is increased in 5-second intervals, up to 1 minute. No weight is used until 1 minute is reached, and then the hold time is reduced, progressing to 1 minute again.

Cocontraction. The athlete tightens both the quadriceps and hamstring muscles at the same time by "digging" the heel downward (Fig. A—3), holds for 5 seconds, contracts the muscles as tight as possible, and then completely relaxes the thigh and rests for 2 seconds. This exercise may be performed sitting up, lying down, or seated in a chair. Cocontractions may be modified by performing each set with the knee bent at a different angle.

Hip Adduction. The athlete lies on the side of the involved leg, places the opposite foot just in front of the involved knee, lifts the involved leg up away from the table, pauses (Fig. A—4), slowly lowers the leg, and relaxes, resting for 2 seconds.

Hip Abduction. The athlete lies on the side of the uninvolved leg, bending the leg at the knee for stability; straightens the top leg; lifts upward toward the ceiling; pauses (Fig. A—5), slowly lowers the leg, and relaxes, resting for 2 seconds.

Hip Extension. The athlete lies supine on the table with the feet off the table

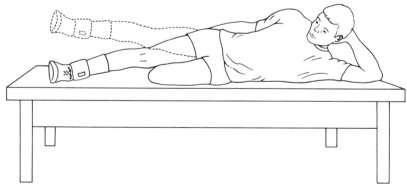

FIGURE A—5

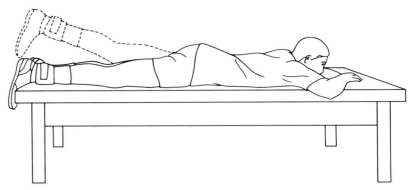

FIGURE A–6

edge; lifts the involved leg straight up, keeping the leg straight; pauses (Fig. A–6), and slowly lowers to rest position, resting for 2 seconds. This can also be performed while standing, lying over the table edge at the waist.

Gluteal Extension. The athlete lies prone on the table, flexes the knee on the involved side to about 90°, lifts the involved leg straight up, pauses (Fig. A–7), slowly lowers to resting position, and rests for 2 seconds.

Hip Flexion. The athlete sits on the edge of a firm surface with the feet resting on the floor, lifts the knee toward the chest, pauses (Fig. A–8), slowly lowers to rest position, and rests 2 seconds.

Heel Raise. The athlete stands with the feet slightly pigeon-toed, using a wall or table for balance (Fig. A–9A), pushes up on the toes, lifts the heels; pauses (Fig. A–9B); slowly lowers; relaxes; and repeats.

90°–45° Knee Extension. In a sitting position, the athlete extends the involved leg slowly to a 90°–45° angle, pauses (Fig. A–10), and slowly lowers the leg to the starting position.

Terminal Knee Extension (TKE). A hard roll is placed under the involved knee, allowing the knee to bend approximately 30°. The athlete extends the leg slowly until straight, pauses (Fig. A–11), slowly lowers the leg to the starting position, and rests for 2 seconds.

Standing Hamstring Curl. The athlete stands straight with the thigh resting against a table or wall, raises the heel slowly toward the buttocks, pauses (Fig. A–12), slowly lowers the leg, and relaxes.

Text continued on p. 513

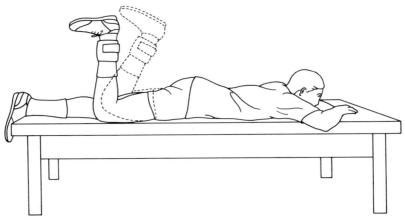

FIGURE A–7

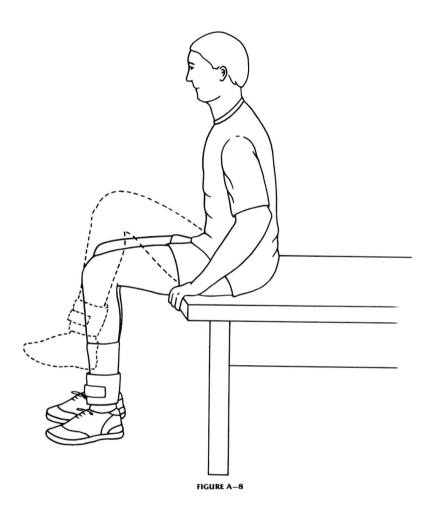

FIGURE A—8

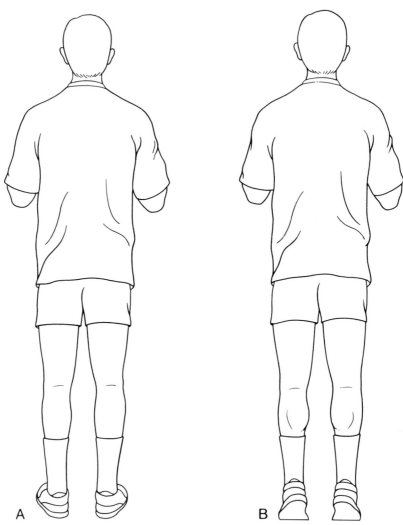

A   B

FIGURE A–9

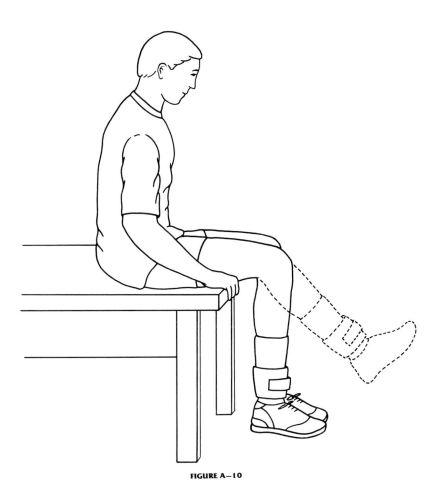

FIGURE A–10

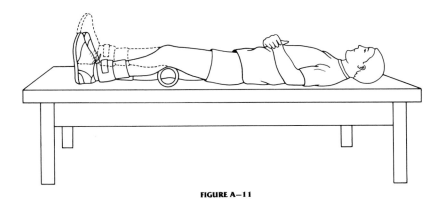

FIGURE A–11

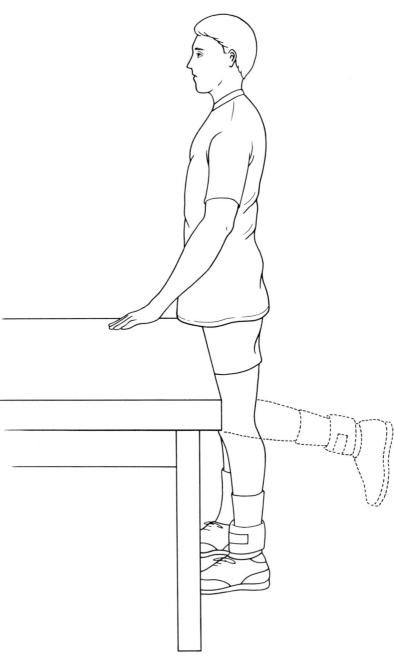

FIGURE A—12

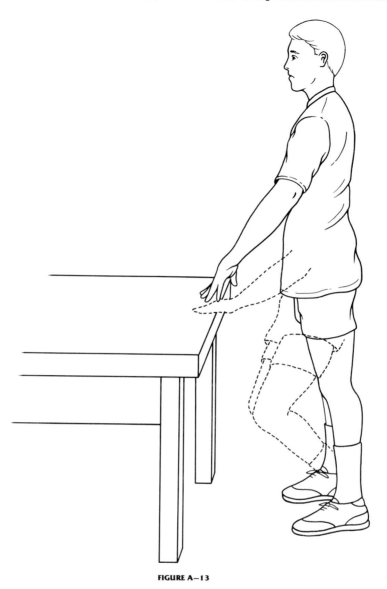

FIGURE A–13

Mini Squats. The athlete is standing, using a table for support; bends at the knees to about a 45° angle; pauses (Fig. A–13); and then returns to the starting position with the knees straight. This can be progressed to no support, back against the wall, and using only the involved leg.

Passive Knee Flexion. The athlete sits in a chair, pushes the lower leg on the involved side as far back as possible with the opposite leg (Fig. A–14), holds for 5 seconds, and then relaxes.

Active Assisted Knee Flexion. The athelte sits in a chair and slides the lower leg on the involved side as far back as possible. Keeping the foot stationary, the hips slide forward (Fig. A–15). The athlete then holds for 5 seconds and relaxes.

Lateral Step-Ups. The athlete stands with the involved leg toward a step, places the involved leg's foot on the step (Fig. A–16A), lifts the body weight with the involved leg (Fig. A–16B). The exercise may be advanced by standing on the heel of the uninvolved leg and lifting the entire body weight with no push-off.

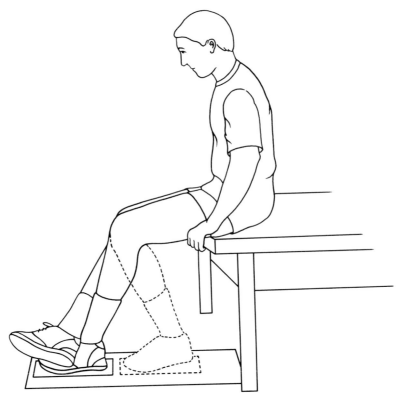

FIGURE A—14

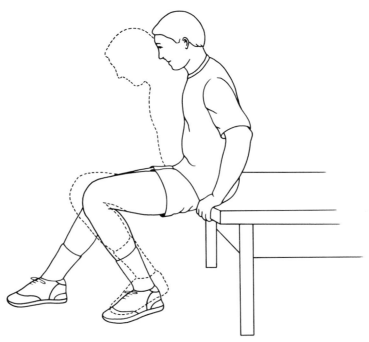

FIGURE A—15

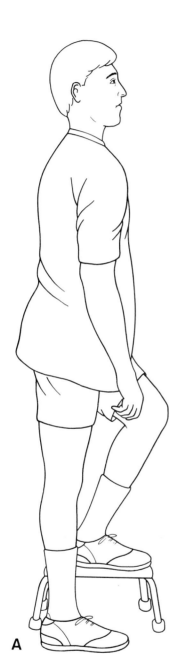

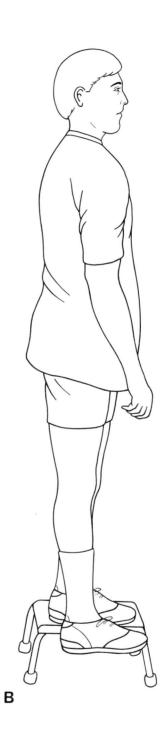

A

B

FIGURE A—16

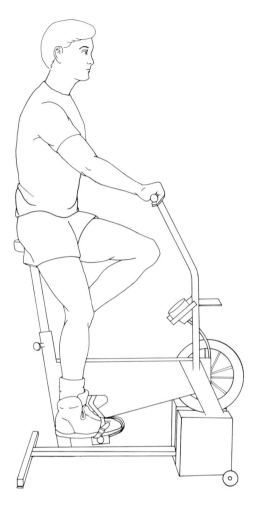

FIGURE A–17

The athlete begins with about a 4-inch step and gradually progresses to an 8-inch step, as tolerated.

Stationary Cycling. The seat height is adjusted so that the involved leg is almost straight when the ball of the foot is on the lowest pedal (Fig. A–17). The tension should be set to allow minimum to moderate resistance.

Hamstring Flexibility. The athlete straightens the supported leg with the opposite leg off to the side, slowly leans forward, keeping the toe pulled back and knee straight, until a stretch is felt in the hamstrings (Fig. A–18), and holds for 10 seconds. This stretch is performed with the chin up, the back straight, and without bouncing.

Achilles Flexibility.

1. The athlete stands and leans into a wall with the weight on the heels and the back knee straight (Fig. A–19). The feet are turned inward in a slightly pigeon-toed position. The athlete slowly leans forward until a stretch is felt in the calf, holds for 10 seconds, and repeats with each leg.

2. The athlete stands and leans into a wall with the weight on the heels and the knees slightly bent, slowly leans forward until a stretch is felt in the calf, (Fig. A–20), holds for 10 seconds, and repeats with each leg.

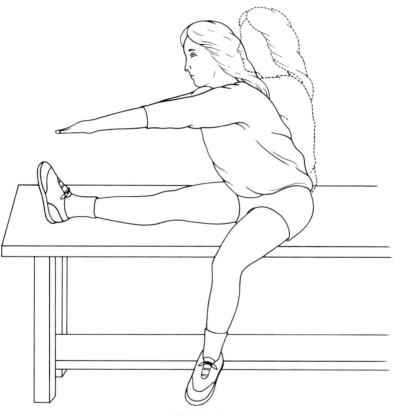

FIGURE A—18

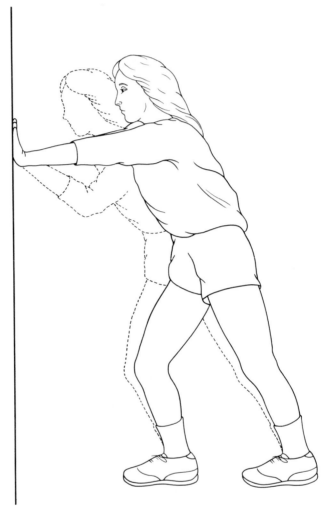

FIGURE A–19

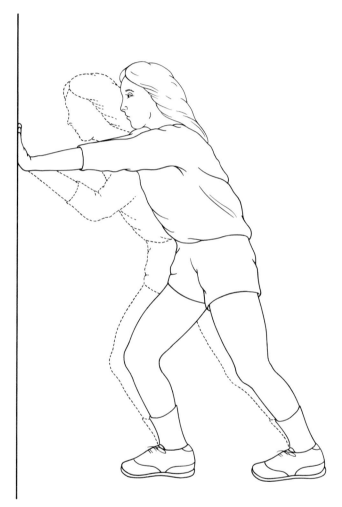

FIGURE A–20

APPENDIX B

———◆———

Interval Rehabilitation Programs

INTERVAL THROWING PROGRAM FOR BASEBALL PLAYERS

The Interval Throwing Program (ITP) is designed to bring about a gradual return of motion, strength, and confidence to the throwing arm after injury or surgery by slowly progressing the athlete through graduated throwing distances. The ITP can be initiated after clearance by the athlete's physician for the resumption of throwing and is carried out under the supervision of the rehabilitation team (physician, athletic trainer, and/or physical therapist). The program is set up to minimize the chance of reinjury and emphasizes prethrowing warm-up and stretching. In the development of the interval throwing program, the following factors are considered most important:

1. The act of throwing a baseball involves the transfer of energy from the feet through the legs, pelvis, trunk, and out the shoulder through the elbow and hand. Therefore, any return to throwing after injury must include attention to the entire body.
2. The chance for reinjury is lessened by a graduated progression of interval throwing.
3. Proper warm-up is essential.
4. Most injuries occur as the result of fatigue.
5. Regard for proper throwing mechanics lessens the incidence of reinjury.
6. Baseline requirements for throwing include a pain-free range of motion of all joints involved in throwing and adequate muscle power and resistance to fatigue.

Because there is an individual variability in all throwing athletes, there is no set timetable for completion of the ITP. Most athletes, by nature, are highly competitive individuals who wish to return to competition at the earliest possible time. Although this is a necessary characteristic in all athletes, the proper channeling of the athlete's energies into a rigidly controlled throwing program is essential to lessen the chance of reinjury during the rehabilitative period. The athlete may want to increase the intensity of the throwing program, but this can increase the incidence of reinjury and may greatly retard the rehabilitation process. It is recommended that the program be followed rigidly, because this represents the safest route for returning to competition.

During the recovery process the athlete may experience soreness and a dull, diffuse, aching sensation in the muscles and tendons. If the athlete experiences sharp pain, particularly in the joint, all throwing activity should be stopped until this pain abates. Throwing should also be discontinued if the athlete's elbow or shoulder becomes swollen. Heat on the shoulder or elbow may help loosen up the joint prior to throwing. Ice alone is recommended after throwing or to treat swelling.

Weight Training

The athlete should supplement the ITP with a high-repetition, low-weight exercise program. The strengthening regimen should maintain a proper balance between the anterior and posterior musculature so that the shoulder is not predisposed to injury. Special emphasis must be given to the posterior rotator cuff musculature in any strengthening program. Weight training does not increase throwing velocity but increases the resistance of the arm to fatigue and injury. If the athlete uses weight training, this should be done on alternate days, with throwing on days in between. Because weight lifting tends to tighten the joints, it must be stressed that weight training is of no benefit unless accompanied by a sound flexibility program.

Individual Variability

The ITP is designed so that each level is achieved without pain or complication before the next level is started. This sets up a progression—a goal is achieved prior to advancement instead of advancing according to a specific time frame. Thus, the ITP may be used for those with different levels of skills and abilities, from athletes in high school to professionals. The reasons for performing the ITP vary from person to person, so the length of time required to complete each step successfully also varies. For example, one athlete may wish to throw on alternate days, with or without using weights in between, and another athlete may have to throw every third or fourth day because of pain or swelling. "Listen to your body—it will tell you when to slow down." Again, completion of the ITP steps is subject to individual variation. There is no fixed timetable in terms of days to completion.

Warm-up

Jogging increases blood flow to the muscles and joints, thus increasing their flexibility and decreasing the chance for injury. Because the length of the warm-up varies among individuals, the athlete should jog until a light sweat develops and then progress to the stretching phase.

Stretching

Throwing involves all muscles in the body. So all muscle groups should be stretched prior to throwing. This should be done in a systematic fashion, beginning with the legs and including the trunk, back, neck, and arms.

Throwing Mechanics

A critical aspect of the ITP is maintenance of proper throwing mechanics throughout its advancement. The use of the crow-hop method simulates the throwing act, allowing emphasis on proper body mechanics. This method should be adopted from the onset of the ITP. Throwing flatfooted encourages improper body mechanics, placing increased stress on the throwing arm and thus predisposing the arm to reinjury. The pitching coach and sports biome-

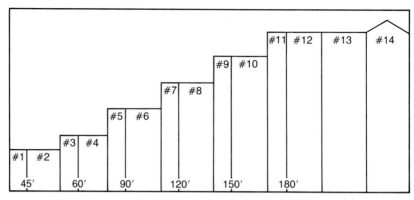

FIGURE B—1   Graduation of the Interval Throwing Program.

chanist (if available) may be valuable allies to the rehabilitation team because of their knowledge of throwing mechanics.

The crow-hop method begins with a hop, then a skip, and followed by the throw. The velocity of the throw is determined by the distance—that is, the ball should have only enough momentum to travel the designated distance. Again, emphasis should be placed on proper throwing mechanics when the athlete returns to throwing off the mound or to his or her respective position to decrease the chance of reinjury.

Throwing

Using the crow-hop method, the athlete should begin warm-up throws at a comfortable distance (approximately 30 to 45 feet; Part I of the ITP) and then progress to the distance indicated for that phase (see Fig. B–1). The object of each phase is for the athlete to be able to throw the ball the specified number of feet (45, 60, 90, 120, 150, or 180), without pain, 75 times at each distance. Athletes who can throw the ball 180 feet, 50 times, without pain, are ready for part II of the ITP, throwing off the mound or returning to their respective position (step 14). At this point, full strength and confidence should be restored in the athlete's arm. It is important to stress the crow-hop method and proper mechanics with each throw. Just as advancement to this point has been gradual and progressive, the return to unrestricted throwing must follow the same principles. A pitcher should first throw only fast balls at 50%, progressing to 75% and finally to 100%. At this time the athlete may begin to throw more stressful pitches, such as breaking balls. The position player should simulate a game situation, again progressing from 50 to 70 to 100%.

Once again, if an athlete has increased pain, particularly at the joint, the intensity of the ITP should be reduced. Readvancement should be under the direction of the rehabilitation team members.

Batting

Depending on the type of injury, the time of return to batting should be determined by the physician. Stress placed on the arm and shoulder during the batting motion is very different from that during the throwing motion. Return to unrestricted use of a bat should also follow the same progressive guidelines as those for the throwing program.

Therefore, by using the Interval Throwing Program in conjunction with a structured rehabilitation program, the athlete should be able to return to a full competition status, minimizing the chance of reinjury. The program and its progression should be modified to meet the specific needs of each individual athlete. A comprehensive program consisting of a maintenance strength and flexibility regimen, appropriate warm-up and cool-down procedures, proper pitching mechanics, and progressive throwing and batting will assist the baseball player in returning to competition safely.

PART I: WARM-UP THROWS

45' Phase

Step 1:
(A) Warm-up throwing
(B) 45' (25 throws)
(C) Rest 15 minutes
(D) Warm-up throwing
(E) 45' (25 throws)

Step 2:
(A) Warm-up throwing
(B) 45' (25 throws)
(C) Rest 10 minutes
(D) Warm-up throwing
(E) 45' (25 throws)
(F) Rest 10 minutes
(G) Warm-up throwing
(H) 45' (25 throws)

60' Phase

Step 3:
(A) Warm-up throwing
(B) 60' (25 throws)
(C) Rest 15 minutes
(D) Warm-up throwing
(E) 60' (25 throws)

Step 4:
(A) Warm-up throwing
(B) 60' (25 throws)
(C) Rest 10 minutes
(D) Warm-up throwing
(E) 60' (25 throws)
(F) Rest 10 minutes
(G) Warm-up throwing
(H) 60' (25 throws)

90' Phase

Step 5:
(A) Warm-up throwing
(B) 90' (25 throws)
(C) Rest 15 minutes
(D) Warm-up throwing
(E) 90' (25 throws)

Step 6:
(A) Warm-up throwing
(B) 90' (25 throws)
(C) Rest 10 minutes
(D) Warm-up throwing
(E) 90' (25 throws)
(F) Rest 10 minutes
(G) Warm-up throwing
(H) 90' (25 throws)

120' Phase

Step 7:
(A) Warm-up throwing
(B) 120' (25 throws)
(C) Rest 15 minutes
(D) Warm-up throwing
(E) 120' (25 throws)

Step 8:
(A) Warm-up throwing
(B) 120' (25 throws)
(C) Rest 10 minutes
(D) Warm-up throwing
(E) 120' (25 throws)
(F) Rest 10 minutes
(G) Warm-up throwing
(H) 120' (25 throws)

150' Phase

Step 9:
(A) Warm-up throwing
(B) 150' (25 throws)
(C) Rest 15 minutes
(D) Warm-up throwing
(E) 150' (25 throws)

Step 10:
(A) Warm-up throwing
(B) 150' (25 throws)
(C) Rest 10 minutes
(D) Warm-up throwing
(E) 150' (25 throws)
(F) Rest 10 minutes
(G) Warm-up throwing
(H) 150' (25 throws)

180' Phase

Step 11:
(A) Warm-up throwing
(B) 180' (25 throws)
(C) Rest 15 minutes
(D) Warm-up throwing
(E) 180' (25 throws)

Step 12:
(A) Warm-up throwing
(B) 180' (25 throws)
(C) Rest 10 minutes
(D) Warm-up throwing
(E) 180' (25 throws)
(F) Rest 10 minutes
(G) Warm-up throwing
(H) 180' (25 throws)

Step 13: (A) Warm-up throwing
(B) 180' (25 throws)
(C) Rest 10 minutes
(D) Warm-up throwing
(E) 180' (25 throws)
(F) Rest 10 minutes

(G) Warm-up throwing
(H) 180' (50 throws)

Step 14: Begin ITP off the mound or return to respective position

PART II: STARTING OFF THE MOUND

All throwing off the mound should be done in the presence of the pitching coach to stress proper throwing mechancis. A speed gun can be used to aid in effort control.

Stage One: Fastball Only

Step 1: (A) Interval throwing
(B) 15 throws off mound, 50%

Step 2: (A) Interval throwing
(B) 30 throws off mound, 50%

Step 3: (A) Interval throwing
(B) 45 throws off mound, 50%

Step 4: (A) Interval throwing
(B) 60 throws off mound, 50%

Step 5: (A) Interval throwing
(B) 30 throws off mound, 50%

Step 6: (A) 30 throws off mound, 75%
(B) 45 throws off mound, 50%

Step 7: (A) 45 throws off mound, 75%
(B) 15 throws off mound, 50%

Step 8: 60 throws off mound, 75%

Stage Two: Fastball Only

Step 9: (A) 45 throws off mound, 75%

(B) 15 throws in batting practice

Step 10: (A) 45 throws off mound, 75%
(B) 30 throws in batting practice

Step 11: (A) 45 throws off mound, 75%
(B) 45 throws in batting practice

Stage Three

Step 12: (A) 30 throws off mound, 75% warm-up
(B) 15 throws off mound, 50% breaking balls
(C) 45 to 60 throws in batting practice (fast ball only)

Step 13: (A) 30 throws off mound, 75%
(B) 30 breaking balls, 75%
(C) 30 throws in batting practice

Step 14: (A) 30 throws off mound, 75%
(B) 60 to 90 throws in batting practice, 25% breaking balls

Step 15: (A) Simulated game— progressing by 15 throws per workout

LITTLE LEAGUER INTERVAL TRAINING PROGRAM

The Little League Interval Throwing Program parallels the interval throwing program in returning the Little Leaguer to a graduated progression of throwing distances. Warm-up and stretching should be performed prior to throwing.

30' Phase

Step 1: (A) Warm-up throwing
(B) 30' (25 throws)
(C) Rest 15 minutes
(D) Warm-up throwing
(E) 30' (25 throws)

Step 2: (A) Warm-up throwing
(B) 30' (25 throws)
(C) Rest 10 minutes
(D) Warm-up throwing
(E) 30' (25 throws)
(F) Rest 10 minutes
(G) Warm-up throwing
(H) 30' (25 throws)

45' Phase

Step 3: (A) Warm-up throwing
(B) 45' (25 throws)
(C) Rest 15 minutes
(D) Warm-up throwing
(E) 45' (25 throws)

Step 4: (A) Warm-up throwing
(B) 45' (25 throws)
(C) Rest 10 minutes
(D) Warm-up throwing
(E) 45' (25 throws)
(F) Rest 10 minutes
(G) Warm-up throwing
(H) 45' (25 throws)

60' Phase

Step 5: (A) Warm-up throwing
(B) 60' (25 throws)
(C) Rest 15 minutes
(D) Warm-up throwing
(E) 60' (25 throws)

Step 6: (A) Warm-up throwing
(B) 60' (25 throws)
(C) Rest 10 minutes
(D) Warm-up throwing
(E) 60' (25 throws)
(F) Rest 10 minutes
(G) Warm-up throwing
(H) 60' (25 throws)

90' Phase

Step 7: (A) Warm-up throwing
(B) 90' (25 throws)
(C) Rest 15 minutes
(D) Warm-up throwing
(E) 90' (25 throws)

Step 8: (A) Warm-up throwing
(B) 90' (25 throws)
(C) Rest 10 minutes
(D) Warm-up throwing
(E) 90' (25 throws)
(F) Rest 10 minutes
(G) Warm-up throwing
(H) 90' (25 throws)

INTERVAL GOLF REHABILITATION PROGRAM

The athlete should do flexibility exercises before hitting and strengthening exercises after hitting. Ice should be used after hitting.

Week	Monday*	Wednesday	Friday
1	5' C & P	5' C & P	5' C & P
	5' rest	5' rest	5' rest
	5' chipping	5' chipping	5' chipping
		5' rest	5' rest
		5' chipping	5' chipping
2	10' chipping	10' chipping	10' short iron
	10' rest	10' rest	10' rest
	10' short iron	10' short iron	10' long iron
		10' rest	10' rest
		10' short iron	10' long iron
3	10' short iron	10' short iron	10' short iron
	10' rest	10' rest	10' rest
	10' long iron	10' long iron	10' long iron
	10' rest	10' rest	10' rest
	10' long iron	10' wood	10' wood
4	Repeat last Friday	Play 9 holes	Play 18 holes

* ' minute; C & P, chipping and putting.

INTERVAL TENNIS PROGRAM

The athlete should do flexibility exercises before the tennis program and strengthening exercises afterward, as well as stretching completely after the workout. Ice is used as necessary.

Week	Monday	Wednesday	Friday
1	10' GS	10' GS	10'GS
	10' rest	10' rest	10' rest
	10' GS	10' OH	20' GS & OH
2	20'GS	20'GS & OH	20'GS
	10' rest	10' rest	10' rest
	10' GS & OH	20' GS & OH	20' GS & OH
			10' rest
			20' GS & OH
3	20' GS	20' GS	20' GS & OH
	10' rest	10' rest	10' rest
	20' GS & OH	20' GS & OH	20' GS & OH
	10' rest	10' rest	10' rest
	20' GS & OH	20' GS & OH	20' GS & OH
4	20' GS	20' GS & OH	20' play
	10' rest	10' rest	10' rest
	20' GS & OH	20 GS & OH	20' play
	10' rest	10' rest	10' rest
	20' GS & OH	20' GS & OH	20' play
	10' rest	10' rest	10' rest
	20' GS & OH	20' GS & OH	20' play

* ', minute; GS, ground strokes; OH, overhead shots.

INTERVAL RUNNING PROGRAM

The athlete should always stretch completely before and after the workout and should use ice when necessary.

Week	Run	Walk	Run	Walk
1	¼ mile	¼ mile	¼ mile	¼ mile
2	¼ mile	¼ mile	½ mile	¼ mile
3	½ mile	¼ mile	½ mile	¼ mile
4	½ mile	¼ mile	¾ mile	¼ mile
5	¾ mile	¼ mile	¾ mile	¼ mile
6	¾ mile	¼ mile	1 mile	¼ mile
7	1 mile	¼ mile	1 mile	¼ mile

The Interval Throwing Program, Parts I and II, the Little Leaguer Interval Training Program, the Interval Golf Rehabilitation Program, and the Interval Tennis Program have been reprinted with permission from Middleton, K., Courson, R., Young R., and Andrews, J. R. (1989): Preventive and Rehabilitative Exercises for the Shoulder and Elbow. Birmingham, AL, American Sports Medicine Institute.

INDEX

◆

Note: Page numbers in *italics* indicate illustrations;
those followed by (t) refer to tables.